Talking Nets

Talking Nets

An Oral History of Neural Networks

edited by James A. Anderson and Edward Rosenfeld

A Bradford Book
The MIT Press
Cambridge, Massachusetts
London, England

First MIT Press paperback edition, 2000
© 1998 Massachusetts Institute of Technology

This book was set in Palatino on the Monotype "Prism Plus" PostScript Imagesetter by Asco Trade Typesetting Ltd., Hong Kong.

Photographs of Gail Carpenter and Stephen Grossberg by Deborah Grossberg. Photographs of James A. Anderson by Philip Lieberman. All other photographs by James A. Anderson.

Library of Congress Cataloging-in-Publication Data

Talking nets : an oral history of neural networks / edited by James A.
Anderson and Edward Rosenfeld.
    p.   cm.
"A Bradford book."
Includes bibliographical references and index.
ISBN 978-0-262-01167-9 (hc : alk. paper), 978-0-262-51111-7 (pb : alk. paper)
1. Neural computers. 2. Neural networks (Computer science)
3. Scientists—Interviews. I. Anderson, James A. II. Rosenfeld,
Edward.
QA76.87.T37   1998
006.3'2'0922—dc21   97-23868
                                                 CIP

The MIT Press is pleased to keep this title available in print by manufacturing single copies, on demand, via digital printing technology.

Contents

Introduction

How does the brain work? What do we want computers to do? Do we want our computers and computer-enhanced systems to act the way we do? If so, how do we want them to mimic the abilities of humans?

Since World War II, a group of scientists have attempted to understand the human nervous systems and to build artificial systems that act the way we do, at least a little bit.

In this book, we have put together a series of interviews of well-known, productive scientific leaders in the important, controversial, mildly glamorous and very high-risk area of science described as "brain theory," "neural networks," or "theoretical neuroscience." The interviews describe how this science is done and how it was done in the words of the scientists doing it.

Many of the early developments of brain theory sprang from the roots of cybernetics. Other theorists took inspiration from neuroscience, physics, electrical engineering, mathematics, and even economics. The neural network field is a hotbed of cross-disciplinary activities, where these messengers from many disciplines and their ideas collide like subatomic particles swirling around a particle accelerator. The interactions, influences, and changes occasioned by these collisions are described in this collection of informal conversations.

One of us (Anderson) is a well-known scientist in the neural network field. The other (Rosenfeld) is a journalist who has chronicled neural net developments for more than a decade. Many of our interview subjects directed specific comments to one or both of us in our roles as a scientist who participated in some of this history and as a journalist who has described some of this history in print, particularly the parts related to practical applications, computer applications, and business developments.

What emerges are fascinating life stories: seventeen people at the center of complex scientific and social developments. Their personal stories include intimate and often touching details about their childhoods and their families that complement the details of their discoveries.

This book contains the words of individuals who agree about some things, but disagree about more. They range in age from the mid-thirties to the mid-seventies and were educated in several continent, although most of them currently live in the North America. Most are academics. However, anyone who believes that academia is an island of serenity populated with tweedy Mr. Chipses instructing the young in the ways of man and the world with wise and prudent counsel has obviously had little to do with a modern university.

Bringing a new field into existence involves the participants in a bitter and sometimes brutal Darwinian struggle for jobs, resources, and reputation. All of our interviewees had been through this process. The first thing they discovered about trying to promulgate genuinely new ideas is that most of their colleagues were not really very interested in hearing about them. The participants' struggles simply to obtain access to scientific communications channels, so that others would hear what they had done, occupy a significant part of several interviews and form an undercurrent in others.

Our interviews present neural network stories—the stories that have been told, referred to, whispered about, and imagined throughout the history of the neurocomputing field. These interviews are a Rashomon-like web of reality slices, rendered by interested parties, raconteurs, and sometimes those who believe that they are, in fact, the central characters. What's more, some of the mythic people responsible for the foundations of modern brain theory, communications, and computing—such as Norbert Wiener, Warren McCulloch, and Frank Rosenblatt—appear prominently in some of the recollections collected here.

One way to view this collection of stories is as a set of candid discussions about how science is actually done, as opposed to how we are told it should be done. Sometime during high school, we get exposed to a bloodless something called the "Scientific Method," which consists of a set of rules for doing science the proper way. First, we generate a hypothesis. Second, we test the hypothesis by doing an experiment. Third, we modify or reject our hypothesis based on the results. Like most things we learn in high school, such an idea has only a vague connection to reality. This book is about the reality.

These interviews were done in hotel rooms, in offices, and, in one case, by telephone over a period of several years. We were interested in the history of the neural network field and of the ideas that formed it as well as in the personal history of the participants. We had a list of topics we wanted to cover, but we often did not need to ask our questions. All of our interviewees have extensive experience teaching and lecturing, and most of them shaped their own narrative, with only modest prodding from us. Looking over the transcripts, almost all our predesignated topics were covered in some form or another during each interview. After a couple of questions to get things going, most interviewees became self-propelled and developed their story as they wished.

Over and over again, we were struck by the drama and passion involved in the stories. The questions these scientists wanted to answer in their work were important because they involved the way the mind works, the way the brain works—the way we as humans connect to and contact the physical world. Surprisingly, they sometimes involved religion, as something both to reject and to accept. None of our subjects fit the stereotype of scientists as cold-blooded, remote intellects. Exactly the opposite was the case. The work they were doing was an obsession and so dominated their lives that often they could think of little else.

Some of our interviewees worked alone, some with a few local colleagues. However, there were two particularly productive centers of work on neural networks and brain modeling. One was in San Diego in the early 1980s, a time and place that had a major impact on nearly half of our interviewees. The famous two-volume "PDP books," published in 1986, summarized the work of the "parallel distributed processing group" at the University of California at San Diego in this era.

However, by far the most romantic center of research in brain theory was the group that formed in the 1940s and 1950s around the charismatic Warren McCulloch and his brilliant, unstable, and ultimately tragic collaborator, Walter Pitts. Jerry Lettvin, Michael Arbib, and Jack Cowan describe this time in some detail and give their sometimes differing perspectives on it. The interviews are arranged in order of the scientist's date of birth so some of these historical themes can become clearer.

We would not want to give the impression that our interviews reflect only dour intensity. There are stories with considerable humor: Bernie Widrow sliding down the hills of San Francisco in his new, leather-soled shoes; Jerry Lettvin's future in medical school being determined by an unusual gross anatomy exam; Michael Arbib's misadventures job hunting in California.

This book will not provide an introduction to neural networks or brain theory, though most of the important ideas are quite accessible. For a formal introduction to the field, let us recommend two collections of well-known papers that we edited: *Neurocomputing* (1988) and *Neurocomputing 2* (1990). Anderson's textbook, *An Introduction to Neural Networks*, gives a systematic introduction. At this time, a number of other good introductions at many levels of complexity are in print.

Some of the interviews contain quite technical material. We have left much of this material in place, although there is no actual mathematics in this book. Mathematics is a powerful tool for working with complex systems, but, unfortunately, it often serves as a barrier rather than an aid to understanding. One way to view mathematics is as a kind of language that very accurately describes some important kinds of complexity. It is a difficult language to learn to speak. If a reader does not happen to speak that particular language, however, many of the basic ideas can still be communicated, often in simple sentences and images. Mathematics makes these intuitions precise and usable, but the essence of the ideas often comes through without the mathematics. In this context, some of the seemingly throwaway comments in the interviews are very deep. Some of these comments may strike resonances in those knowledgeable in the field, but the basic issues should be quite clear to everyone. Real science is often like this: it starts with simple questions; insights often begin as fuzzy pictures or vague verbal descriptions; and deep intuitions are communicated offhandedly, using metaphor and analogy.

Interviews that touch on such deep issues include Carver Mead's discussion of analog versus digital processes and Jerry Lettvin's comments on the role of discrete and continuous processes in the thinking of Walter Pitts and on the way Leibniz influenced both Pitts's thinking and indirectly the entire McCulloch group. Many interviews touch on the important distinction between engineering ("it works") and science ("it works like the brain"). Often, what seem like far-fetched connections turn out not to be: Jack Cowan's discussion of the forms that hallucinations take and the underlying functional cortical neuroanatomy is a striking example.

These talks also mention the controversies that surrounded the rise and fall of public and scientific interest in Rosenblatt's perceptron, as well as the influence of Marvin Minsky and Seymour Papert on the loss of interest in neural networks during the 1970s. Robert Hecht-Nielsen addresses this history during his interview and also describes some of the history of the momentous IEEE neural net meetings that took place in the late 1980s, a subject also addressed in detail in Bart Kosko's interview.

Another controversy raised in a number of the conversations is the scientific "credit assignment" problem related to the backpropagation algorithm, discovered by a number of different researchers seemingly independently. There is also a highly charged area related to the tremendous public attention brought to the field in the early 1980s by two of John Hopfield's publications in the *Proceedings of the National Academy of Sciences*.

We hope that some of the excitement and power of the ideas about brain function and intelligent systems discussed in this book come across to others as powerfully as they did to us during the actual interviews.

Let us make a few technical comments. These interviews were tape-recorded and expertly transcribed by Dr. Emily Pickett of the Brown University Department of Cognitive and Linguistic Sciences. We owe Dr. Pickett a great debt. No one speaks grammatical English when talking out loud, even Ph.D.s, even for the record, so we edited the raw transcripts in order to make them reasonably grammatical, to eliminate repetitions and hesitations, and to tighten them up when interviewees started to ramble. We also eliminated much of the redundancy that characterizes a long conversation. We also had to work within length limitations forced upon us by the economics of book publishing. The editorial assistance and publishing guidance provided by Betty Stanton was invaluable. In addition, our editor-shepherds, Jerry Weinstein, Wendy Drexler, and Katherine F. Arnoldi made sure that these interviews successfully completed the journey from manuscript to published book.

In editing the interviews we tried hard to retain the distinct personality of each speaker and let them convey their ideas as clearly as possible. The speakers were offered the opportunity to make corrections, check spellings, and, rarely, to make additions.

Jim Anderson
Providence, Rhode Island

Ed Rosenfeld
New York City
March, 1998

References

J. A. Anderson. 1995. *An Introduction to Neural Networks*. Cambridge, Mass.: MIT Press.

J. A. Anderson and E. Rosenfeld, eds. 1988. *Neurocomputing*. Cambridge, Mass.: MIT Press.

J. A. Anderson, A. Pellionisz, and E. Rosenfeld, eds. 1990. *Neurocomputing 2*. Cambridge, Mass.: MIT Press.

J. L. McClelland, D. E. Rumelhart, and the PDP Research Group. 1986. *Parallel Distributed Processing*, vol. 2: *Psychological and Biological Models*. Cambridge, Mass.: MIT Press.

D. E. Rumelhart, J. L. McClelland, and the PDP Research Group. 1986. *Parallel Distributed Processing*. vol. 1: *Foundations*. Cambridge, Mass.: MIT Press.

Note: John Hopfield is mentioned in many of the interviews in this collection. Though we were unable to meet with Professor Hopfield in person, we did conduct an interview with him in 1996 by telephone. However, due to technical problems that interview could not be transcribed. We asked Professor Hopfield to redo the interview by telephone early in 1997, as this book was going into its final stages of production. Unfortunately, he declined. We regret the loss.

Talking Nets

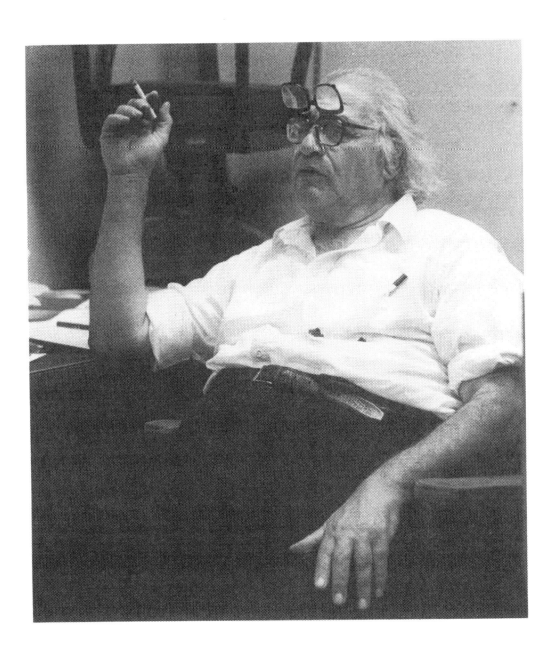

1   Jerome Y. Lettvin

Jerry Lettvin is Professor of Electrical Engineering and Biomedical Engineering, Emeritus, at MIT, Cambridge, Massachusetts. Professor Lettvin is well known for his classic 1959 paper with Humberto Maturana, Warren McCulloch, and Walter Pitts, "What the Frog's Eye Tells the Frog's Brain," Proceedings of the Institute of Radio Engineers *47: 1940–1951 [reprinted in* Neurocomputing 2*]. Some of the history and implications of this influential paper are discussed in the interview.*

June 2, 1994, Cambridge, Massachusetts, at MIT [Some material added in 1997]

ER: I want to find out how you grew up and how it was you happened to get interested in the brain. What's your date of birth and where were you born?

JL: I was born in 1920, February 23, so I am now seventy-four.

ER: Where were you born?

JL: In Chicago, grew up and went to school there.

ER: What did your parents do?

JL: My father was a lawyer. My mother was a piano teacher. I was the oldest of four children, and my youngest brother became a concert pianist. He's now professor of music at Rutgers University. My mother failed with me because she wanted me to be a pianist. I gave my first concert when I was eight and then retired from the field and decided to write poetry. That's what I wanted to do, to become a poet.

When I graduated high school, mother made it clear to me that either I would go into medicine or all funds would stop. She had a whim of iron, so I agreed to study medicine. I eventually entered University of Illinois Medical School in 1939 and graduated early in 1943 because of the war. Then I came to Boston City Hospital to the Harvard Neurological Service under Denny-Brown.

But my interest in nervous systems started in my premed college years at Lewis Institute, a working-man's school. Fifteen dollars per course. There I was exposed to psychology by David Boder. He had worked with Pavlov before becoming the psychologist for the prison system in Mexico. He bragged that it became the most advanced prison system in the world, with conjugal rights and an educational program.

He was a remarkable teacher who started me thinking about psychology as an interesting field, so I began reading. By the time I got into medical school, I was already committed to study the nervous system if I couldn't escape and become a writer. I was very lucky to have Gerhardt von Bonin as my teacher in brain anatomy. You want me to ramble on?

JA: Absolutely.

JL: I was a first-year student and I told Gerhardt I wanted to be a poet, that I really hated medicine. He read some of my poetry and said, "You're absolutely right; you'd make a better poet than a doctor."

So, comes the final practical examination in anatomy, and Gerhardt approaches the table. There's the cadaver. He looks me in the eye. He says, "You know, you want to be a poet, and I think it's right that you should be a poet. Let me put it this way. I will pick up something out of the cadaver. If you name it, you pass and you go on; that's your fate. If you can't name it, you fail, and then, by God, you can became a poet."

So he picks out something from the abdomen, deep in the abdomen. He holds it up without looking at it and says, "What is this?"

At this point, you know, it's a very weird choice. I decide to take the middle ground. So I say, "Cerebellum."

He looks at me with disgust, drops it back in without looking at it. "You named it. You pass." He was a very civilized guy, wonderfully civilized.

The year before I had gone to medical school, I had spent at the University of Chicago. There I met Walter Pitts, who became and remained my best friend. Walter was an autodidact. He taught himself logic and mathematics, and was able to read a fair number of languages, including Greek and Latin.

He already had a peculiar history. At the age of twelve he was chased into a library by a gang of ruffians, and took refuge there in the back stacks. When the library closed, he didn't leave. He had found Russell and Whitehead's *Principia Mathematica*. He spent the next three days in that library, reading the *Principia*, at the end of which time, he sent a letter to Bertrand Russell, pointing out some problems with the first half of the first volume; he felt they were serious.

A letter returned from Russell, inviting him to come as student to England —a very appreciative letter. That decides him; he's going to be a logician, a mathematician.

He went to University of Chicago, which is where I met him; but he never registered as a student. The two of us met at a Bertrand Russell lecture, and for some reason or another we became fast friends. I knew no science whatsoever, no mathematics at all. I was only interested either in literature, or if I was going to have to go to medical school, medicine. The two of us became inseparable. During that year at the University of Chicago, Walter had gotten hold of Carnap's new book on logic. This was in 1938. He walks into Carnap's office with his own annotated version of the book, pointing out some flaws. And he gives it to Carnap, talks to him a while, then goes out, but doesn't introduce himself. Carnap spends the next couple of months hunting high and low for that "newsboy who knew logic." In the end, he did find Walter and persuaded the University of Chicago to give him some menial job. Walter had no funds, had separated himself from his family, so that was good.

We stayed fast friends, even when I'd gone to medical school. We met often, would have long conversations together. He was a wonderful teacher. When I was in the third year of medical school, McCulloch came to University of Illinois, and Gerdhardt, who had worked with him once before at Yale, took me over to meet him. I remember, when I was about fourteen, I had read Buckle's history of the Scotch mind in the seventeenth century [Henry Buckle, *On Scotland and the Scotch Intellect*. Chicago: University of Chicago Press, 1970; orig. pub. 1857]. It set up in me a morbid fear of the Scotchmen. So when I first meet McCulloch, who carries himself as a cavalier, a Scotch cavalier, he scared the hell out of me.

Nevertheless, I settled in, and I became absolutely committed to the notion of working in the nervous system. I didn't do any experiments at the time. Walter then came over, and Warren was enchanted with him. Walter was homeless, and I had to escape from my family because the supervision was incredibly intense; it's very hard to say how intense it was. And so early in 1942 Warren invites Walter and me to live with him and his family. Warren and his wife, Rook, were always enormously generous. We settled in, and it was in the evenings then that Walter and Warren got together on "A Logical Calculus of Ideas Immanent in Nervous Activity" [the famous 1943 McCulloch-Pitts paper, reprinted in *Neurocomputing*]." Walter at that time was, if I remember correctly, about eighteen, something like that. Walter had read Leibniz, who had shown that any task which can be described completely and unambiguously in a finite number of words can be done by a logical machine. Leibniz had developed the concept of computers almost three centuries back and had even developed a concept of how to program them.

I didn't realize that at the time. All I knew was that Walter had dredged this idea out of Leibniz, and then he and Warren sat down and asked whether or not you could consider the nervous system such a device. So they hammered out the essay at the end of '42. Now, from fall of '42 I, in effect, dropped out of medical school, that is, formal medical school. I didn't appear at classes. What had happened was that a lot of personnel had been taken away by the war. At that time, the military was short on doctors and nurses, so I became, as it were, intern, resident, and nurse, depending upon what was needed, at the Neuropsychiatric Institute, the basement of which housed Warren. The upper floors were dedicated to psychiatry on one side of the building, neurology and neurosurgery on the other. I would appear for examinations in the various courses, but otherwise didn't go very much to class because it was sometimes close to twenty-four hours a day that I had to work. Walter very decently used to come over and keep me company when I was exhausted and had to rest.

The hospital gave me residence quarters so that I wouldn't have to go home, and Walter still lived with Warren, but he would come in, and the two of us would talk together. I graduated from medical school to everyone's surprise because I'd only appeared for examinations. But now I was really passionate about neurology. I had written a criticism of some stuff that had been put out at Harvard on the Argyll-Robertson pupil, and gave an alternate explanation for it. I sent this to Harvard, along with my application. I was immediately accepted, to my family's astonishment, in Harvard neurology. So I went there.

In 1943, I was working part time in neurology and part time in medical wards because I had to have general medical experience. My co-intern had a relative, a second uncle or something of the sort, by the name of Norbert Wiener, and said we should go over and visit him sometime. OK, so we go over and visit, and I meet Norbert Wiener for the first time. Wiener had just lost his right-hand man to a skiing accident, and was desolate; he couldn't find anybody else of that quality.

So I said, "I happen to know a young man from Chicago a mathematician, who's extraordinary" and so forth, and I described Walter Pitts.

Wiener said, "There doesn't exist such a person."

So I called McCulloch, and I remember the two of us chipped in together and got Walter a round trip train ticket to Boston.

It was very funny. If you don't mind an image occasionally, I remember Walter walking into Norbert's office, and Norbert says, "Hello," and no introductions, "Come, I want to show you something," and takes Walter next door, where there is a blackboard on two walls, and Wiener says, "I want to show you something; I'm going to prove the ergodic theorem." He starts out, and a short distance down the board, Walter begins some critical questions or asking for clarifications, and by the time they'd finished the first board, with Walter going along making commentary, it's sort of obvious what's going to happen. By the end of the second board it's definite, Walter's going to work with Wiener.

Now this was a wonderful thing. When Walter moves to work with Wiener everything is quite nice, except now I have to go off to the wars. After basic training in January of 1944, I have to report to New York, Bellevue Hospital, for a few month's training in neuropsychiatry. Walter at this time is hired by Kellex Corporation, which is part of the Atomic Energy Project. They're over in the Woolworth Building, and so we move to New York together.

We take a room together in the Village. He goes in the morning to Kellex, I go over to Bellevue, but meanwhile we're having a ball because I keep sending him at Kellex postcards written in German: "Enclosed you'll find the secret documents." They never got to him, you know, and we wondered what happened to them, whether people were dissecting the periods, or whatever.

Any rate, he also used to have fun there. He tangled with General Groves in a mischievous way. There were two wastebaskets in every room, a red wastebasket and a green one.

The red wastebasket was for sensitive material, anything in it had to be taken down, burned in the presence of two witnesses. So one day when the General is coming down the hall, Walter's sitting there, feet on the desk, cracking peanuts, throwing the shells into the red wastebasket, and the General screams, "What are you doing?"

Walter says, "Look at the shells," and on each shell he had inscribed alpha or beta, the magic Greek letters used in formulas, so the peanuts had to be taken down and burned in the presence of two witnesses.

In any case, the people there at Kellex were not allowed to talk to each other. Our apartment was one of the places to which they would come in the evening so as to be able to talk. If anybody had known this, I'd never have been allowed to go overseas, even though I understood nothing of what they said.

You want anecdotes, so I'm giving you some. At this time, the Atomic Energy effort was being embarrassed by the fact that the draft laws gave no exclusion of scientific personnel. The result was that good technical people were being drained from Kellex. They didn't know how to stop it. The 42nd Street induction station was an important place.

Now I always wondered whether the solution occurred by design or accident. There was a particular psychiatrist, Sam Wortis, whom I accused of arranging it. He refused to deny it, but he also refused to affirm it at the time. Installed as senior psychiatrist in the 42nd Street induction station was A. A. Brill, the fellow who had translated Freud. Now, Brill was a nut. He had the theory that schizophrenia had to do with symbolism, and since mathematicians dealt with symbols, etc.

So once Brill was put in office, and mind you, nobody had instructed him, it was his own meshugas that kept things going, scientists and engineers were being turned down right and left for being preschizophrenic, prepsychotic. It was highly demoralizing to the physicists and mathematicians who took seriously this schmuck's diagnosis. At any rate, the morning that Walter was supposed to appear, I decided, "I'm not going to go." It happened to be my turn, I've got to be there, but I call off sick; and it was fortunate I did, because the story came back to me.

Walter at that time wore a beard. He walks in, Brill looks at him and says, "Young man, why do you wear a beard?" And Walter says, "Old man, why do you?" And you can imagine that from this point it was straight downhill. Walter came out with a diagnosis of frank schizophrenia. Now, this upset him considerably. In some respects, he was fragile, and he tried his best to go back and volunteer. It took several people, including myself, to talk him out of it.

Then I go off to the wars and I'm overseas till the fall of 1946. I come back, I'm sort of demobbed, and Walter and Wiener had decided it was about time that I should learn some science.

So Wiener admits me single-handedly here at MIT as a special student. I hadn't had the calculus yet, and here I am, late on, twenty-six years old, and what the hell, what am I going to do? At any rate, I'm signed up for courses 18.01 and 18.02 [elementary calculus], analysis with Franklin, 8.01 and 8.02 [elementary physics], and that's my first term.

Now, I've got to put it to you, I had second-hand contact through Walter with this stuff, but you don't learn it when you are aged, and twenty-six is advanced age. Anyhow Oliver Selfridge, Hyman Minsky (the future economist), Walter, and I all move in together in one room on Beacon Street. The VA has taken me on as psychiatrist, and that pays a good part of our cost of living. I'm trying to make my way through MIT at the same time as doing part-time psychiatric work at the VA. It's not an easy job.

So I managed to survive the first term, passing everything. And then the second term is 18.03, 8.03, differential geometry, a third course in physics, and something else that I've since forgotten. Halfway through the term, Walter manages to lose one of Wiener's manuscripts, which he was supposed to look at. So I say to Walter, "Listen, I'm not cut out to be a scientist even if I've learned something. Let me take the blame." It's clear that Wiener's going to kick me out if that's the case. So I took the blame and got kicked out, and that was it.

So now I was on my own. One of the things I encountered was a weird prejudice. I had graduated from Harvard, internship in neurology; and that was the field I was really interested in. All of a sudden, my New York training and army experience had made me into a psychiatrist, and I went overseas, and became the head of neuropsychiatry at the 237th General Hospital.

I don't regret any of it. It was the busiest goddamn time I ever had, that oversea stint. But once I got out of the army, I come to visit Denny-Brown. Denny-Brown almost doesn't want to talk to me.

I ask, "What's wrong?"

He says, "You became a psychiatrist."

I said, "I didn't become a psychiatrist. You know I'm a neurologist. They forced me."

He said that was no excuse. Looking back, I agree with him. I wanted to go back into neurology, but one thing was true in medicine at that time. Once you were classed as a psychiatrist, forget it; you're never going to be able to get out of it. That classification makes you untrustworthy for anything else. I'm not joking. That was true back in those days. I didn't want to do psychiatry although I had some flattering offers. So I decided to hell with it, and went back to see McCulloch.

He says "Look, the easiest way to get out of this bind is to tell people that you're a physiologist, and see who bites."

I say, "I'm not a physiologist."

He says, "You'll become one."

He was a sweetheart. So I hired out and went to the University of Rochester, and Walter visits me often and we get back together again. At Rochester, they put me in charge of a very strange project, which is "How do you abort cats by using an elevator?" It turns out, a very little known fact today, almost all of the high rides in the amusement parks in the United States were used by women who wanted to have abortions. You see, motion sickness is a well known way of producing abortions. One of the reasons women used to sign up for cruises in the winter is that in the rough seas you get seasick so you abort.

Here's the psychologist who at Rochester says we've got to find out if this works for other animals. So he builds an elevator that moves up and down in square waves, sine waves, triangular waves. Anyhow I'm hired on for that. Warren doubles up with laughter, says, "It serves you right."

At any rate, there were also some extraordinarily good people in the neurophysiology of the ear at Rochester. And when the project director is not looking, I'm over there and I'm doing work on the vestibular system of cats, doing, I think, a damn good job. I had discovered some things already, but the boss forbade me to publish it because the data were electrical records. He had no confidence in electrical records, would not allow anyone in the department to publish such data.

So at the end of the year, I got an offer to go to Utah. Gee, that's nice. Meanwhile, I had got married just as I came to Rochester. I had met Maggie in Chicago while I was visiting Warren, and three dates later decided to be married. So Maggie's pregnant now, coming to term, and we're passing through Chicago, and I send a telegram to Utah, "Maggie's having a baby," and I get a telegram back. "We were trying to get in touch with you. Don't come because the funds didn't come through."

Let me describe Maggie for you. She was one of the most beautiful women I ever met, in both appearance and character, utterly unpretentious and with great native intelligence. My family looked down on her, my friends did not. She had had only a high school education, and my mother stayed angry for years.

One evening, shortly after we came to MIT, we visited Giorgio de Santillana, the historian of ideas and an old friend from my student days, at MIT. Giorgio was an adept at interpreting the Tarot. Scarcely a month would go by but Wiener would insist on having his Tarot told. Giorgio vainly explained that the Tarot should be consulted only at times of important choice. Wiener claimed he always had such a crisis and needed counsel.

At any rate Giorgio was charmed by Maggie and offered to read the Tarot for her. She was now about twenty-five. He read the cards with a faint air of disbelief. They told that by age forty she would become a figure of renown, an author and an innovator. Maggie still remembers that evening with some awe, for all came true. In her early thirties, after we had forged our three kids she was back-ended by a hit-and-run driver. For months she could scarcely lift here arms. Refusing surgery, she studied *Gray's Anatomy* and worked out what sort of mechanical regimen would restore her. Recovery was slow but steady, and within a year she was symptom-free. Others came to her for their mechanical disabilities and she worked out from here newly gained knowledge of anatomy and kinematics some remarkably successful conservative treatment. She charged nothing, was only interested in helping.

Several students, after being helped, persuaded her to hold fitness classes at MIT. Within a year there were about two hundred people per day taking those classes. Then Channel 4 in Boston picked her up, then PBS. For the next seventeen years her program, *Maggie and the Beautiful Machine* (everybody's body), was a PBS standby and her MIT classes stayed crowded. She published four books in her forty's and gloried in the fact that medical practitioners approved of her approach. One book is still in print after twenty-five years. Now she is beginning a new career on the Web, giving counsel on how to relieve back pain without medicaments.

The only pity is that Giorgio could not know that all this happened. He began failing before her ascent picked up steam.

We are still in love, though I am seventy-four and she is sixty-seven. She has not ever changed in my eyes and I cannot, in retrospect, imagine a luckier choice. (Nor, she claims, can she; I had all the luck).

So going back, there I am, high and dry in Chicago with Maggie, and I ask myself, "What am I going to do?" I don't want to be a psychiatrist, but what the hell. So I go to Manteno State Hospital, near Chicago. The head of the hospital is a very decent guy. I say, "Look. I'm willing to trade you psychiatric work if you'll give me a place to put up a laboratory."

So he said, "Sure, no problem. We have a shortage of physicians."

So I moved to Manteno State Hospital, where I was for the next three and a half years. Now what happened was that von Neumann, whom I had met via Warren, heard that I was doing this. He was very decent; and arranged that I get five thousand dollars for equipment. By this time I'd learned enough electronics, so I was able to build my own apparatus, and I started building my own amplifiers, remaking old oscilloscopes, and so forth. Within a few months I had a decent lab going. Some of the work I had done in physiology at Rochester had prepared me. McCulloch was a very good friend, so the laboratory got some attention. I was visited by some remarkable characters, like Pat Wall from Chicago, who became a collaborator.

We formed a little enclave down in Manteno, and it was a delight. Walter would come and stay with Maggie and me for weeks at a time. I worked in Manteno for three and a half years. By this time I've developed my own reputation. At RLE [the Research Laboratory of Electronics at MIT], Wiener convinces Jerry Wiesner that it's about time he got some physiologists of the nervous system.

Warren was a distinct catch because he had gotten tired of Chicago. So Warren, Walter, Pat Wall, and I sat together and decided that if they would take us as a quartet, we were willing to go, so we came to MIT. That was in 1951.

By this time I had gotten some sophistication in circuit design. I had to because it was the only way in which I could work, and in fact, I had built some things that had already attracted some comment. I had no problem settling in here and getting started. Walter and I now were more or less inseparable; Maggie was as fond of Walter as I was.

At MIT McCulloch became seduced into what can be done theoretically with nerve networks. A number of people gathered around and tried to see what could be mined out of this.

Walter by this time had more or less set himself against the concept of doing only abstraction. To him it was much more important to come up with notions of how automata were to be devised. He wrote a thesis, a very long one, on the properties of nets connected in three dimensions. Others like Caianiello had already done two-dimensional nets. Walter had come up with some very strange properties of the three-dimensionally connected net. He was in no uncertain sense the genius of our group. He was absolutely incomparable in the scholarship of chemistry, physics, of everything you could talk about history, botany, etc. When you asked him a question, you would get back a whole textbook. You sat back and listened for two or three hours because he would go on and on. To him, the world was connected in a very complex and wonderful fashion.

At the same time he was strongly opposed to having his name known publicly, so much so that when they offered him an advanced degree at MIT if he would just sign his name or translate a page from the German, which he did very easily, he refused. Later on, when they offered him an official position if he would just sign his name to a document, he refused.

In many respects, he was like the eccentrics you read about in England. He had exactly that quality. But he was a most winning person. I mean, almost everyone who knew him was fond of him. He was in a sense almost pure thought, thought personified, but with a delightful understanding about things generally, and was a most amiable companion.

At any rate, there was a sudden violent turning of Wiener against McCulloch due to Mrs. Wiener, who hated Warren, and Wiener cut off all relations with McCulloch and anybody connected with McCulloch, which meant Walter as well. Now Wiener was what Walter never had, a father figure, and that threw Walter into a decline from which there was no pulling out. He burnt the manuscript for his work on three-dimensional nets. Jerry Wiesner offered me a fair amount of support for the lab if I could just recover bits of it, but I couldn't. Walter was quite complete in destroying his own past work.

From that point on, we had no way of getting him interested in things. He did one major piece of work with Bob Gesteland. Bob Gesteland's first work on olfaction published in the *Journal of Physiology*, a really prestigious work that started a new branch of study, was done in collaboration with Walter. That was it.

When Humberto Maturana and I did the work on the frog vision, Walter was a little appalled by the results, which were very different from what he expected. That is, here were the qualities sought, but not as you would have them. There were invariances that were not formally tractable, or at least not in any ordinary logical way, and that were of a nature different from anything that anyone expected. They looked more like black magic than anything else.

Walter had an interesting response to these results. It's hard to characterize, but let me try to do it. On the one had, he believed the results wholeheartedly, and he approved vastly, but on the other hand, it was an index to him that logic was not the right approach to the brain. See, up to that time, Walter had the belief that if you could master logic, and really master it, the world in fact would become more and more transparent. In some sense or another logic was literally the key to understanding the world.

It was apparent to him after we had done the frog's eye that even if logic played a part, it didn't play the important or central part that one would have expected. And so, while he accepted the work enthusiastically, at the same time it disappointed him. He would never admit it, but it seemed to add to his despair at the loss of Wiener's friendship.

Warren, as I say, had committed himself to two-valued and three-valued logic. Walter lost interest in that. He was perfectly willing to be amiable about it but he didn't want to spend too much thought on it. He became more and more introverted. It was difficult to find him. He would try to escape from all his friends. We'd go hunting for him night after night.

Watching him destroy himself was a dreadful experience for several people who knew him very well. Warren, at the same time, also began having trouble. He had developed an inability to eat solid food. He had had two lung episodes, blowing out a hole in the lung and getting a pneumothorax. They stitched him up, and then finally attached the lung to the wall of the chest. But in doing so they set up what appeared to be a vagovagal reflex. Every time he would eat solid food his cardiac T-waves would undergo reversal, indicating coronary insufficiency. He would only take liquid food. It was clear that he felt that he was decaying in his physical powers. To the end, he always was enthusiastic, but you felt that somehow or another you weren't touching him. So Pat and I and Humberto worked more or less independently.

ER: Could you discuss the beginnings of artificial intelligence?

JL: Let me now say that I know nothing about artificial intelligence, which is a separate discipline from nervous physiology. I have admired the effort since Marvin Minsky and Seymour Papert began it at MIT, but I never tried to study it and have as little grasp of it as anyone not directly involved. I do

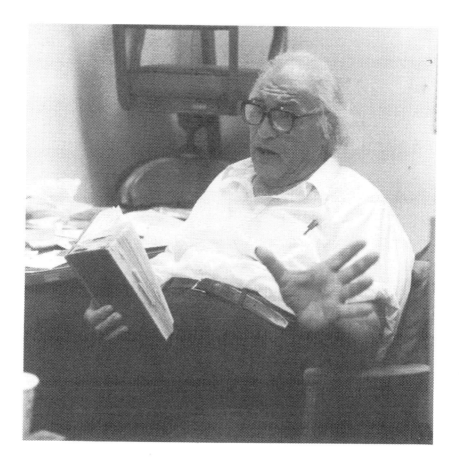

know a little about the history of the problem that they propose to solve and I can talk about that.

When Walter and I went to live with Warren and Rook McCulloch in 1942, Walter introduced Warren to Leibniz's remarkable work in the latter part of the seventeenth century. First of all, Leibniz showed long before Boole that logic reduced to arithmetic. The demonstration was incomplete but went far enough to establish the plausibility of the hypothesis.

Leibniz was an engineer as well as mathematician, scientist, and philosopher. Early in his career he designed and built the first calculator that did all four arithmetical operations in decimal and thus superseded Pascal's adding machine that could only add and subtract numbers. Leibniz's method of multiplication and division was ingenious and remained in use for hand-powered calculators till the end of the nineteenth century.

But then he invented the binary number system whereby multiplication and division reduced to addition and substraction. He was unable to build a hand-powered calculator in binary because of the friction between the many parts, and the technology of the time could not support alternative designs (e.g., there were no reliable valves).

Nevertheless he pointed out that if a binary calculator was possible, so was a logical machine which could perform any finite task that could be expressed completely and unambiguously in logical language. That was the proposition that Warren and Walter adopted. If a neuron could be axiomatized as a device that performed elementary logical operations, then a nervous system would be regarded as a computer.

The thrust of their original paper on "The Logical Calculus of the Ideas Immanent in Nervous Activity" (and of their elegant but less often quoted second paper, "How We Know Universals") [both in *Neurocomputing*] was to apply this concept.

Half a decade earlier Turing had issued his fundamental paper on the universal logical engine. Half a decade later, at the end of WWII, von Neumann and Bigelow, would begin to design the first electronic computer in this country. So in that magical decade the great effort began to realize Leibniz's concept.

Now Leibniz had also developed the ideas of negative feedback control. The practice of this control goes back to antiquity, but Leibniz abstracted the idea, and expressed it in intelligible form. Wiener's "Cybernetics," appearing in mid-decade was, as he says in the book, also in the tradition of Leibniz. And so too was the concept of information that had appeared at the hands of Szilard in the 1920s and was to be elaborated wonderfully by Shannon and Weaver and other mathematicians beginning in the '40s.

What with information theory as analyzed and logical machines as synthesized it was certain that Leibniz's logical automata would appear, machines that performed tasks and acted as if animated by intelligent purpose.

While I could not but be aware of these potential developments by close association with Warren and Walter, it wasn't till about five years later, after we had come to MIT, that I began to suspect that logical machines may not provide useful models for perception. Von Neumann had voiced his doubts in his Hixon Symposium Lecture (1949). Certainly I had not the competence in logic or mathematics to consider the issue myself. But it seemed to me that before you considered a mind that would perform combinatorics on perceptions there had to be some qualifications on how perceptions represented the world. Everything I had found so far and had read about suggested that the world was reported by natural language rather than logical language, that is, in terms of things and their relations rather than sense data to be processed into the concepts of things. There was no feedback from brain to retina, so that whatever synthetic a priori [genetic programming] was involved in vision had to be indwelling in the retina itself, a five-layer device alternately connected vertically and horizontally in the layers. That a fixed five-layer system of elements, laterally interacting, gave the content of perception to a frog suggested that we were dealing with a system of active complex analogue filters rather than a system of logical elements. Each cell in the array was a complex processor of local spatiotemporal relations in the images, and was modified by remoter influences.

For this reason I had my doubts about artificial intelligence based on logical processing. I realize, of course, that any continuous function can be represented by a logical program, but also that combinations of such functions, themselves modulating one another, are not so easily represented in real time. But then, my ignorance of computational arts is unsurpassed at MIT and I doubt if I could word a satisfactory argument.

Having delivered this apology let me say that artificial intelligence as a way of understanding and realizing purposive action and even reasoning is entirely in the Leibnizian tradition. It is a noble effort to develop by synthesis new principles to guide the analysis of animal and human activity. Furthermore, it is in the spirit of biology to discover functional laws as well as composition of parts and the programs encoded in DNA. In short, AI becomes an adjunct to psychology in the normal course of events.

I would like to put it that AI and computer science are one and the same were it not that this would incur the wrath of my colleagues who see a great difference between their science and psychology.

But the changes in thought brought about by the scientific revolution in the seventeenth century have not only persisted but been sharpened. Everything observed must be explained in terms of mechanism alone, everything but the knowing observer. What we call process, the strategy of performing a task, has to be explained by the state-history of the mechanism, that expresses the process. In the modern biological view it is a vulgar error to imagine Big Blue as playing chess with the purpose of winning a game. The state-history of the mechanism, which includes the changes made by the opponent's moves, provides a determined sequence that explains how the end-state of the board resulted from the initial state. Nothing is added to our knowledge by the concept that Big Blue is playing chess.

This may sound like a caricature, but any review of modern biology shows preoccupation with mechanism even in the study of brain and nervous function. Whatever studies of process there are, they appear as speculations in clinical journals. And you only have to read the Harvard version of Darwinian evolution to see the lengths to which academics go to avoid the concept of an evolutionary process; or else read the current neurobiology literature to marvel at the utter lack of interest in process.

Ever since biology became a science at the hands of biochemists it has carefully avoided or renounced the concept of purpose as having any role in the systems observed. Purpose in observed nature was once and for all anathematized by science in the seventeenth century. Only the observer may have purpose, but nothing observed is to be explained by it. This materialist article of faith has forced any study of process out of science and into the hands of engineers to whom purpose and process are the fundamental concepts in designing and understanding and optimizing machines.

Leibniz showed beautifully at the end of the seventeenth century that in any system provided with a flow of energy there were two aspects of energy. One explained interaction in mechanical dynamics. The other explained how an interaction would be represented by an independent "spontaneous" flow. E.g., if you cut the cord suspending a weight (in his example), the weight

Jerome Y. Lettvin

falls of its own accord; the cutting only removes the impediment. Cutting does not act on this weight, the weight does not act on the cutter. The only relation between the cut and the fall is that the fall represents the cut. The same is true for a flow of water from an elevated tank through a valved outlet. The flow represents the position of the valve. Thus switches and analogue amplifiers are responsible for process.

Once representation, as the essence of spirit, is given an energetic explanation as information, the structure of an automaton as the mechanism sustaining the processing of information becomes intelligible. Logical engines, computers, are possible, and, if possible, cannot be excluded from reality. So far as Leibniz was concerned, if automata would be manufactured, animate things could be regarded as automata.

An automaton, thus, must have two explanations, one in terms of mechanism and accounted by efficient cause, the other in terms of process and accounted by final cause. Thus, to deny purpose to living creatures is foolish, it is tantamount to denying what you don't choose to explain, a peculiar stance for a scientist. Logical computers can be built by the arrangement of switches. Analogue processors can be built by the arrangement of amplifiers. What is the problem? Every process must have a mechanism to sustain it. And this holds even for thinking about a process. The spirit has no subtle action (such as thinking abstractly) which is not accompanied by the action of devices in the brain which is part of the body.

All this is part of a longer essay I will write sometime, organizing all the relevant material out of Leibniz's essays. He felt that living automata differed from manufactured automata in that the elements in living automata were themselves machines while those in manufactured automata were not. Thus analogue computations were possible to living machines; manufactured machines did logical computations.

In the modern case artificial intelligencers took the strong engineering position. Tell us, they say, in unambiguous terms the tasks you want performed, including the task of designing task-performing programs, and we will design them. Even better, we will design them to optimize themselves to the purpose, to learn. We will even build a program that will discover theorems of which it hasn't been informed. That was the salutary beginning. But the difficulties were soon apparent. For example, the world as it appears to us is not unambiguously described anywhere. Idealizations that are natural to logic are unnatural to me as an animal. Every attribute of a definite object of perception, such as color, shape, size, form, order, whatever, is known by relations with other things and changes as they change. Attributes are not as we speak of them, predicates of things in themselves, they are relations. Furthermore, we perceive things in terms of the uses we make of them rather than as what they are intrinsically as things alone.

Yet the current doldrums of AI are far more laudable than the cop-out of biology's anathema on purposive process and its self refinement. It is obvious by now that the immediate future of biology is in mechanism only.

It will classify programs and then explain subassemblies of mechanism as shorn of purpose. Strategy and process will remain, as always, the forte of engineers who are not at all self-conscious about not being scientists.

You see, to me, biology is a dead end now. Current neurobiology is like somebody coming in with shelves and shelves of transistor manuals and saying, "See, this is how, this is what the world reduces to." And you say, "But tell me how to put them together."

At this point, I part company with biologists. I find the artificial intelligencers, the nerve-net people, and their colleagues far more clever. It doesn't matter that they are wrong in some sense; they are right in spirit, and whatever they discover, it's going to be useful in the end, whereas so far as I'm concerned, whatever the biologists are discovering tells you nothing about the nature of the system. I mean, the components don't tell you anything about what the system does, only how it works.

So, from my point of view, I'm a strong supporter even if I'm not a sympathizer or participant in artificial intelligence. Forget about biological preoccupation with receptors and transmitters and magic molecules. You take that for granted as mechanism, but the process of a system is a different thing from its mechanism.

As I say, Walter held this view, but at the same time, by holding that view he partly sterilized himself. The economy that we have encountered in nervous system operations drives us up a wall. Most of that stuff I haven't published, and I'm not likely to publish. But the economy is so fantastic that at times you almost sort of believe Leibniz's notion about the infinity of operations. Somewhere in between the logical approach of artificial intelligence and the semilogical approach of nerve nets lies the possibility of VLSI of analog devices with variable connections. Let me give you an example.

Consider the eye. You have a very interesting item from Pascal's memoirs in the seventeenth century. He buys a telescope. This is only a few years after Galileo introduces it. He's looking up at Venus, and sees it has a phase, like the moon, just as Galileo remarked. He calls over his mother, who is a very intelligent woman. She knows a great deal about science. She looks through the telescope and says, "But Venus is the wrong side to. It's reversed."

Pascal is startled, and says, "How do you know that?" She says, "Because I can also see it with my naked eye."

Now, there's a very interesting point here because people had claimed to see things by naked eye that ordinarily you would say it was impossible to see. You certainly have the identification of the largest moon of Jupiter, Io, by a Chinese astronomer in the third century A.D. There were people whose ability to resolve double stars was quite fantastic. So you look at Pascal's story, and you're not willing to dismiss it for two reasons. First, the *Scientific American* didn't exist then telling you about the phases of Venus. Second, you know that telescopes invert. That doesn't come to mind usually when you're looking up at the stars.

So the question arises, would it be possible for Madame Pascal to see what she did? It's an interesting question. Now, the angular size of Venus at its closest approach is a little over the diameter of a foveal core. It's bright enough that you can use your fovea. At its farthest distance, it's a little less than a cone in diameter. So how are you going to issue a statement that it's flattened on one side?

I looked at this, and then I said, "Well, suppose we imagine the initial layers of the retina as a Wiener filter" [the rods and cones along with the horizontal cells]. Let me specify what I mean.

For a normal young person with a four-millimeter aperture pupil [the optimum aperture for the eye as an optical instrument], a point spot of light at infinity goes into a Gaussian distribution on the retina of about four cones, five cones in diameter, maybe a little more. This is a blur. Furthermore, when you consider the rods and cones, you find that they are resistively connected at their bases to each other in such a way that the space constant of the resistance away from a photoreceptor is even larger than the space constant of the Gaussian distribution.

So you say, God is playing games with us. Here's this woman sees this thing, and you're giving me one form of crapping it out by the optical image and a second form of crapping it out in the receptor arrangement and this is ridiculous.

But there's an interesting point. If the resistive connections are between the cones and the cones are taken as voltage sources, then the current flow into each cone is the Laplacian of the voltages. The Wiener filter consists of a Laplacian applied to a Gaussian, you get super-resolution out of it. With this super-resolution, you now have a sharpening of the image in a satisfactory way. Helmholtz said about the human eye, "If somebody brought me this as an optical instrument, he would be fired on the spot." To put it bluntly, it doesn't even have the optics of a Brownie camera. So far as Helmholtz was concerned, this was very bad optics, but he did not know of image-processing in this way. If you're going to do resolution on the basis of a Wiener filter, wait a minute, that's a better way to do it because if in fact I have a discrete manifold of the cones, I don't want to limit myself by discontinuity of receptors in determining the resolution of the image.

I want to be able to get honest-to-God sharpness, which means that I must process at the first layers before I ever go through any nonlinear synapse. Now I haven't published this. I'm looking for a graduate student who's willing to work on it. It's not a very challenging topic, and image processing experts who say, "Oh, come on, this is obvious," But I'd have to reply, "Well, if it's obvious, let's set up a synthetic model of the receptors on the computer, and let's see what we come up with."

You don't want to try for something that's going to restore the image because that's a different problem. You want to know, "Is the information that I get sufficient to be able to say that I can resolve such and such?" That's all you want to know, for the point is to account for expert vision and how it is possible.

If what I said is true, then the notions that we have of image processing in the eye are going to have to undergo a major change. You would have to stop working with the computers and start building instead the arrays of coupled analog devices that are capable of giving you this sort of operation. Because if Madame Pascal spoke the truth we had better use the process to tell what to look for in the mechanism rather than the other way round.

JA: That's a wonderful example. You have all these receptors electrically stuck together. They're all interacting, and they should make a mess out of everything.

JL: Which is precisely what they do if you follow ordinary visual physiology. The moment you bring in any sort of additional hints of process, it begins to look tasty. But I'm seventy-four years old. You know, I'm not an adept. I've seldom used computers. I'm not going to learn programming. But the problem is straightforward and any reasonable student should be able to sit down and grind this out in a few months. After all it is now accepted that the human eye has super-resolution, and this has to be accounted in the first layers of the retina for it would be impossible to do later.

The problem I mentioned is the sort of thing that you would say is meat for any engineer. The difficulty is, it's so trivial formally that nobody wants to pursue it, and on the other hand, at the level of the physiology it's at odds with all the received wisdom.

JA: This sounds a lot like ideas I've read of yours along the lines of when the nervous system does something, it really does it right. It's just a question of finding how it's doing it right.

JL: And how to do it economically.

JA: That's a very profound way of analyzing the system.

JL: Let me give you another example. Humberto and I described the bug detectors [in "What the Frog's Eye Tells the Frog's Brain," 1959]. What we did not report, and what to me is still the most astonishing thing about the bug detectors, is the following property which I explored with Arthur Grant. You have a central region of a bug receptor three degrees in diameter, a three-degree visual angle outside of which you get inhibition of response.

So working strictly within this three-degree angle, by masking off everything else, you find the following property. You bring one spot in, move it into the field, and as long as you move it around, wonderful response.

You bring in two spots; if they're rigidly coupled in their motion by a fixed distance between them and are moved around, you get a good response almost as if they are only one spot.

You bring three rigidly coupled spots in, and it doesn't matter their size or their disposition or their distances from each other: move then around as a rigidly coupled triad and there's no response at all.

"Wait a minute," you say "Just a second. You're telling me that this thing is able to separate four phases from three phases?" If you have a white background and two black spots, OK; three spots, forget it. You connect any two spots of the three by a barely visible black line, and all of a sudden it's a two-spot system. It becomes visible. Or else you move any one spot with respect to the other two, now there's a response.

How do you build in a system such as the retina, a device that distinguishes between four and three phases? That to me is a delightful problem. I've been worrying about it for a couple of years, not seriously, you know, not devotedly, but how would you go about it?

But I don't have any students, and I cannot take on graduate students. Because of my age, taking on a graduate student is equivalent to asking him or her to take a chance. If I die, the student's left high and dry. Who else is going to take him on?

What I'm saying is that if you're going to look at visual form even in a frog you're also going to have to use notions of topology not geometry.

Those three spots, if they move translationally, rotationally, it doesn't matter how they move, how big they are, how separate they are, whether they are the same size or different sizes: three spots, no response, providing they move rigidly together. Now that, I consider that to be a lovely find, but I can't publish it, you know, so what's the point? I can see an editor saying, "So big deal. So what does this tell us about vision?" It tell us that in the analysis of vision, if we stick to conventional methods and conventional processing, we're not going to get anywhere.

JA: Is there any work on theory that you've particularly liked recently? You mentioned that you talk to Marvin Minsky.

JL: Oh, yeah. Gad Geiger and I are working on something quite different, top-down sort of stuff. Eight years ago we showed that dyslexia is learned, not genetic or neurological. And we also devised visual tests by which you could demonstrate this. Then we went in and showed that we could teach dyslexics to read. The theory is what our colleagues have jibbed at. If we had only presented the results, everybody would have said, "Oh yes, very interesting." But what we have is evidence that there is an internal feedback of intended action onto the perception of the objects to be acted on. It performs a weighting function, not on anything related to contrast or anything else, but on some operation that switches between the distinctness of form and the indistinction of texture.

You can demonstrate lateral masking in yourself by experiment. On a clean sheet of paper make a small X in the middle as a fixation point. About an inch and a half to the right or left print a capital letter such as N, about a quarter-inch high. When you gaze at the X you have no trouble in seeing and identifying the N. So your visual resolution is sufficient. Now print two more capitals of the same size on each side of the N to make a five-letter word, e.g., TENET or SANTA or FUNKY. Now when you gaze at the X most of you will not see the N identifiably even though you know what you printed. It is not as if the N is blurred. It has become nonidentifiable—it has texture but not form. You see clearly both the beginning and ending letter of the word, and surprisingly, the end letter is clearer even than the beginning letter. But it is as if the other letters somehow interfere with seeing the middle letter. Since you can recognize the N by itself, the problem is not in resolution. Instead the order has departed from the form, leaving only a statistical impression rather than a distinct set of relations. It is this conversion from form to texture that is controllable, but not by the will directly, rather by choice of task. It is an unusual concept, but we have evidence to support it and can even demonstrate an appropriate mechanism in the variable receptive field sizes of single cells in frog texture.

In any case, the concept suggested a measure for diagnosing dyslexia and a treatment to alleviate it. What we showed is that lateral masking applies to whatever in the field of vision is not directly relevant to the task you want to perform. It is as if when you decide on the objects of the task, those objects take on distinct foreground form, and everything else is reduced to background texture. This is what is meant by attention. The point, of course, is that attention is not confined to the direction of gaze. It can wander over the whole visual field. If you mislearn where to attend for a task, the region that should be attended is laterally masked and so there is a barrier to correcting misattended task performance.

So we've used that, you see, and now our latest paper has just been published in *Vision Research* about the work we did in Tuebingen [G. Geiger, J. Lettvin, and M. Fahle 1994, "Dyslexic Children Learn a New Visual Strategy for Reading: A Controlled Experiment *Vision Research* 34; 1223–33]. We did it there with grammar school kids. There they let us take a batch of grammar school kids who were dyslexic, and within eight months they were reading within three quarters of a grade of where they should have been reading. The method works. But the theory behind the method, namely, this concept of task-determined later-masking operations, goes against the grain of every psychologist. And yet now there is evidence that this occurs with all forms of perception, for example, audition. We've played our game out, and we wrote sort of a manifesto. Now I would like to switch to some other stuff.

ER: Where would you point people just entering the field now, and what do you think the difficult problems are?

JL: Well, to me, the difficult problems are how to go from an image to its content. The important thing that you realize, for example, in perception is that just as in mathematics, lines are imagined, so they are in vision. You argue from phase boundaries; boundaries are the things that are important in vision. A line is a doubly bounded area. Line drawings are sets of doubly bounded areas.

JA: I get the feeling you aren't too impressed by the very empirical nature of neuroscience now.

JL: I think much of it is beside the point if you want to relate mental activity to nervous activity. Don't misunderstand me. I've great respect for you if you say, "I'm going to find out how this thing is or what the elements are in building it." That's a legitimate project, and if people who are doing it confine themselves to that, if those were the only claims they made, I would be delighted and show intense respect. But the pure nonsense that comes out as if, for example, particular feelings, things, ideas, images were functions of particular chemical compounds, you know, I have no use for that.

JA: I get the impression that neuroscience is far more empirical now now than it was twenty-five years ago.

JL: It is. Twenty-five, thirty years ago it was still imaginative on a systems level. Now unless I were interested in chemistry, I don't think I would go into it at all.

JA: You know, when I was a graduate student at MIT, I found your approach to doing science really inspirational. You did stuff that you thought was important and not what other people thought was important.

JL: Yes, it's going barefoot. You see, I'm lucky. I'm one of the few people who managed to be on the outskirts of everything at the right time. So, in a certain sense, wherever I walked barefoot, I would pick up some things. I don't think that sort of liberty is going to be anything that you get anymore, so I was very fortunate in being a hanger-on in the right places at the right time.

JA: I remember they had the faculty come in and give talks to us incoming students. We had a number of very earnest talks about biology. Then you came and made it sound like a lot of fun. You did interesting problems and had a lot of fun doing it. It was wonderful.

JL: Actually, there are a huge number of delicious problems in biology on a macroscopic level that are going begging because, in the first place, NIH [the National Institutes of Health] will not sponsor anything that doesn't sound like careful science, and in the second place, it's very difficult to get people to be interested in naturalist approaches. It's not deep technical stuff that appeals to them. There's this intermediate range in which I operate sort of solo, simply because I'm not learned enough for one group, and am not enough technically sophisticated enough for the other.

JA: There should be more people like that!

JL: There's a big hedonistic element in looking at individual problems and asking, just as a first-order pass, "What could I do quick and easy before going into it deeply?" These first-order and second-order passes are themselves informative, much more so than people think. The Pascal's mother story, that's a first-order pass at an image-processing system. But it suggests that if you're really going to do image analysis, you could do worse than design yourself a receptor region that is a discrete manifold but in which you use operations of the sort I described, where you're not precise in image down to single points and where you must use something like a Wiener filter. It's a trivial thing to design in analog computers because all you have to do is replace every cone by an op-amp, and you have a voltage governed by the light while the lateral resistor connections between op-amps gives you the current. Now, it's trivial to build such a thing, and behold, if you monitor the currents, you now have a resolution that is very good indeed. It may seem a mess, but it's a sort of mess that tells you what to look for.

So.

Jerome Y. Lettvin

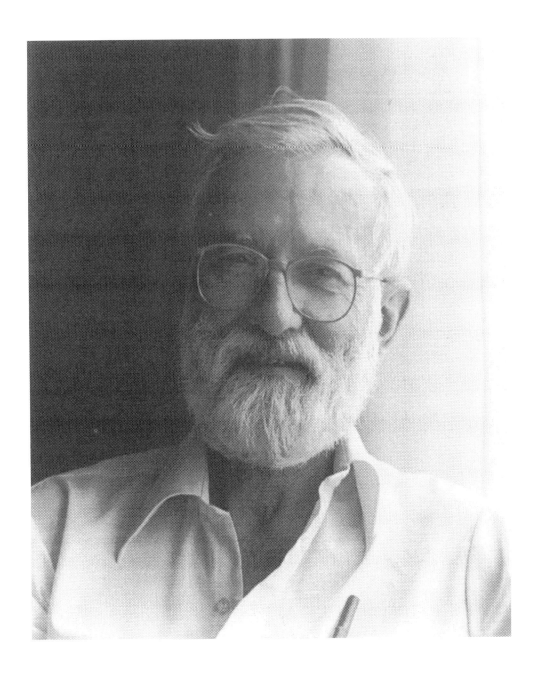

2   Walter J. Freeman

Walter J. Freeman is Professor of the Graduate School, Division of Neuroscience, Department of Molecular and Cell Biology, University of California at Berkeley, Berkeley, California. A good source for more information on his research is in his 1995 book, Societies of Brains: A Study in the Neuroscience of Love and Hate, *Lawrence Erlbaum Associates.*

June 1993, Baltimore, Maryland

ER: Why don't we start with your date of birth and place of birth?

WF: January 30, 1927, Washington, D.C. The year Lindbergh flew the Atlantic.

ER: Could you tell us something about growing up and about your early education?

WF: I was born in Georgetown in a growing family, which moved out into what were then suburbs in Chevy Chase in Washington, D.C., where I went to grade school, junior high, and high school. We lived across Connecticut Avenue from the Bureau of Standards, now called the National Institute of Standards and Technology. I spent many happy hours rooting through their trash and finding the most amazing pieces of discarded equipment and devices. I started exploring early. One day a worried-looking streetcar conductor met my mother at our front door and asked, "Do those babies belong to you?" My twin brother and I at the age of five months had crawled out and sat on the tracks with two or three streetcars lined up behind us. Home was where I did my first scientific experiment. I'd heard that cats always land on their feet, so I held the family cat upside down by its paws, releasing it lower and lower to find out how much space it needed. The tests ended when she scratched me and ran off, but I learned that it had to be at least above its normal standing height.

My ancestors were a mix of foreigners. My mother's folks were Irish from County Cork and an Ulsterman from County Fermana. On my father's side were political refugees from the War of the Roses in Dorset, Huguenots after the revocation of the Edict of Nantes, a deserter from the Hessian mercenaries in the revolution, and a former captain from the Swedish army that lost the Thirty Years War. Family legend has it that one of our Mayflower descendents was raped and scalped by Narragansett Indians. She survived in a hollow tree on rainwater for ten days, contributed to the family gene pool, and wore a cap ever after.

Times were hard in the depression, and some of my earliest public memories were of seeing bums and hoboes going from door to door for handouts. I graduated at the age of seventeen, went to MIT, and spent my first two semesters there before going into service. Gladly, I might say, because I came to detest the place for all the reasons that the Berkeley students came to detest the Berkeley campus in the 1960s. I went into engineering initially as a prospective way to make a good living as a civil engineer because I wanted to build bridges and pipelines and dams, things like that. But I found very quickly that there wasn't much intellectual content, and besides, I had a course in surveying, which involved standing around on street corners in Cambridge, Massachusetts, in midwinter, which was very unpleasant.

So I switched my major to physics and then went into the Navy and did service in the South Pacific. They trained me as a radar technician, so I learned basic electronics, and when I got into research, I could design circuits with vacuum tubes, though I never mastered transistors. I was out there fairly late in the action, so I was shot at a couple times, but it wasn't anything you'd want to make a story out of.

But what did happen that was of interest was that I was stationed in the Marshall Islands at the time of the Bikini tests and was evacuated along with most of the other inessential personnel because the hypothesis then was that when the atomic bomb went off in an underwater explosion, this would rip the coral atoll in pieces, and they would slide down the top of the undersea mountain and create an immense tidal wave, which then would essentially wipe out all the people in Oceania. Knowing that this was a possibility, they went and set off the bomb anyway. But nothing happened. I did see the illumination, the blast, from a distance—the mushroom cloud. So that was my introduction to the atomic age. At the time I was rather grateful for the existence of the bomb because it meant that something like a projected million casualties, which I would likely have been one of, in the invasion of Japan didn't take place.

So I went back to MIT with the conviction that I would get out of the place as soon as feasible. But at the time, with all the veterans coming back, there was no place else to go. A turning point came when I went with my fraternity brothers to a meeting, which was set up by ONR [the Office of Naval Research], of people who had done war research and who had an invitation to continue on, to see what new weapons could be developed. Norbert Wiener was the key speaker in this. His speech consisted, essentially, of the statement that he had regrets that he had carried out the kinds of activities he had done. He thought that further weapons research was immoral, and he was getting out. He advised all his colleagues to get out, and a good third of the audience got up and left. To my regret, I did not. I was puzzled as to what was going on. But having thought about it for the next several months, I decided that physics had no future. What it was going to be was making weapons. I went to see the dean to talk this over, and he said, "Education is either qualitative or quantitative. Which would you prefer?" I would find something else. I left.

Not knowing what that "else" was, I dropped out, essentially left the sciences and went into English and mathematics at a place called Hamilton College in upstate New York, a small liberal arts college. And that was like going into a monastery. It was very isolated—a long, long, winter in upstate New York. So by the time spring rolled around, I consulted with the dean of students, after having had more than one run in with him, and he very quickly said, "Yeah, go to the University of Chicago; that's where all the other misfits go."

And so I arrived and spent two very interesting years there studying philosophy under Richard McKeon. He was an Aristotelian and responsible for the architecture of the University of Chicago undergraduate system, based on his philosophy of education. He was very difficult as a teacher. He was abusive, attempting to be challenging, but in the process, leaving people behind. The history of his teaching—well, of his style, I should say—is well documented in Robert Pirsig's book, *Zen and the Art of Motorcycle Maintenance*, where the chairman of the Committee of Methods and Ideas is modeled on McKeon. In fact, Pirsig left Chicago to go to a mental hospital for treatment, which was the motif of his book, and I left to go to medical school.

While I was in Chicago, I read an account in *Time* magazine of the work of Warren McCulloch, and I was impressed with his approach to neurons as switches, binary switches doing Boolean algebra. So I left Chicago without ever getting an undergraduate degree because I changed majors too often. I chose to go to medical school at Yale because John Fulton was the leading neurophysiologist at the time. He was one of the last students under [Sir Charles] Sherrington, and the thought appealed to me of being a scientific grandson of the old master, who was still alive then. I wanted to go into neurology and biological psychiatry in particular. In this I was very strongly influenced by my father, who was an eminent neuropsychiatrist and who had introduced a number of innovative techniques in psychiatry, most notably the use of prefrontal lobotomy, which was widely practiced in the era before the introduction of chemical treatment for psychotic and neurotic disorders. We were proud of the medical heritage of our family, which went back to a physician at the time of the revolution, John Morgan, who studied medicine in Edinburgh. My great grandfather, W. W. Keen, was the first surgeon to succeed in removing a brain tumor. When I was growing up, our house had visitors from around the world, with talk about the battles between the psychoanalysts and the neurosurgeons. The mental hospital at St. Elizabeth's, where my father worked as the neuropathologist, was a childhood playground for me.

Yale is where I got to know some neurophysiology and was very quickly informed in my studies in physiology, in my first year of medical school, that McCulloch did not have a valid picture of the nervous system, however fruitful it might be in other ways. McCulloch was, I think, really the originator of automata theory, of self-organizing systems, using digital logic. He was the godfather of the digital computer since von Neumann relied upon him so heavily for his neural metaphors. But it was clear to me that that's not how the nervous system worked.

I did my second experiment on cats in my freshman year. I attended a lecture by Bob Livingston and José Delgado, the guy who made history in a bullring in Madrid by fighting a bull after he put electrodes into its diencephalon. He used a radio transmitter instead of a cape to make the bull turn. Anyway, they described all the reactions you can get by electrical stimulation in the diencephalon, the sort of thing that Hess had done for his Nobel prize, so I went up afterward and asked whether they had ever seen panting or shivering because that was the topic of the lectures in physiology that week. Livingston said, "No, but would you like to try?" I said, "Sure," and spent the next three years trying and eventually got cats with thermodes chronically implanted in their hypothalamus to pant. The cats also showed some interesting postural adaptations to heat and cold. That way I disproved the old dual-center hypothesis of temperature regulation that Magoun and Ranson had proposed, by showing that the anterior hypothalamus was sensitive to both heat and cold.

Well, the reason I went to medical school was to go into practice, not into research, so after I graduated, I did an internship in pathology at Yale, doing autopsies, frozen sections for surgeons, that sort of thing—getting into the basic science of medicine. Then I did a year of internship on the Osler Service at Johns Hopkins. It was a pretty demanding time being on twenty-four-hour call for an entire year, and the standards of patient care were extremely high, but after some rough spots in the first three months, I got really good at it and enjoyed that sense of real professional competence. You didn't expect to save everybody, but you knew what to do, no matter how bad things were. The turning point came when I drew an old lady, unconscious, with total paralysis on her right side. She was old and had a history of a bad heart and weak kidneys, so I wrote orders on her, "No fluids, no antibiotics, turn every two hours, and call me when there's a change." Well, that blew the lid off. My resident took me off the case and did the whole heroic thing—tracheotomy, positive pressure respirator, levophed drip, urinary catheter, and so on—and he pulled her through, sort of, though she couldn't talk or get out of bed or recognize her family. Then I got called into see the chair of medicine, who held a kind of court martial with some of his senior people, and the upshot was that I was not to be punished, but, as the chair put it, "If you cannot accept the prevailing ethics of the profession, Dr. Freeman, you are advised to seek alternative employment." I thought about it for a few hours and then decided that that was good advice, so that night

I wrote an application for a postdoctoral fellowship from NIH [National Institutes of Health] to study neurophysiology under Bob Livingston and Ted Magoun at UCLA. I had my licence, and I kept the door open to go into practice as a kind of safety net, but after I got tenure at Berkeley, I let it go because the only practice I had was on my growing family. But that's another story. I've always considered myself to be a good scientist, but first and foremost a good father.

I came to study olfaction by the back door. I started with my medical school thesis doing temperature regulation and decided after my departure from clinical medicine to go into a study of feedback regulation by the brain in what were then called psychosomatic diseases—hypertension, hyperthyroidism, hyperhydrosis, that kind of thing—and in particular to study fever as a resetting of the body thermostat and to do this by recording the unit and EEG field-potential activity of the hypothalamus with local heating, first with diathermy and then with various bacterial toxins to induce endogenous fever. I'd done some of that work already in medical school. Well, you can heat the hypothalamus to the point where it's been cooked, and it doesn't change its field potentials. The unit activity, of course, is gone. That led me to search for the origins of the field potentials in the hypothalamus, which turned out to come from the hippocampus, from the thalamus, but most strongly from the olfactory cortex, the prepyriform cortex. And that then led to a study of the mechanisms of origin—how the dendritic field potentials were generated and what their behavioral correlates were—and to the study of these mechanisms in waking animals with implanted electrodes. It was obvious that they were dependent on the degree of arousal, but in other respects there were no clear behavioral correlates of the time series. They were dependent on respiration, as a driving input, and on the level or degree of arousal, but virtually nothing else.

This was a period when, as I look back on it now, there was the emergence of a virtual obsession with unit recording. The techniques for that had been developed by C. G. Phillips in England and by Richard Jung in Germany for recording single cells intact in the CNS in behaving animals and for studying sensory processing using single units. Of course, the people who became most widely known, Hubel and Weisel, established a kind of methodology for doing these studies in which theory was virtually abolished. That led eventually to the emergence of cellular neurophysiology. And although I was interested in unit recording and used it extensively, it was mostly in conjunction with recording of the dendritic potentials at the same time. This was from a conviction that the single neuron embedded in very high-density synaptic connections with other neurons couldn't function as a single element like a transistor—or a vacuum tube, for that matter—in a discrete connection system.

Networks were becoming increasingly elaborated, and this was, of course, when the perceptron was in vogue and a dozen other network type of devices, like the Ommatidiac, which I looked upon as, well, interesting gadgets, but they had nothing to do with how nervous systems work. I think that I became somewhat isolated from the main flow of activity—not ever to the extent where I had difficulty getting funded, though, mainly because there were some very helpful journal editors like John Fulton and Bill Windle, who maybe didn't understand the work, but saw that I could write well, and because the program directors at NIMH [the National Institute of Mental Health], real idealists, had faith in me and what I was trying to do, so I never starved. But I had difficulty in establishing ties and working relations with any one of the three or four main camps, if you count the physiological psychologists who were doing evoked-potential studies, which I had very little interest in or use for.

There were people doing unit analysis in the style of Vernon Mountcastle in the somatosensory system—Jerry Lettvin and Horace Barlow—and Steve Kuffler in vision, unit studies. There was the prevailing development of perceptron theory, which again was irrelevant to what I was doing. What I was interested in was dynamics—how a system could work in the context of feedback control. I was very impressed with Larry Stark's work, opening the loop of control of the iris by shining a very narrow light beam into the pupil, too small to be influenced by the pupillary contraction. When I looked at the oscillations in the olfactory system and the beautiful ringing, sinusoidal kinds of activity, I was very quick to see that these were not due to oscillations of single cells being coupled together, because when I looked at the spike-interval histograms, they were essentially Poisson distributions. They couldn't come from coupled oscillators at the single-cell level. And when I applied chelating agents to remove the calcium, which is the way of boosting oscillations in single cells, it didn't bring out oscillations at all. But when my student Maria Biedenbach and I applied synaptic facilitators like acetylcholine to the prepyriform, we got enhanced oscillations, so they had to arise from synaptic interactions.

On the other hand, in 1965 when I looked at the relationships between the single-unit firings and the field potentials, I found that if I recorded units from the same cells that were generating the field potentials, the unit firings and the EEG waves were in phase, just as the feedback equations required. But there was another class of units that showed a ninety-degree phase lag, which had to be the units coming from the inhibitory interneurons. I got comments when I published this or sent it off for review; I got comments back from the editor, "Well, this phase difference here, the difference you're talking about, is only a few milliseconds. Why get excited about it?" People were looking at it in terms of a time delay of 5 or 6 milliseconds for an oscillation with a period of 25 milliseconds, and they thought that was insignificant and didn't look at it as a phase delay, which was ninety degrees. Well, you see, the distinction is between looking at the activity in terms of a logical net as distinct from a dynamical system, and I think that that difference in perspective still persists. It relates to how you look at this intervening process of integration of the dendritic current between the incoming pulses and the outgoing pulses. It's a kind of a multifaceted difference between my way of looking at the nervous system as masses of neurons and most other groups around looking at it as nets of neurons. I think that this difference still to a large extent persists now. But, for me, the 1960s were really a time of laying down some basic principles. One of them was the negative feedback loop, which I modeled using differential equations and Laplace transforms.

JA: I remember hearing you speak in, I guess it was 1968, at the Salk Institute, where you discussed some of your linear systems analysis approaches. I thought it was just wonderful. I was really impressed by it.

WF: Oh, I wish you would have said something; I would have felt better!

JA: I went and looked for all your papers because I thought, "Wow, this guy's doing something really neat."

WF: It's a different way of looking at brain activity, so I had the negative feedback loop early. In fact, you know, you don't have to look for how the cells couple together selectively. It emerges as a simplifying principle: the notion that there's not just negative feedback, but there are mutual excitation and mutual inhibition. At that time, mutual inhibition had been demonstrated by Hartline and Ratliff for Limulus eye, and it was widely used to model Mach bands and lateral inhibition, but mutual excitation, especially, was regarded as a no-no, along with reverberatory circuits, because these were unstable, abnormal, epileptic. Cajal himself had said that feedback couldn't exist in brains because then a neuron couldn't tell the difference between its input and its own output. So this is in the nature of a simplifying principle because you have excitatory neurons and inhibitory neurons, so why restrain/restrict the action of each onto the other? In fact, if you have the mix, and you have each type acting on both other types, then very quickly you come to the conclusion that there are these three types of feedback. I started to play with what are called Mason diagrams, which show the relationships between different boxes in a linear circuit where you can rearrange things. I had the feeling of having broken into a space which was so big that I couldn't see the other side. I remember thinking to myself, "Hey, if I go into this, into this area, I'm going to get swallowed up and may not come out again." In fact, it was some seven or eight years later that I finally came out the other side, so to speak. This is when I had this marvelous comment from Marcel Verzeano. Mike was a biophysics professor at UCLA and a senior statesman at the time. He came up to me after I'd given a talk on the use of impulse responses and root locus techniques, and he said, "Walter," he said, "I've got some advice. You've got to give up this 'mademadics.' People won't understand your papers, and they won't read you, and you'll be ignored." And he was quite right, in a way, though not the way that counted.

This was the time in the mid-1960s that I discovered the sigmoid curve. I called it bilateral saturation because it showed upper and lower limits on neuron firing. If you use the evoked-potential technique and the poststimulus time histogram, you can't see the upper limit because you can fire the neurons—you can drive the frequency up as high as you want—and they have time for recovery during the inhibitory rebound. It's only when you look at the ongoing spontaneous activity and use a statistical measure—the probability of firing conditional on the EEG amplitude—that you can begin to see the upper limit, which shows that the cells can't go over the top of the sigmoid. It's a static nonlinearity because the firings of the neurons in the populations are uncorrelated. In fact, I had trouble publishing that. I found an oddball journal in '67. They finally took it, but the journal subsequently went out of business, so the original paper is hard to find. It was called the *Logistics Review*. It's not carried by most libraries.

JA: Never heard of it.

WF: Yeah, I'd like to get it republished sometime, reprinted sometime, because I look on that as a seminal paper, which contained most of these ideas about cortical systems with feedback, multiple-loop systems, and the bilateral saturation nonlinearities, about piecewise linearization and the root locus technique with Laplace transforms, and about the importance of opening the feedback loops, to get the open-loop rate constants. You do that with deep anesthesia, either local or general. You can't do feedback analysis unless you find ways to separate the forward and feedback limbs. Also, the idea of amplitude-dependent gain changes, of changes with learning, which was identified with the mutually excitatory synapse, that was also discovered by you, Jim, among others, in terms of the connection matrix, where there's a reciprocal connection among the excitatory elements. In fact, Anderson and Amari and Hopfield and Kohonen—all have that connection matrix. I discovered this change with learning, identified it there in the prepyriform in 1968, which I think preceded most of you.

That was done in a very simple, elegant experiment where I placed electrodes into the olfactory tract of a cat and used electrical stimulation to get the monosynaptic synaptic evoked potential and then trained the animal to respond to the stimulus. As the animal learns, during the learning process, there is some magnificent wave activity that's going on, which is so transient that it's not possible really to measure it because it's too chaotic. But once the learning process is completed, then you see this change emerging. Out of a roiling activity you see this evoked potential coming out. The initial amplitude is no bigger, so it's not the first synapse which is doing this, but the duration of the wave is a little bit longer. Again, it's not much longer, only a couple of milliseconds, but what it tells us is that the synapse, which has undergone a change, is between the excitatory neurons rather than the input ones, where LTP [long-term potentiation] takes place, for example. All these findings came out in the 1960s, and I went on into the 1970s to build on these studies, to connect them all together with the root locus techniques. Most of that work was done on the prepyriform cortex.

I went on then to look at the olfactory bulb—working that way outwardly toward the periphery, instead of inwardly, as is more commonly the case. I did some studies on the self-exciting populations and the input to the olfactory bulb, and here again I ran afoul of the establishment because the prevailing dogma is that the external interneurons, the periglomerular cells, are inhibitory because they are small and they're GABAergic [GABA is a neurotransmitter], and they're supposed to carry out surround inhibition. My studies showed that not only are they mutually excitatory, but they're also excitatory to mitral cells, and they don't have the need for inhibitory neurons to stabilize them because they're stabilized by saturation. I demonstrated this by using root locus techniques. But, as you can understand, physiologists don't understand root locus, and engineers don't understand physiology. So it's a beautiful study, but it's just not easy. In fact, it took six papers to put the study itself out and I couldn't get the papers all in the same journal. So two of them are in *Brain Research*, and two of them are in *IEEE Biomedical Transactions*, and the other two are in the *EEG Journal*. I put it all together in a book as a kind of an overview. I did that on invitation from Ilya Prigogine, who invited me to lecture in Brussels. I gave a series of half a dozen lectures as "Titulaire de la Chaire Solvay," so I was able to summarize the linear analysis of neural dynamics in one book, using piecewise linearization. Later on, at my suggestion, Joachim Wolff and his group at Göttingen showed that these GABA cells, the periglomerular cells, accumulate chloride ions, which explains why they are excited by GABA.

JA: That was a very interesting book. What was it, '75 or '76? [Walter J. Freeman. 1975. *Mass Action in the Nervous System: Examination of the Neurophysiological Basis of Adaptive Behavior through the EEG.* New York, N.Y.: Academic Press.]

WF: Yes, in fact, it's on display in the Academic Press booth here [at the conference]. It's still hanging on. Going to Prigogine's group gave me an opportunity to learn nonlinear dynamics, and that was when I started off doing dissipative structures. I pushed linear analysis as far as it would go. I was introduced to this new field by Aharon Katzir-Katchalsky, who was a frequent lecturer at Berkeley. He organized a workshop because of his insight into the possibilities for hierarchical organization of neural populations. This came out posthumously. He was killed on his way home with the notes for this congress, this NRP [Neuroscience Research Program], an MIT think tank, which meant that it had to be done by others who really didn't understand what he saw. He was incredibly quick, had an incredibly well-informed and broad mind. I sent him a paper which essentially was a summary of what I'd been doing, and he called me up; he wanted to talk about this. I went up, and he asked me a few questions, and then he got more and more excited, and I got more and more excited, and we had this kind of intellectual orgasm together as he began to explain to me what this work meant. So that was how I got introduced to Prigogine because one of the last things he said to me before he went back to Israel was, "You've got to go and see Prigogine." And I said, "Who?" and he explained to me who this Belgian theoretical chemist was and what he had to offer. And so that is where I learned to formulate differential equations with nonlinearities and to find some way of solving the problems of state transitions.

JA: That was Katzir-Katchalsky who was killed in the airport massacre in Israel, right?

WF: Yes, he was devoted to dissipative structures and state transitions, which I think people haven't really picked up on even now. I asked him for some background, and he sent me to Alan Turing's 1952 paper on chemical morphogenesis, which was really the origin of Prigogine's thinking on dissipative structures.

JA: Those were the unknown Turing papers, the ones that were not on computers, but on biological dynamical processes.

WF: When Turing essentially got out of computing, he figured that the really important work was in biological dynamics and especially the growth of form, the geometrical shapes of trees and flowers. And that's what led to the emergence of nonlinear dynamics as a major way to study brains now. So that was also a time that I had finished putting together a system with sixty-four preamplifiers, a multiplexer, and analog-to-digital converters for doing spatial recording because I wanted to get back to this old question of where's the sensory information. It was obviously not in the time domain. There wasn't a wide enough frequency band, and it wasn't in frequency modulation, and it certainly wasn't in any small number of pulse trains in a network. I had developed a system for recording from up to ten microelectrodes simultaneously and for taking multiple units from each one. I placed this array in the mitral cell layer and did simultaneous recording of wave and unit activity. It was strenuous, trying to watch ten oscilloscopes at the same time, to balance them all. It was obvious to me that the variability of the unit activity was so great that only a small fraction of the variance in each pulse train was covariant with the other pulse trains, and that small fraction was the crucial information to extract because the output tract of the olfactory bulb to the olfactory cortex, the prepyriform, has no topographic order to it. It does have some kind of operation, but it's in the nature of a spatial divergence and integration, not topographic mapping. This is another key feature overlooked among people as diverse as anatomists and engineers. There are some pathways in brains which have topographic order in them, but the majority of pathways have this wide divergence. There's got to be a reason for that. It's not simply that there's some kind of specific wiring of relatively small numbers of neurons. There are literally tens of billions of neurons. The only thing that can survive that kind of real-time, on-line integration is activity that is common over the whole surface—that has the same instantaneous frequency.

So that led me to looking at the spatial patterns, regarding the olfactory bulb as Lord Adrian had postulated a half century before, as essentially a spatial-coding mechanism. But Adrian had thought that this was a coding in

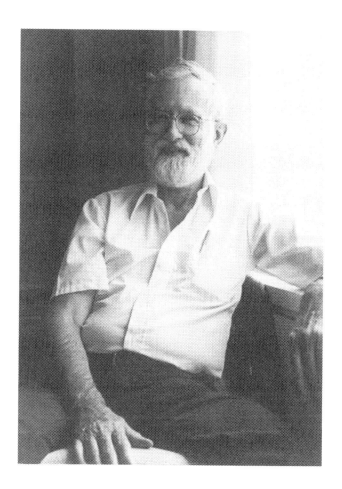

which each odor would have a certain location in the bulb, and that maybe one location would fire whenever an active odor was presented. This is essentially the perceptron model of olfaction. But the patterns occupied the whole bulb, like the kind of interference pattern that Karl Lashley looked for, and the patterns weren't related to the stimuli, but to the context.

I think the most compelling demonstration was to train the animal to respond to two odors—one rewarded, the other not—and then simply reverse the contingency. And we got new patterns. Not only that, but the pattern for the control state changed too. Well, in a true associative memory, this would have to be the case because in making an association to a new input, you change the existing store; everything has to change, and that is basically what we see. Of course, it raises the question, "How can you still have stimulus-response [SR] invariance when this intervening store is subject to continual modification, a change with everything that's put in?" And the obvious answer is that when you change the input side, you also change the output side. So the SR invariance is maintained through the environment, that part of the loop where it belongs, and not on the inside, where in fact it can't hold if you have a true associative memory. We came to the conclusion that what we're looking at then is not a record or not an image of the odor itself, but rather of its meaning for the animal, its significance—what a stimulus will imply for the animal in terms of what it will have to do about the odor. Again, this is something that very strongly diverges from existing views of how the nervous system is operating.

JA: An associative computer is a very different kind of computer than a nice, clean, digital computer. Things are really a mess, and you have to view it in a very different way.

WF: I think that's why Horace Barlow, for example, has such difficulty with mass action. He was in my department; in fact, I hired him when I was department chair in physiology. He, of course, has a conviction that the only thing you can know about the nervous system is what comes out of a microelectrode. EEGs and populations are all part of what Jerry Lettvin once described to me as the "Sherringtonian ooze."

JA: I've heard that called microelectrode myopia.

WF: Very good. So that's how I got into neurodynamics and then more recently into chaos, with the realization that these patterns are not periodic, temporally or spatially. For a while I thought that brains couldn't work if they were chaotic. In fact, when I was modeling the olfactory system with what I called Katchalsky sets, I stumbled onto chaos without knowing what it was, and I changed the design so that sort of thing just wouldn't happen. What a mistake!

JA: Sort of an interesting evolution from linear to nonlinear dynamics to chaos.

WF: Kind of going along with the field. I've had an occasional look into the history of psychiatry by reading the first chapters in textbooks from the 1850s, 1880s, on into the 1920s, and it's very clear that psychiatry and neurology under Hughlings Jackson and Freud, was dynamic. They thought in terms of nerve energy, resistances. In fact, Freud has a marvelous passage in his "Prologue to a Scientific Psychology," in which he describes the importance of the contact barriers between neurons as the site of the changes with learning and changes with degree of will or energy or whatever. It was two years before Sherrington and Foster came out with the word "synapse," but there it was, as Freud said, the contact barrier—that's where the action was.

JA: It's always amazed me how knowledgable people were about neurophysiology in the nineteenth century. You read William James and Freud and some of the other early work, and it's remarkable.

WF: John Dewey is another of my favorites; he wrote this essay in 1892 in which he says that the concept of the reflex isn't scientific; it's a religious idea.

JA: Do you have any thoughts about where the field is going to go in the next few years?

WF: I think increasingly it will go in the direction of the emergence of a new class of machines which are truly dynamic and not symbol processors. I've been urged, for example, to take my system and put it into a form like a Hopfield net, where it can be operated on by logical tools. But of course that's throwing out the baby with the bath. The initial approach that I thought was optimal would take the equivalent of hardware, using operational amplifiers to take advantage of continuous-time dynamics for solving the equations, because the big problem you come out with is how slow the digital simulation is. But I encountered serious problems in trying to do it that way. I think the nervous system essentially solves the same problems by using pulse frequency as an analog variable. Basically, that's what we do in numerical simulations. Within a few years I think we'll be on real time, using fully parallel processing and using big machines which are going to be operating in the gigahertz range, and then probably go in the direction of dedicated hardware involving large numbers of DSPs [digital signal-processing chips]. Then we'll replace not the single neurons, but rather the local neuron pool, which really I think of as the functional unit. Self-organizing dynamics will be increasingly used as means for designing feature extraction.

In other words, when you have a problem of scene reading—a problem of defining what's figure and what's ground, what things to look for—this is a high-level cognitive problem, even philosophical, because it concerns what is important for an animal, what it needs to see in order to stay alive. You don't just look for angles, edges, and write digital code to specify these things; you turn the system loose and let it do its own thing. And we do that already with our KIII model, as we call it. Just turn it loose, and it decides for itself from examples, generalizing over a few samples for a class. And we don't know what it's looking at. In fact, the first thing you do is what the eye and the ear do: take a transform of the input. We can do that most simply with a Fourier transform because that's easy to code, but almost any one will do. In that case, you disseminate the information; it's all there, but it's not in a form that we can, as individuals, hear or see. It's what our brains do inside. It takes a fully parallel system to operate on that stuff.

JA: It sounds as if you're saying that parallel hardware is nice, but the software is going to be extremely odd in a parallel domain. You have to worry about these dynamical systems, these nonlinear systems. And the whole idea of knowledge will be different in a parallel dynamical system.

WF: Well, it will certainly be different from what is currently conceived as knowledge in a conventional digital computer. Knowledge arises from actions that people take with their brains—to make a move and try to see what happens when you do that. When we design machines to learn from their own mistakes, knowledge in machines will be, I think, more akin to knowledge in the sense that we understand the world around us with our own brains. And what brains create and process is not information. It's meaning. That's the big difference between man and machines, meaning versus information.

For example, the device that we are currently developing, which is the basis for a couple of patents that I hold, is essentially used to identify or to classify small industrial objects. The classification is either acceptable or unacceptable. It's good or bad. What's extracted, essentially, is the meaning of the object and not anything having to do with the specifics of the object. This kind of system can be trained to operate on any number of classes or kinds of things, just with a couple of examples. Given an example, it takes a simulated time of a couple of seconds, and then it's off and ready. It's like having a worker on an assembly line. Today it's going to be sorting apples from oranges, and tomorrow it's going to be something else. I view this as a kind of interface between a finite brain and essentially an infinite-dimensional outside world. I mean, if you think of it in terms of what's coming in to us all the time, it's a collection of photons, of phonons, of molecules in the airflow, of whatever. All of this collection of physical energies can be subdivided or restructured in an infinite number of ways. And what we do, essentially, is to take this massive inflow—what William James is said to have called the "blooming buzzing confusion"—and replace it with something that we generate inside. That replacement is chaotic in its finite dimension, which is manageable for this finite-state machine inside. Now I see the role for this kind of dynamical system as providing the interface, which is preprocessing the inflow from the infinite outside and reducing it into something that's more manageable, like the dimensions that come with the raw letters on a printed page. But I don't see that happening very quickly, not so much because of the technology, which I think is there already, but because a reorientation of thinking has to take place.

JA: It's a painful process.

WF: In some respects it's painful, if it means that you have to learn whole new kinds of disciplines. For example, we have learned that digital computers work well in simulations for point and limit-cycle solutions of our equations but not for chaotic solutions. This is because of attractor crowding. As the number of first-order equations is increased, the number of attractors also increases, and the size of their basins decreases. Over a hundred or so, the size of the basins approaches the size of the digitizing step. Numerical solutions are like a drunk trying to walk a straight line. Sooner or later the projection for the next value falls outside the desired basin, and the model goes awry. Basically the problem is that digital computers work with rational numbers, not with real numbers. They truncate, and this is incompatible with modeling chaos. We have found that we can stabilize chaotic solutions with additive noise, but we don't have the mathematics that could tell us how this works. The implication is that we should use analog hardware to model chaotic brain dynamics. So the study of brain dynamics leads us right to the frontiers of mathematics and of analog devices.

ER: Could you describe your current work?

WF: That might get a little too technical, but maybe I could simplify. As I say, one of the critical problems is trying to play with the parameters in the system as we have it now to get some clearer idea of the nature of the chaotic dynamics. The chaotic process has certain obvious properties in the nervous system, like spatial coherence and stability, and we can't fully control them. We need to be sure that the kind of process we're looking at is in fact a global process and not a capture of the system by some local part of it that is dominating it, which I think is antithetical to the way in which the nervous system's operating.

I'm continuing to work with animals. I'm trying to develop an alternative measure of a chaotic process, which depends on spatial-pattern measurement of the phase, rather than the amplitude pattern, because of what we've seen in the olfactory bulb. Each burst of gamma oscillation has a phase gradient in it over the surface. But, you see, when a stimulus comes and a burst of oscillation happens, this is not the spread of a synaptic wave; this is spread of a state transition, and it's what physicists call anomalous dispersion. It's like when you hit a metal bar on one end with a hammer, and the sound wave gets to the other end before the impulse does. Anomalous dispersion involves a separation of the group velocity of the spreading state transition from the wave velocity of information transmission. If you put a stimulus into one part of the olfactory bulb, then by synaptic transmission presumably ultimately the stimulus would get to where it's going, although it dies out much faster. But when the bulb undergoes a state transition from one level to another, making this jump essentially involves undergoing a major global change in its spatial pattern, and that has its own velocity. It's like what happens when water is supercooled. That crystal falling into it forms the site of nucleation, and the state change will spread the crystallization throughout the whole system. It's that kind of a process. And the velocity that it travels out at is about two meters per second, which is the velocity of the mitral cell axon collaterals. Most of the collaterals go only a millimeter or so, but there are some which go longer distances, and that small number is sufficient when the system is brought close to the edge of a basin for a state change. When it's close to a separatrix, then a very small stimulus will carry it over.

This is where the sensitivity to initial conditions comes in. When a chaotic system is brought close to its transition state, then any small event can flip it over. This is why people talk about the flapping of a butterfly's wing in the Caribbean causing a hurricane in New York. It's a statement of the sensitivity of the system. It's what Hermann Haken, who worked on lasers, described as the expression at the macroscopic level of a microscopic event. I think that that's a good way to describe a sensory transformation, which often starts with a very weak stimulus. A small twitch of the visual field or a faint whisper, whatever, can lead to this galvanic change of the whole nervous system. It's that macroscopic state change over a global piece of cortex, which has been primed appropriately by past experience and by present sensitization to a small input to realize that change as an appropriate global pattern. That's an excellent reason to go and look at chaotic dynamics.

JA: Makes good biological sense, too. It's big and it's fast. That's exactly what you need for an animal response. A big behavioral response. Not graded.

WF: I gave a talk on this to a group of statisticians a year ago. I went to a summer symposium of the American Mathematical Society. It was supposed to be on statistical modeling in biology. I thought I might talk about brains and their chaotic dynamics, but that seemed to make them somewhat uneasy. They were not happy about this. The reason is that invoking a deterministic model to describe these essentially unpredictable phenomena, which you can look at with statistics, sort of put them into a secondary role. Their interest in modeling was stochastic equations, and chaos puts them simply in the journeyman position of having to do the janitorial work of cleaning up after the fact. So I asked this one guy, "Did you find it interesting?" and he said, "Once you see it, it's so obvious, it's not interesting anymore. What else could it be?"

JA: The same is true among psychologists. They love random noise. And of course you know most of the models in psychology have huge amounts of random noise in them, so immense the poor brain would never be able to function.

WF: Well, the brain makes its own noise. In fact, when a transition of this kind occurs, it's not that there's signal emerging from noise or embedded in noise. It's that the noise generator is now generating a signal, but the properties of the signal have such a noisy appearance that oftentimes you can't tell that it's a signal.

JA: It looks now as if they're finding waves all over the cortex—these "new" oscillations.

WF: Yes, in fact, Wolf Singer says he did what I told him: he opened the pass band on his amplifier, and the waves fell right out. We've found the same dynamical patterns as in the olfactory system in the visual and auditory and somatosensory cortices. But they're still interpreting the process in terms of coupled single cells. They characterize it as "the binding problem"—how to get together a bunch of feature detectors. They're not thinking of the processes in terms of a dynamical systems approach.

JA: People got quite exotic, saying this is the basis of consciousness and all that ...

WF: Christof Koch and Francis Crick.

JA: That's who comes to mind.

WF: I have thought this, too, and there are some others now that think that waves are the basis for consciousness. You might as well say the same about action potentials. People have done that, too—in fact, Sherrington and his "magic loom," though he was actually a dualist when it came to consciousness. It's an old story that goes back to—well, it's this pattern of attempting to fix onto some lower level some higher-order property. Like Holger Hyden came to the conclusion that because he was seeing changes in RNA, it must be the molecule of memory, which led to that infamous flatworm story. A whole generation of young people were misled by cannibalizing flatworms. The idea was that you train a flatworm by electric shock to go to one side or the other of a T-maze, and then you grind it up and feed it to the cannibals, who remember which way to turn.

ER: In the *Journal of Irreproducible Results* ...

WF: The *Worm Runners' Digest*. Well, for a good twenty years I was getting students who would come, and they wanted to study memory, and this was how they got started. In fact, high school science fairs featured this. Nobody could reproduce it in a scientific setting, but it was easy to reproduce in high school fairs. Melvin Calvin was a Nobel prizewinner in chemistry for having solved the problem of photosynthesis, and, like an even dozen other Nobel prizewinners, he decided that he was going to get a second prize in the nervous system—that he was going to solve the problem of memory. He had an enormous laboratory with highly coordinated, skilled technicians, Ph.D.s and so on, working under his direction. So he hired a couple of guys from Michigan to come out and train flatworms, and then he set up everybody else to study the brains. These guys spent an entire year trying to reproduce their own results with Calvin breathing hot fire down their necks. But they couldn't reproduce their own results, and they went to other people's places to try and reproduce their results. Finally, Calvin had to come to the conclusion that the only animals that were learning were the investigators. A great defeat.

ER: Is there other work that you think has importance for the neural net field that you haven't touched on?

WF: Well, in terms of dynamical systems, the most important structure to study is the limbic system—the part of the brain that puts intentional behavior together, the part that creates emotional behavior and orients it in time and space—especially the entorhinal cortex, which is the main source of input to the hippocampus and the main target of hippocampal output. This area is kind of wide open.

As far as applications are concerned, the carryover of these studies to humans is really important. I'm engaged in a joint program with Alan Gevins and Vinod Menon to try and find these patterns in EEGs from human volunteers, and I'm doing some in my own lab, trying to extend the methods. But there's a major problem, which is to screen out the EMG [electromyogram], which rather badly obscures what it is that we'd like to look at. We haven't solved that problem.

I see this whole area of nonlinear dynamics as of major importance in the future development of psychiatry. They have enormous quantities of data that they don't understand. When you think of it, every transmitter has a certain level that is maintained by regulatory feedback of the enzymes, which are manufacturing it on one side and upgrading it or re-uptaking it on the other side. And the enzymes themselves are subject to regulatory feedback through the genome, and the set point is subject to modification under regulatory control. Well, then there's the interaction. It just balloons out. To approach that kind of a problem with the same tools that were used by Sir Henry Dale makes no sense. It's obvious that they have data which they can't interpret, and a dynamical systems approach is the only way to solve that kind of a problem.

You go to meetings, and you see the more sophisticated people presenting the slides in which they've got these boxes with arrows going here and there. It's not a model. Not a dynamical model. It's a description of the parts. It's like a collection of parts that you want to put together to make an airplane. Unless you put them together in a functional way, which can only be done with an understanding of dynamics, you can't understand the system. You can't really interpret your results. I foresee the emergence of a whole new class of residents and medical students who have the facility in the information age of working with computers, so they can handle the problems in enough detail and still apply the theory. I don't think math is the barrier here because you don't need a higher degree in mathematics to understand enough about, let's say, solutions to ordinary differential equations when they're studied by numerical techniques. I foresee an enormous expansion in that domain, and I think that the INNS [International Neural Network Society] can play a very important role in helping to fuel that enterprise if the right connections are made among people.

JA: If you were counseling your students about what courses to take and what areas to get into, what would you tell them to do?

WF: I'd tell them to take—well, we already tell them to take a basic course in calculus. I tell them to take a good course in C-language programming and a good course in numerical techniques for solving differential equations.

JA: The more mathematics the better?

WF: Only as much as they can handle. And then be prepared to learn enough now so that you can teach yourself, basically, because there is a tendency to take too many courses. You're taking too much material that somebody else wants you to learn, which is not relevant. But if you have a year of calculus, a year of differential equations, and then a year of some form of systems analysis or linear algebra, well, that's three years already. That's enough to get started. And after that, be prepared to learn some more. I had, in fact, to go back. I had three years of mathematics in undergraduate school, but I had to go back and learn linear algebra and learn engineering mathematics, learn multivariate statistics, and then learn some nonlinear dynamics. It's just a continuing process of education. But I have to say that the most important undergraduate courses for me were in English and philosophy. It's satisfying to be a good technologist, but it's more important to have a sense of where you came from, where you are, and what you think the next direction you ought to take is.

ER: Could you talk a little bit about your own thinking style? Do you think visually? Do you think in symbols?

WF: Yes, I would say that what I'm best at is putting a large amount of data on the wall and gestalting it, and just sitting on it and looking at it and thinking about it and puffing on a cigar now and then, and getting a kind of large database in mind, which will ferment there in some way. Then gradually things will start to emerge, pop out; connections will start to form. Simplifications will begin to emerge, which I facilitate by using pencil and paper sketches, making little flow diagrams. It's a lot like writing poetry. You have to turn your mind loose and then be prepared to take down in shorthand whatever it tells you. I'm adept at algebra, which I use for shorthand. That's also why I like Laplace transforms because they can algebrize equations; I can do a lot of manipulation that way.

But most of it is a kind of geometrical flow, taking this amorphous stuff and filtering it down. And eventually, when I come to these new insights, I don't even know where they came from or how they were formed. I know a crucial part of it is that I get, "Aha, I think I have something." I then start looking for the illustration which will exemplify it, and I can't find it, so I have to go back and do the experiment over again. Then I typically will have changed the conditions. I can't even remember what the controls were, and this time it comes out the way it's supposed to. But now, you see, the experiment has already been changed by the theory. So it's very much an inductive, data-driven process in which the theory that was originally set up to do the experiment typically is already very quickly proven wrong, but there isn't anything to replace it yet. And it's very helpful to have a good "forgettery," to flush your mind of the old data before you start taking in new stuff. My father used to say that there are far more people in mental hospitals because they can't forget than because they can't remember. You have to unlearn what you used to believe.

ER: You had mentioned a couple of your patents, and I wondered if you could describe whether you're still actively trying to go forward and exploit those intellectual property rights.

WF: That has to do with trying to develop these filtering techniques. Two of the patents have to do with spatial filtering and spatial imaging of EEG activity, which involves decomposition using Fourier and PCA [principal component analysis]. Another has to do with chaotic dynamics in pattern recognition. I don't regard the patents as any more than a kind of source of pride that I got there first—like it's an ego trip. And I have some documentation that some patent attorney recognized a certain priority, but I'm not intent on doing any commercial development of these. That's not my bailiwick.

ER: So you're not interested in the commercialization of your own work?

WF: Well, I'd like to see it done, but I don't expect to make any money out of it, don't in fact really feel the need for it. What's really important can't be patented—like applying dynamics to understand epilepsy, neurosis, and psychosis, where the task is to educate, not commercialize.

ER: Aside from the new machines that are coming on line, how do you view the commercialization of the whole neural net field?

WF: I think it's remarkable the number of applications which have emerged, the great utility of this whole approach, but I don't see the neural network as a fundamentally new kind of machine. I see it as more of an extension of some existing ideas. I foresee the dynamical systems approach and how that will transform psychology and psychiatry from empirical trial and error to a biologically based science. That should fulfill Freud's nineteenth-century dream, which he abandoned because he thought it was premature.

I would say that we can only barely glimpse some of the implications of that new approach and that these really will be fundamentally different machines. They'll be unimaginably more competent at certain tasks but also maybe unreliable. We were talking only the other day about a neural network that can do routing of phone calls in a mobile phone system—you know, cellular phones—and I raised the question, "Well, how about using this for air traffic control?" But, well, it's not reliable enough. I wouldn't expect that this kind of device that I'm talking about, at least for the foreseeable future, could be used for that kind of task—something where high precision, high reliability, and crucial fault-free performance are required. If you're really interested in artificial intelligence and going beyond the current meaning of the term and the creation of forms of intelligence that truly have biological capabilities, this is the way to do it. And what are you going to do with them when you've got them?

ER: Get out of the way.

WF: One computer guy in Silicon Valley said, "We'll be lucky if they keep us as their pets!" I find that expression amusing in a cynical way. But we humans have the advantage of millions of years of biological and cultural and social evolution, and I'm sure that it will stay the other way around. Though they may beat us at chess and suchlike games, we will always be a couple of steps ahead of them, philosophically speaking. Anyway, we need to be aware of the risks as well as the advantages.

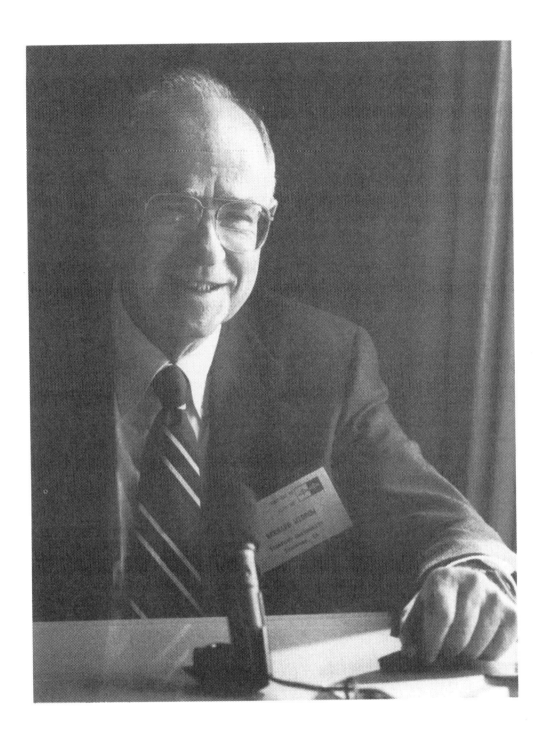

3 Bernard Widrow

Bernard Widrow is Professor of Electrical Engineering at Stanford University, Stanford, California. The best single source for an introduction to his work is his paper, "Thirty Years of Adaptive Neural Networks: Perceptron, Madaline, and Backpropagation" in the Proceedings of the IEEE, 78: 1415–1442, 1990.

March 29, 1994, San Francisco, California

BW: I was born on Christmas eve in 1929. I didn't know anything about the depression because I was too little. The city was Norwich, Connecticut. It's a small town with about 35,000 people, where people have lived for generations. My grandfather came from Russia around the turn of the century and settled in New York City for a while. He sold from a pushcart and saved every penny and was eventually able to bring his wife and children to the U.S. They lived in New York City and again saved every penny and finally had enough money to get out of New York City and buy a farm in Connecticut. On the farm there was an icehouse. There was a river there. People were cutting ice from the river, and they filled the icehouse in the wintertime. Then they'd pack it with straw so that throughout the whole summer they would have ice. My father found himself in the ice business. In the '30s, in the depths of the depression, my father built an ice plant to make artificial ice. Natural ice became unavailable because they had warm winters for a couple of years in a row. He eventually bought another ice plant. He prospered with it and was able with that little business to send four kids to college.

I became fascinated with all the electric machinery in the ice plant. I used to build things. During the Second World War, when I was a kid, I would take old radios and mix the parts together and make one that worked. You couldn't get radio parts then; everything was dedicated to the war. If a radio got sick, it got sick, and that was it. But if you had a couple of sick ones, you could pull the tubes out and pull the parts out and make something that worked. That's how I began working on radios.

I was interested in everything electrical. I was browsing in the school library one day through an encyclopedia that looked interesting, called the *World Book*. I just happened to have the R volume, and I was thumbing through it and came across "Radio." The article was so simply written that I picked up the idea right away. There were a few details that I didn't get quite right. I didn't realize how important it was to have a few hundred volts of B-plus to make the tubes work correctly. I thought the electrons just boiled out of the cathode and went all by themselves straight to the anode, just from the heat, by thermionic emission. I didn't realize that you have to have a high voltage to get a decent flow and make it operate properly. So for several years I was trying to make radios, and none of them worked. Finally, I got on the right track by reading some more things and talking to people, and I made a radio work.

It wasn't so easy to make a radio work because there was no radio station in our little town. The nearest radio station was either in New York City or Boston, which were about a hundred miles away in each direction. You had to have a pretty decent radio to pick up the signal, and I didn't. I made a one-tube radio. I was able to listen with a pair of earphones. The first successful one began working on my sixteenth birthday. I called my father. He came down, and he saw this workbench all covered with wiring and parts, tubes, everything glowing, and he just stood there shaking his head. He said, "I never taught him this."

ER: Did your parents expect you to go into the ice business?

BW: My father did not expect me to go into the ice business and did not expect any of his kids to go into that business. His idea was that all four kids go to the best colleges that they could possibly go to and become professionals. A person that I had very high respect for was an electrician who came to do wiring or fix things in the ice plant. I always watched everything he did. I worshipped the guy. I told my father that I wanted to be an electrician when I grew up.

My father said, "No, you're not going to be an electrician; you're going to be an electrical engineer."

I said to him, "What's that?"

He said, "I can't describe it to you, but that's what you're going to be."

Then we were talking about school, and he said, "And you're going to go to MIT."

And I said, "MIT, what's that?"

He said, "Never mind, you're going to go to MIT."

So when I was a senior in high school, I came home from lunch one day, and my father said to me, "The physician of MIT wants to know about your health."

So I said to my father, "Why does he want to know about my health? Why does he care?"

And my father said, "You dope, they accepted you." That's a quote.

So I went off to MIT. I started out as a freshman, and I ended up as a faculty member. I was there for twelve years. After that I went off to Stanford and became a faculty member there. I've been at Stanford since 1959.

I had a bachelor's, master's, and doctorate from MIT. A bachelor's degree in '51, master's degree in '53, and the doctoral degree in '56, all in electrical engineering.

ER: Were there specific faculty members at MIT who were influential in the future path you took?

BW: Yes. The man who turned out to be my doctoral thesis advisor was William K. Linvill, Bill Linvill. I took a class from him. The course was called "Sampled Data Systems." Today, you would call it digital signal processing. I liked that course so much, I liked him so much that I wanted him to be my thesis advisor.

Usually I had to work very hard to get an A. I really had to work my butt off. The reason is that my mind works very slowly. It's very, very hard for me to learn things. What I do is fight with everything. I don't just accept things. I try to recreate things. What I was doing all throughout my early life was practicing for the point where I wouldn't have to learn from someone else, where I have reached the frontier of knowledge and I alone must push byond. I always fought when someone was trying to teach me something. At MIT, it was an incredible struggle because of the rate at which information came. Someone described an education at MIT as like trying to get a drink from a fire hose. If you just accept, if you just relax and accept that everything is right and just give back what you're taught, you're going to do very well. I could do that too, but I refused to do it. Struggle, struggle, with every subject.

So with Linvill's subject, my mind just seemed built for digital signal processing. I was the one who had the highest grade on the final exam. After that, I asked if he'd supervise my master's thesis, and he said he'd be delighted. And then to go on beyond that for the doctorate was what I wanted to do.

I took a class from a man named David Middleton at Harvard. We were able to take at that time up to 10 percent of all of our courses at Harvard, so I took Middleton's class. Middleton was a stochastic signal processing guy. He literally wrote the first book—a huge, huge tome. The man was prolific. Trying to learn from him was very difficult. Learning from Linvill was very easy. Linvill said that he always liked to take a horse-and-buggy approach. Linvill was born and brought up on a farm. He appreciated the simple horse-and-buggy approach. Linvill would fight with things to make them simple. To me, this was a great inspiration. If you'll look throughout almost all the work that I've ever done, you'll see how simple it is. Make it simple, make it read clearly, make it easy for somebody to read so that they can just pick it up and walk away with it, so they don't have to fight with it, so they don't have to struggle with it. This attitude came from studying with Bill Linvill.

ER: So the converse was true of Middleton?

BW: Middleton was encyclopedic, difficult, extremely analytical. But I learned from Middleton. What I did for a doctoral thesis was a combination of what I learned from Linvill and what I learned from Middleton. I put the two together, the statistics and the digital signal processing, and made a theory of round-off noise. Round-off is quantization. If you digitize the signal, you sample it in time, and you quantize it in amplitude. These are two different kinds of quantization. But the sampling in time is linear; the quantizing in amplitude is nonlinear. What I was able to show was that you can analyze this precisely. Even though it's nonlinear, you can use linear theory to analyze it by analyzing not the signal, but the statistics of the signal, the probability density. That was really my first major piece of work.

I stayed at MIT for three years after finishing the doctorate. And then left to go to Stanford.

JA: While you were at MIT, did you talk at all to the people interested in brain theory, like Warren McCulloch or Jerry Lettvin?

BW: I had known about McCulloch and Pitts. Not so much Lettvin. I had met him a few times when I was on the faculty. I never did know McCulloch and Pitts, but I had friends who had taken classes with them, classes that were very difficult to learn from. I also had friends who took classes from Norbert Wiener, also not the easiest classes to grasp things from.

When I studied Wiener theory, I learned it from a man named Y. W. Lee, who was a disciple of Wiener. Lee was in the electrical engineering department. Wiener was in the math department. I took the class on Wiener theory in the EE department from Y. W. Lee. It was interesting, but I didn't think it was very useful. But it turned out to be incredibly useful for me later on when I got into digital filtering. The way I began working on learning systems was to make a digital filter. I was able to make a filter that could adjust itself. For what purpose? The purpose was to minimize mean square error. So it became possible for all the Wiener problems to be done, but not the way Wiener did them.

Wiener said, "You need to know the statistics. Given the statistics, you can design the filter." But if you don't know the statistics and all you have is signal, what do you do? That was the problem that I became interested in. Given the signal, let the filter optimize itself.

I got my doctorate in June of 1956. There were, I think, twenty of us who got doctorates that year. It was a good crop. I think about ten of the twenty stayed on the faculty. If you were an assistant professor then, it was more like a postdoc. You're going to go somewhere else after a couple of years.

A friend of mine was doing work at our lab at MIT. There was a seminar going on at Dartmouth College that somehow he had found out about. The subject, he told me, was called artificial intelligence.

I said to him, "What's that"? So he explained to me a little bit about artificial intelligence, and so we went to Dartmouth College. We just got in his car, and we took off and drove to Hanover, New Hampshire. We decided we were going to spend some time there. We didn't know how much time. We spent a week, listening to what people were saying. It seems to me Minsky was there, and McCarthy was there, and a man from IBM named Rochester was there. He was doing some very early work on neural nets. I think Clark and Farley were there from Lincoln Lab. It was an interesting collection of people, and the seminar was ongoing. We went there and asked questions and participated. It was open. Anyone can come, and whenever you want, you go. The principals involved were planning to stay there for the whole summer, just talking about artificial intelligence. There was a book that was already out, by Shannon and McCarthy, called *Automata Studies.* We all had read that and knew about it before Dartmouth. I was fascinated by the things that I heard about artificial intelligence. I knew that I was going to dedicate the rest of my life to that subject.

I came back to MIT, and I began to think about thinking. I was trying to think about how to build a thinking machine. I spent six months thinking about building a thinking machine—the parts that we had available to build things and the complexity that you need—and my interest in being an academic, and the problem that you know that you're going to have to do something useful in the relatively short term ... Because decisions about whether or not you're going to get tenure were coming up, and if you don't get that, you're not going to be an academic. If you want to be able to do research and do the things you like to do, you do have to play the game according to the rule book.

So I realized after six months of thinking about thinking—it was very interesting, and I felt the time was well spent—but I'm going to have to do something useful, something in the near term. So what did I know about? I knew about digital signal processing, so I went back to digital signal processing. I could easily have made a career out of the theory of quantization, but I became more interested in intelligence and learning.

In going back to digital signal processing, I make things adaptive. I had the idea of Wiener filter theory. I had the idea of signals coming in. Wiener theory requires that you know the statistics of the input signals. One of my objections to Wiener theory was that you're required to know beforehand what the statistics are. When you have a real problem to solve, how do you know what the statistics are? You don't.

What you'd like to do is to have something that can automatically optimize itself, adjust itself. Suppose you experiment with the design of the filter, you make changes in the parameters of the filter, and see if the performance is getting better or worse.

A typical Wiener filter problem was the prediction problem. You have a time series, a sequence of signals over time. Take the Dow Jones industrial average. Several times a day you can get readings on the Dow Jones Industrial Average. What you'd like to do is predict some time steps in the future, what the value of the Dow Jones is going to be because it might have something to do with the way you are investing. You want to use a system and let it predict. And then, because it's going to predict, you can let it predict and wait a little while and see what happens. You get an idea of what the error is. What you're going to do is adjust parameters to make the error as small as possible. When you do that, you've got the best predictor in some sense, whatever your error criterion is. The one that Wiener used was mean square error. That seemed like a good one, so I began to work with the mean square error and developed procedures for minimizing mean square error. What I found was that mean square error was exactly a quadratic function of the weight values at the taps of a tapped delay line. The filter was a tapped delay line, a series of delays with coefficients attached to the taps. The determination of those coefficients allowed control of the impulse response—in other words, the basic characteristics of the filter.

When you Fourier transform the impulse response, you have the frequency response. The filter responds differently to different frequencies. The way it responds is obtained by the architecture of the filter and the adjustments of the adjustable parameters, the weights.

I was developing an automatic means for adjusting these parameters. I was using the method of steepest descent. I realized early on that the mean square error is precisely a quadratic function of the weights. When you have two independent variables, you can draw a picture of mean square error as a function of these two parameters. It's a paraboloid. The idea is to use its gradient to go down to the bottom of the bowl, where mean square error is minimized. You just roll down the hill; that was the whole idea.

We were measuring the gradient by taking the values of the weights and pushing them forward and then pushing them backward, and taking the difference in mean square error and dividing by how much you have changed that weight. That would give you the partial derivative of mean square error with respect to that particular weight. Then you do it with the next weight and the next one. Eventually, you get all the components of the gradient. Then you make a jump in the direction of the negative gradient and that takes you down the hill.

ER: Tell us about your transition from the East Coast to the West Coast.

BW: In '59, after three years at MIT, I went to Stanford. I was presenting a paper at WESCON about a year or so before I went from east to west. [WESCON is a famous and long-established West Coast electronics conference.] I had never been west before. The title of the paper was "Adaptive Sampled Data Systems." I was talking about the tapped adaptive delay line and an adaptive method of adjusting it. I was measuring gradients very crudely by the method of elementary calculus—in other words, rocking each weight forward and backward. That's an extremely inefficient way to do it, not only computationally but also very inefficient in the use of the data.

WESCON alternated every other year between San Francisco and Los Angeles. I attended the conference in the San Francisco area. They held the meeting at the Cow Palace, which is a good name for it. It was quite an experience. This was the first time I'd ever really gone to a big meeting and tried to present a paper. It was the first time I'd been away from New England.

I planned to spend a week after the conference driving around in California to find out what California was all about. Since I knew it was a big place, a week of driving seemed like a reasonable time. After the conference was over, I got a Hertz rent-a-car. It was a 1957 Chevrolet, Bel Air model. It was a great car. We made good cars in those days.

I was staying at the Mark Hopkins Hotel in San Francisco. There was a bus that took us every day out to the Cow Palace for the conference. I remember being impressed with San Francisco. I had never seen anything like it before. Such a clean, pretty city. I remember walking up and down on the sidewalks near Nob Hill and having to grab onto cars parked on the side to pull myself up because I had new leather shoes with leather soles. The leather was so slippery on the sidewalk; without having rubber soles, it was impossible to get up without grabbing onto the cars.

You see the cable cars running up and down the hill, and you understand why you have to have cable cars to get up and down those hills. I was amazed. I couldn't get over San Francisco.

I left the hotel, went down to pick up the rent-a-car, and walked down this steep sidewalk, holding on for dear life, and finally got to the Hertz rent-a-car agency and got the car. I went back to the hotel and got my luggage and then took off. Started driving. I had no idea where I was, where I was going, didn't have a map. All I wanted to do was to see California. I got in the car and drove.

Leaving the Mark Hopkins Hotel and driving in the city—what an experience, driving up and down those hills. When you start driving at the crest of the hill and start going down, you can't see where you're going. You have no idea what's in front of you. I just couldn't believe that people could drive like this. I went down the hill and took off. In wandering around in the city, I saw big green signs that said 101, Highway 101. And I thought, you know, that's probably like Highway 1 on the East Coast. It probably goes north, south. Probably goes between Mexico and Canada, up and down the spine of California. That should be a good road. So I said, "OK, I'll go on 101." I just got on the first entrance to 101 and I found I was going south, instead of north. I said, "Gee, that's interesting, let's go south."

So I went south, and after a little while, I was noticing signs to Palo Alto. I said, "Gee, Palo Alto, that's where Stanford is. I'd like to see Stanford."

So I got off the highway at Palo Alto and drove down University Avenue. I said, "How can you go wrong with that?" I drove right through the town, and I said, "God almighty, what a pretty little place this is." It was just beautiful driving on University Avenue, the shopping area; the homes, the residences along it are just gorgeous. They're old and stately.

I kept on going right through the town, right through the downtown area, and kept on going. I went under an overpass, crossing El Camino Real. I'd heard about El Camino Real, the famous road that the ancient padres traveled. I went onto the Stanford Campus and drove down Palm Drive, and I saw a road lined with palm trees and thought, "My God, I'm in the tropics." I went down onto the campus, and I just was completely taken by it. So beautiful. I said to myself, "This would be a fantastic place to spend a career at."

The brother of my thesis advisor was John G. Linvill, who was on the Stanford faculty there. So I called on John Linvill when I made that first visit to Stanford, after the WESCON conference.

The chairman of the Electrical Engineering Department at Stanford was a man named Hugh Skilling. His field was electric machinery and power systems and electric transmission lines. He was what you would call a classicist. At the time, research in those subjects was pretty well done. He had written his books and done his teaching and now was chairing the department, an excellent man. His real emphasis was on quality of teaching. He went along with research more or less, but John Linvill was completely research oriented, and John Linvill was his right arm. I visited with Professor Skilling when he attended a conference some time later, in New York City.

I wanted to go to Stanford. They made me an offer, and I was delighted. I got a 50 percent pay raise over my MIT salary.

Then I had a problem. I'd been going out with a girl who I met at MIT. She was a secretary, and I bumped into her in the elevator one day. And it was good. Like it says in Genesis, you know, this was done and that was done, and "it was good." I started dating her, and this was going on for a couple of years. Then all of a sudden, I was going to be leaving and going to Stanford. She made it plain that although I'm a young fellow and having a very nice life being a young faculty member and not worrying about a damn thing, that if I go to California, I better be planning to take her too. Had I thought about that? So I thought about it, and we got married.

We came to Stanford, and I began research on adaptive filters once again. The first year that I was there, no one knew me. The students didn't know me. I began teaching a course in adaptive systems in 1959. I taught a class in digital signal processing called "Sampled Data Systems." This went quite well. I had students coming to me.

The first doctoral student that I had was a man named Ted Hoff. John Linvill was advising him on his course program. John called me up one day and said, "I've got this student who's my program advisee, and I've been trying to interest him in some of my research, but it doesn't seem to do it for him. He's looking for something else, and he doesn't know quite what he's looking for. He's a very nice young fellow, awfully bright guy. Would you be willing to talk with him?"

I said, "Certainly, I'd be delighted."

So he sent over Ted Hoff, and the two of us began talking. I was telling Ted about research. I had several sessions with him. One day I had a session with him, and out of this session came the LMS [least mean squares] algorithm. I don't know how it happened, but it just popped right out. I was at the time explaining to him how we're measuring derivatives and getting the gradient and following the gradient with steepest descent. I was showing him the theory of how this thing learns and how you determine learning rate. Somehow or other, the idea came for a different way of getting the gradient, and that was the key to the LMS algorithm.

The idea was to get the gradient not by taking many many samples of data and measuring mean square error over a long period of time. The idea was to be able to get the gradient from a single value of error—a single number, square it, and say that's the mean square error. Then when you work out the gradient of that error with respect to the weights, it's really simple. You get an algebraic expression and you realize that you don't have to square anything; you don't have to average anything to get mean square error. You don't have to differentiate to get gradient. You get this all directly in one step. Not only that, but you get all components of the gradient simultaneously instead of having to make measurements to get one gradient component at a time. The power of that, compared to the earlier method, is just fantastic.

1959 was the date of the algorithm. The first publication about it was at another WESCON conference. I liked WESCON because you could get things out quickly, and you could do a significant paper. It had a convention record, so there was a written record of your paper. But you could also present it and get some feedback. I did many things through conferences at the time. Today, if I were coaching a young faculty member, I would tell the person not to do it that way. As far as academic careerism, those papers aren't worth much because they're refereed, but only slightly. They don't get three referees like a journal paper, and they're much more difficult to find in libraries than journal papers.

ER: When you and Hoff were working in 1959, were you aware of the significance of what you had?

BW: I knew it. I think he knew it too. There was no way we could have anticipated what was going to happen with that algorithm and the uses that would be found for it. I knew it was something in adaptive research that was extremely significant. The instant I was at the blackboard writing it, the two of us were talking together, and I think I said, "Jesus Christ!" or something like that.

Within a half hour of the time that the algorithm was written on the blackboard, Hoff had it working in hardware. One of my colleagues, Jene Franklin, had a large analog computer in the building, right across the hallway. There was nobody in the computer room. We just went in, picked up a plugboard, and Hoff wired the algorithm together. We made a single neuron without the quantizer, just the weights and the sums, so it was a linear combiner. We were adapting it with the LMS algorithm right on the spot. This happened on a Friday afternoon in the autumn of 1959.

We wanted to build this thing up in hardware, compact enough to move around. We needed potentiometers to make weights. We decided that the inputs should be not 1s and 0s, but +1 or −1, because we're not doing binary arithmetic; we're doing something more like usual arithmetic. It's a symmetrical thing. What we didn't know at the time was that it had something to do with convergence, and convergence works better with +1, −1. It'll converge just fine with 1s and 0s, but it's better with +1s and −1s.

Everything was there on the analog computer so that we were able to wire it together and form a single adaptive linear combiner. We were adjusting the weights with ten-turn Heliopots. They were very precise potentiometers, good to three decimal places. We didn't really need that. All we needed was approximate changes, but we were making those changes on the Heliopots and adapting this thing. By the time we were done fiddling with the analog computer, it was about 5:00 in the afternoon, and the stockroom was closed. The next day was Saturday, so the stockroom was going to remain closed. The two of us were just beside ourselves. We couldn't wait. I'm not an early riser, but I was that Saturday morning and the same with Hoff. We went down to Zack's electronics shop in downtown Palo Alto on High Street, and we bought all the parts. We bought an aluminum chassis to mount everything. We bought rotary selector switches. The first one we built had ordinary potentiometers. The second model had rotary switches. The first one had just knobs and pots. That night we figured out the parts list, and we were ready to go next morning. We bought everything, and we put it together on the aluminum chassis.

We had little switches to put in +1 and −1 inputs. The input pattern was put in through on array of switches. We arranged the switches in a four-by-four array. You'd be surprised how many different geometric patterns you can make with a little four-by-four array of switches, where each pixel is only binary.

We fed those signals into the weights, and the summation was done by bringing the current together at one solder point. There was no electronics in this at all. We just took the solder point and connected it to ground through a microammeter. There was enough current to operate the microammeter without an amplifier. All we had were the switches, a battery, potentiometers, and a meter. We were able to train that thing with LMS algorithm. The algorithm didn't have the name "LMS" at that time. That came about a year later.

ER: When you built the first Adaline, were you calling it an Adaline?

BW: We called it an Adaline. It was an adaptive linear neuron.

ER: Do you still have the first model that you built?

BW: I still have the Smithsonian model in my office—not the very, very first one, the one with potentiometers on the aluminum chasis. That one unfortunately is in Adaline heaven. But the next one after that. The first little portable one that you could carry around. When you operate the switches, you can see a pattern in lights, so it lets you easily see what the pattern is.

Right after that, Hoff and I became interested in trying to develop electronic circuits to implement this. We were only aware of Rosenblatt because of newspaper stories about his work. This was sensationalized in the press. After a while, our work also became sensationalized in the press. Some of the people doing publicity at Stanford arranged a press conference for me one time. There was a whole room full of reporters, and I was demonstrating a learning machine. Now this was pretty amazing stuff back in 1960. Nobody knew what the hell it was or what you could do with it. We didn't know what you could do with it.

We knew it would be impossible to turn all these knobs by hand. So the question was what to do to make knob-turning automatic. I was talking with a colleague at the time, Norman Abramson, who's now on the faculty at University of Hawaii. I was chatting with him one day and he made the suggestion, "Why not do it chemically, electrochemically, the way it's done in the brain?" So I came up with a circuit diagram to do it. I had the device laid out. I gave the device the name "Memistor" because what I wanted was a resistor with memory, the element that we needed to make an adaptive circuit.

I was envisioning a jar full of electrolyte, with two electrodes sticking in it, and I'm going to vary the impedance between the two electrodes. To make this happen, put another electrode into the jar, a third electrode, and by putting current in and out of that electrode, you can affect the chemistry of the solution, and that would affect the impedance. I didn't know what chemicals to use or what kind of reaction to depend on or how quickly you could change the resistance.

Ted Hoff spent that summer working at SRI [Stanford Research Institute]. I maintained contact with him, even though he wasn't at Stanford every day. I showed him the circuit that I'd drawn up and told him what kind of element I needed. I knew that when he was a kid, he was just as much interested in chemistry as he was interested in electronic things. He knew a lot about chemistry. He knew a lot about everything, this kid. He's not a kid anymore. He's got grey hair like me.

So he said, "It's going to be very difficult to change the impedance of an electrolyte. The electrolyte, no matter what you do with it, is a liquid and salts, and it's going to be a short circuit no matter what you do." He said, "How about if we use the phenomenon of electroplating?"

We took a piece of paper and took a soft lead pencil, and wrote a line on the page, and put an ohmmeter on one end of a few inches of the line, and measured a resistance of something like 10 megohms. Then we put some solution—copper sulfate and sulfuric acid—on top of the line, and just by putting the electrolyte there, the resistance went from about 10 megohms down to about 10 kilohms. Then we took the third electrode, a piece of copper, and dipped it into the solution, and we were able to plate a little bit of copper onto the pencil line on that piece of paper. That took the resistance from about 10,000 ohms down to about 100 ohms.

You can reverse the current and remove the copper. At first, it didn't remove very well. By the time we fiddled with it a little more, it was very erratic, and the acid had eaten through the paper and the whole thing fell apart, but at least we'd established the principle.

I started to work on this thing. I went over to the Stanford bookstore with an ohmmeter. I went up to the counter, and I said to the lady working behind the counter, "I'd like to buy some pencil leads."

She says, "Yes, sir. Look at the showcase full of all different kinds of pencil leads."

So I said, "I'd like to buy the one with the highest electrical resistance."

She said, "I beg your pardon?"

I explained a little bit, and she pulled them all out of the case, and I took the ohmmeter out and started measuring pencil leads. The winner was Fine-line Type H, meant for a mechanical pencil. It measured nine ohms from one end to the other. That was the highest impedance I could find. So we took it back and got some copper sulfate and sulfuric acid, and put a clip lead on one end and dipped the other end into the solution and plated a little bit of copper onto the tip of the pencil lead. We pulled it out, rinsed it off, and had a nice coating of copper right on the graphite, right on the pencil lead, solid as a rock.

We turned it around the other way, put the clip lead on the place we'd just plated, and put a little plating on the other end. We had the two ends with nice plating. We got some light-gauge wire with plastic insulation and stripped the ends and soldered the wire onto the two ends. Then I got some fingernail polish from my wife, and I used that to coat the solder joint because I was afraid that the solder would dissolve in the sulfuric acid. We put this thing in a test tube and put a piece of number 14 copper wire, like a rod, into the test tube. We tied the plastic wire to the copper rod for support and pulled the wires out of the top of the test tube.

It was a three-wire device. One was the copper rod. The others were the two wires soldered to the ends of the pencil lead. So when you measure these two wires from outside, you get roughly nine ohms from the pencil lead with no plating on it. You put plating solution in there and turn on the plating current between the copper rod and the graphite, and you can copper-plate the pencil lead. You can take it from 9 ohms down to about a quarter of an ohm. You can easily get a thiry to one ratio between no plating and fully plated.

We used that to build an Adaline and designed a circuit to implement the LMS algorithm. It was a very simple circuit, easy to build, and it was working. You begin putting in training patterns and you teach it to respond to the training patterns as you like. You can feed in a whole bunch of patterns, one on top of the other. When you train in new ones on top of the old ones,

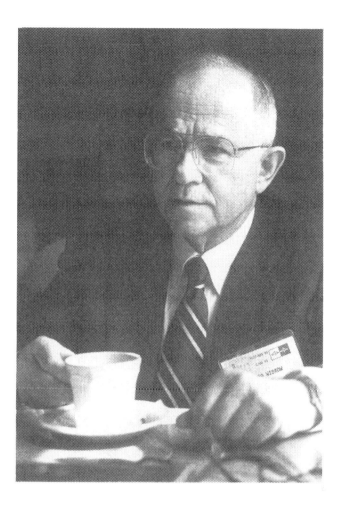

the new ones tend to disturb the old ones, but you repeat them over again until the whole thing sinks in.

You really get a feeling for a learning system because you got a machine here that's learning. The information that's stored in the neuron is stored in terms of the thickness of the copper on the graphite. You have a substrate, which is the graphite that you're going to plate on. That has a certain conductance. As you plate on top of it, the conductance increases over time if there is a constant plating current. If it plates uniformly, as pretty much it does, the conductance increases linearly over time. The weight value is the conductance.

We started a company to manufacture these devices. This began a humongous learning process about everything under the sun, how to make a reliable device. We sold a lot of these devices for fifty bucks apiece. That was a typical selling price for a transistor in those days, an experimental transistor. Any kind of experimental device sold for fifty bucks.

We almost had a big customer, General Telephone. They were going to use it, not in a neuron, not as an adaptive device, but as an automatic gain control in an AGC circuit for a telephone repeater amplifier. It would give a nice dynamic range for gain control. It was very, very stable because you could plate this thing, and when you stopped plating, the plating stayed right where you left it. With the Adaline I have in my office today, which has Memistor devices in it, I can train in a pattern classification problem and come back months later, and the training is still in there.

At first you think it's easy to make a reliable device, and then when you get into it, you realize the difficulty of making something that really works well. We hired a glass-blowing technician, and we bought a glass lathe. He was making little glass vials the size of tiny light bulbs. The resistor that we were using was an alloy made out of platinum and rhodium. We were able to get special wire that was very finely drawn. This little wire was about a half-inch long, and we'd put it inside this little glass vial. You have to make contacts through the glass, so you have to have glass-to-metal seals. The materials have to be impervious to sulfuric acid. They also have to have the right temperature coefficient to match the glass because if you go through temperature cycling, you have to keep a perfect seal between the metal going through the glass envelope and the glass itself.

The glass sealed devices measured about 10 ohms with nothing plated on them, and they'd go down to about an ohm. They were quite reliable. I still have some in my office. We haven't made them for more than twenty-five years, and they work just like brand new.

ER: What was the name of the company?

BW: Memistor Corporation. We were selling Adalines, we were selling Memistors, all sorts of adaptive circuits. The people from General Telephone were going to have Memistors in every manhole all over, wherever GTE is. At the time, I think it was about 10 percent of the United States. Then they decided not to do it. Some people just couldn't accept liquid-state electronics. Everything had to be solid state.

We took that little thing with three wires coming out and spot welded the wires to what's called a TO-5 header. This was the first form of base for a transistor. It plugs into a TO-5 socket, so the Memistor was a plug-in unit. I was able to pick those things up and slam them down with my hand, just as hard as I could, slam them down on the concrete floor, and they bounced twenty-five feet up in the air. Then plug them in, and they'd just adapt like crazy, like nothing ever happened. The trouble was that the Memistor was all handmade. There wasn't anything you could integrate.

I found that it's difficult to make adaptive circuits and make neural nets with analog apparatus. I think people are finding the same thing today with solid state. My own view, and I think the view of Ted Hoff, on neural circuits is that instead of doing them in a politically correct way—meaning that because the brain is analog, if you're to build artificial neurons, you have to do it like the brain and make them analog. I think the two of us are pretty well convinced that this is not the way to go. Do it with digital, all digital. That doesn't mean that there isn't any room for analog because if you need extremely high-speed operation, you're probably going to have to use analog.

I was going to tell you about Rosenblatt and the perceptron. I finally did get to know him. I was attending many conferences where he and I were there on the same program, presenting research. There were a number of followers of Rosenblatt. I was never really convinced that Rosenblatt was doing things in the right way. I felt the perceptron was a disaster. I thought the Adaline was the right way to go. What people today are calling the perceptron, Rosenblatt would not call a perceptron. I know, I talked with him.

I'll tell you an interesting story. The little Adaline in my office uses Memistors. The reason why it's little is you don't need all those potentiometers with the knobs all over it. I was making a trip to the East Coast and wanted to make a visit to Frank Rosenblatt and the guys at Cornell. I went up to Cornell University for the first time and found what a beautiful place it is. I had that little Adaline with me. I went to see Rosenblatt, and for the first time I met the perceptron. I can't remember whether it was in one rack of equipment or two racks. It was a whole pile of gear, and he was making adaptive weights with electric motors driving potentiometers. So he had small electric motors driving the pots, and we had the Memistor getting the effect of a motor-driven potentiometer electrochemically. I noticed in the back of the room a whole lot of chemicals, so I knew they were trying to make Memistors. I could see what they were doing, and I gave them some hints.

So we fed a pattern into the Adaline, and we fed a pattern into the perceptron, and I just put the pattern in and the Adaline went "phut," and the needle was reading to the right or to the left. So I just held the adapt button down so some of the cells are plating while others are deplating, depending on the direction of the error signal.

Rosenblatt's students put the pattern into the perceptron. You could see it in the lights on the perceptron. You could hear the potentiometers grinding away. We put another pattern into the Adaline, and it went "blip," and there it was, adapted. They put it in the perceptron, and it's still grinding away. We put in a couple more patterns. Then we test the Adaline and test the perceptron to see whether the patterns are still in there.

They're in the Adaline. In the perceptron, they're all gone. I don't know whether the machine was temperamental or what, but it was difficult to train.

I argued with Rosenblatt about that first random layer. I said, "You'd be so much better off if you just took the signal from the pixels and ran them straight into the weights of the second layer." He insisted that a perceptron had to be built this way because the human retina is built that way. That is, there's a first layer that's randomly connected to the retina. He said the reason why you can get something to interpret and make sense of random connections is because it's adaptive. You can unravel all this random scrambling.

What I was trying to do was to not model nature. I was trying to do some engineering. I've always been very interested in what the neurobiologists have to say because I think we can learn some things, but I don't think that we should feel obligated to take things literally when we're trying to solve engineering problems.

When the Minsky and Papert book came out, entitled *Perceptrons*, I somehow got a copy of it. Publishers send me zillions of books, so this one came into my office one day. I looked at that book, and I saw that they'd done some serious work here, and there was some good mathematics in this book, but I said, "My God, what a hatchet job." I was so relieved that they called this thing the perceptron rather than the Adaline because actually what they were mostly talking about was the Adaline, not the perceptron.

I felt that they had sufficiently narrowly defined what the perceptron was, that they were able to prove that it could do practically nothing. Long, long, long before that book, I was already successfully adapting Madaline [Madaline = many Adalines], which is a whole bunch of neural elements. All this worry and agony over the limitations of linear separability, which is the main theme of the book, was long overcome.

We had already stopped working on neural nets. As far as I knew, there wasn't anybody working on neural nets when that book came out. I couldn't understand what the point of it was, why the hell they did it. But I know how long it takes to write a book. I figured that they must have gotten inspired to write that book really early on to squelch the field, to do what they could to stick pins in the balloon. But by the time the book came out, the field was already gone. There was just about nobody doing it.

I think where that book actually came into its own is with the second coming of neural nets, when they came back again. Then people began to look back on that book, and some people of faint heart were discouraged. That doesn't mean that the book isn't interesting and isn't valuable. It is. But they had only a few little examples of multiple neurons. I think most of it had to do with a single neuron. What I found was that, certainly, the single neuron couldn't do everything, but the things that it could do were God damned interesting. The single neuron can't learn everything, but so what?

ER: You said that you had stopped doing neural nets? Was that because of the GTE decision not to use Memistors?

BW: No, no, no. We had failed to develop algorithms beyond what we now call Madaline 1, the first algorithm that we developed for the Madaline. The Madaline had an adaptive first layer and a fixed-logic second layer. What Rosenblatt had was a fixed-logic first layer and an adaptive-logic second layer or output layer. Now, it is easy to adapt on output layer. But it's very difficult to adapt a hidden layer. We didn't call it a hidden layer; we called it the first layer. We could adapt an adaptive first layer with a fixed second layer as long as we knew what the second layer was. But we never succeeded in developing an algorithm for adapting both layers, so that the second layer is not fixed and both layers are adaptive. It wasn't that we didn't try. I mean we would have given our eye teeth to come up with something like backprop.

Backprop would not work with the kind of neurons that we were using because the neurons we were using all had quantizers that were sharp. In order to make backprop work, you have to have sigmoids; you have to have a smooth nonlinearity, a differentiable nonlinearity. Otherwise, no go. And no one knew anything about it at that time. This was long before Paul Werbos.

Backprop to me is almost miraculous. The first exposure I had to backprop was around 1985 at a meeting at Snowbird, Utah, the first Snowbird conference. Something funny happened on the first day of the first Snowbird conference. Someone gave a paper in the first morning session, and during the question period at the end of the paper someone got up and said, "You know, something like that was done by Widrow back in the early '60s."

They began to have this big discussion about what Widrow did and Widrow didn't do, and I'm just sitting there, listening to all this stuff. You know what I was? I was like a dead man. I was a man who'd died, who was sitting up on a cloud somewhere, looking down on the Earth, watching what happened after he died. So I let them have their little thing, and then I just stood up. I didn't know a soul there. I stood up and introduced myself to the assemblage. At coffee break, everybody was crowding around. Some people just wanted to touch me to see that I was alive.

We hadn't published anything for all those years in the neural net area, but the neural net people don't know about adaptive filtering and adaptive signal processing. That's where I've been doing my work. We stopped doing neural nets because we'd hit a brick wall trying to adapt multilayer nets. On the other hand, in adaptive filtering and adaptive signal processing, we were making great strides.

We had done work on adaptive antennas. When you have an antenna, you can plot the directivity pattern, the sensitivity pattern of the antenna. The antenna acts like a filter. It filters spatially. There's a direction that you can point the antenna that has maximum sensitivity. But even though you point the antenna in a given direction, it doesn't mean the antenna receives only signals from that direction. It also receives signals, with some attenuation, from other directions. If you make a polar plot of sensitivity versus angle of an antenna, it has a main lobe and then many, many so-called side lobes that give finite sensitivity in other directions than the main direction of the antenna. These side lobes are potentially troublesome. A big problem in trying to receive a signal occurs when a nasty person nearby is trying to jam the transmission. The military is concerned with that.

If there's a strong jamming signal, even though it's not coming in the main direction, it will still come through so strong that it will destroy your ability to receive the signal of interest coming from the direction that you're trying to receive. Usually, the signal that you want is a faint signal coming from far away.

In any event, if you take an antenna that has many dipole receiving elements, instead of just connecting them together in a fixed way like the TV antenna up on your roof, you can take the individual signals from the dipoles and put each signal through a weighting device that can weight it and then form a sum. By doing that, you can control the pattern of the antenna; you can control the direction in which it looks, the maximum sensitivity. Also, if an unwanted interfering signal is being received by the antenna, you can adjust the weights to minimize the reception of that unwanted signal. When the antenna rejects an unwanted signal, you can look at the directivity pattern and see that there's a notch, a spatial null in the direction of the interference. It's put a null in the direction of the bad guy and thereby gotten rid of it.

We published the first paper on adaptive antennas in 1967. That year I was on sabbatical in Belgium. We didn't have Federal Express in those days, or fax machines. We started the manuscript while I was at Stanford, and then I worked on it in Europe. I had several students as coauthors, and back and forth it went by airmail.

When the paper was finally done, it was sent in to the *Proceedings of the IEEE* for publication. A very interesting thing happened. There were three reviews. One reviewer said, "Reject it." Another reviewer said, "Publish it." The third reviewer, the middle-of-the-road guy, said, "Well, there may be some interesting things in here, but overall it doesn't look very interesting." He was on the fence about whether it should be published. The editor himself made the decision to publish it, but it was so close to being rejected and not published.

When that paper came out, it became what's called a "citation classic." I saw a list of citation classics once. I think at that time, Stanford University had about thirty of those in all fields of research, from the founding of Stanford. I think MIT might have had twenty-five; Bell Labs might have had about thirty. It was an amazing thing that this was a paper that was so close to being rejected.

I've had papers rejected, but this one I knew was an important piece of work. The objections that the reviewers had to it just showed that they didn't really understand the paper, and they didn't understand the significance of it. I think the easiest paper to get published is one that's an epsilon change over everything that existed before—epsilon being the well-known very small quantity.

JA: It's easiest to get funded, too.

BW: It's the easiest. But if you've got something that is novel and different, you're going to have a tough time.

I remember one of the strongest objections to this paper was from one of the reviewers who you could see was an old RF [radio frequency] guy and an old antenna designer. He was concerned about using variable weights on the signals of the antenna. When you use a potentiometer on those signals, what you're doing is losing some of the signal. No self-respecting antenna designer is going to design an antenna where you're going to lose some signal in a variable weight.

Now, of course, you could have amplified the thing, and then you can throw away all the signal you want. It's all just scaling. The point is that you can have a receiving array that's picking up the signal nicely, but you're picking up the interference, the jamming signal, much more nicely than the signal you're looking for. It isn't a question of being able to get signal. You've got plenty of signal. You've got plenty of signal, but you've got a hundred times as much interference. The problem is to get rid of the interference, and to do that you have to play other kinds of games.

We did adaptive noise canceling too. It's the idea of adding noise to a noisy signal to come up with a signal with less noise. It's dangerous; you have to do it right because if you add noise to a noisy signal, it's pretty easy to come up worse off than you were in the first place.

We first got started in this stuff when one of my students was interested in doing a doctoral thesis in pattern recognition. He got interested in biomedical pattern recognition, particularly electrocardiograms.

I'd done various biomedical problems over the years, lots and lots and lots of them. That has been a most satisfying experience. During the depths of the Vietnam War, when students were having sit-ins and shutting down buildings, my building, the one my office is in now, every single window in that building was broken. Stanford couldn't keep windows in that building. Eventually they got tired of replacing the glass, and they used masking tape to just tape the glass together. Every night in the springtime, when the weather was nice, the kids would be out there with rocks to break windows. They wanted to shut down the School of Engineering because they thought the School of Engineering was responsible for the war in Vietnam. They were angry, the kids. I think if they hadn't protested the way they did, we probably would be still fighting a war in Vietnam because it's easy for the old guys to be off on some holy mission; it's the young ones who have more sense, especially when they know that they're the ones who have to fight it.

That was a stupid, terrible period. But we were just beginning to work on biomedical problems. Engineering students were really beginning to question themselves. Like, what are they doing? What kind of careers are they going into? They were beginning to listen to the students from the English department and the history department, the humanists who were breaking all the windows.

I felt very strongly about doing the medical work and was able to enlist many young engineering students. The Stanford University Medical Center, which is a major research medical center, is located about five minutes away by foot from my office. I began teaching a course in computer applications, and almost all the applications were biomedical. Sometimes I'd have as many as thirty students at a time working on various research projects. Ted Hoff, who lives nearby, was helping me supervise. The students were working on projects at the hospital, and the doctors were delighted. They had engineers in their labs that they never had before. There was more computer and electronic equipment in the medical center than we had in the School of

Engineering. The kids got experience that they never would have gotten otherwise, and they were supervised by both engineering and medical faculty at the same time.

The first noise-canceling project that we worked on was a biomedical one. The problem was with the electrocardiograph. In those days you couldn't get notch filters. A cardiologist was having trouble with 60-hertz interference from the power line. He was German born and a stickler for detail. He wanted things precise. I mean, he had the mentality of a Mercedes Benz, you understand? He was complaining to me about his EKG equipment. He said he had to roll it off at 30 hertz so that at 60 hertz he was about 60 dB down to get rid of the 60-hertz interference. In Europe, of course, he had the same trouble with 50 hertz.

I took a look at his recording setup. He had a nice Faraday cage. He had copper screen mesh all over the inside walls of the place where he's taking the EKGs. Right in the middle of the room, he's got a 60-cycle wall plug, where the EKG equipment plugs in. The interference comes right inside the Faraday cage. The patient's body acts like an antenna picking the stuff up, and when you amplify the signal from the patient, you also amplify the 60-hertz interference.

Well, today you can put a notch filter right there. In those days, you couldn't just go in the store and get a notch filter. If you designed one, it was built out of analog apparatus. There were no chips, no op amps, no nothing. It was something that was difficult to build, and it wasn't all that precise.

I thought about this and thought about it some more. I had a couple of students taking my course in adaptive systems. The students were supposed to do research projects and write a paper. There was no final exam; they just did that paper. I had a few students who were interested in doing some circuitry. I got this crazy idea, and I decided we'd build and make the recording set up work at 60 hertz. We were going to build a circuit to cancel the 60 hertz.

Here's the way the crazy idea went. The patient is in the room getting an EKG taken. Sixty-hertz interference is amplified and would normally appear on the chart recording. Suppose that you go to the electric wall outlet, and you get 60 hertz right from the wall outlet. You can introduce that 60 hertz attenuated to get it down to low voltage, adjust the phase and magnitude just right, and you can take that small signal, with the right magnitude and the right phase, and subtract it from the signal coming from the patient. Then you can exactly cancel the 60-hertz interference, and you won't need this low-pass filter that cuts out so much of the electrocardiogram. Two students built up the circuitry and made it work. They were able to eliminate the 60-hertz interference.

It's really funny when students study sampling theory in signal processing, and they know about Nyquist sampling theory, and they know that you have to sample at least twice as fast as the highest-frequency component in the signal to capture it. So they say, "Well, what's the bandwidth of an electrocardiogram?" And I tell them, "I don't know."

And they look at me and say, "What do you mean, you don't know? You're the professor." So they come to grips with the idea that not everything is cut and dried, that there just isn't a simple answer. So you then use a method called the method of futz; you futz around with the sampling rate until you get something that looks pretty good. That's how you find the sampling rate.

Today, the students all want to work on neural nets, so I only have a few working on adaptive filters.

ER: You mentioned that you were drawn back into the neural net field in the mid-eighties when you went to the first meeting in Snowbird, Utah. I was curious, what other work going on now in neural nets do you think is of the most importance?

BW: The Snowbird meeting for me was a landmark. You know, we had a lot of controversy in the early days. It was due to publicity that Rosenblatt had in the news media and publicity that I had. I found that this kind of publicity infuriates colleagues. It's not just that they think this is a stupid thing to do; they get furious. That helped also to make the field controversial. You see, you raise the red flag when you've got things that are in development, and you talk to the press when something isn't thoroughly developed. It creates a whole lot of antagonism and anger on the part of fellow scientists. They like to see things published in refereed journals, not in the *New York Times*. That's the problem.

I learned a lot from publicity. Don't do it.

What I found about Snowbird was that the atmosphere was incredible. Here you had a couple hundred people who were crawling all over each other, not to dig knives in, but to praise each other. It was a love fest. People were supporting each other, and people were enthusiastic. They were excited. The other thing was backprop. I never saw that before. I was astounded. I was so pleased to see that. It was such a good feeling.

I knew that some day I was going to go back into neural nets. Neural nets are very, very difficult to deal with, analytically. It's very hard for faculty committees to approve a doctoral thesis in neural nets. There has to be science, not just tinkering. Or another way to put it, it shouldn't be just substituting different values of resistors to try to make something work.

To do research with neural nets with nonlinearities, with threshold devices, and with combinations of these things is difficult. The mathematics is difficult. To do work with an adaptive filter that doesn't have the nonlinearity is the equivalent of doing work with a single neuron instead of a net. You can do remarkable things with it—noise canceling, antennas, control systems. The mathematics for it is really pretty clean stuff, not like the math for a neural net. It was easy for me to stop neural nets and do things that are productive, have great engineering value, and are solid scientific work. But I knew when I left the field that some day, I'm going to come back, when I have more time. It still would have been many years before I'd gone back into neural nets if the field hadn't flared back up.

Once I was at Snowbird, I caught the spirit, the excitement of that group of people. There was no way I could stay away from that field, so I went back in. As soon as that happened, I found that many doctoral students wanted to work on this. I've got fifteen doctoral students right now; that's a lot. If I wanted fifty, I could have fifty Ph.D. students working on neural nets. They're there; they all want to work on neural nets. They don't know what the hell it is, but they want to work on it.

Well, over the years we've had some remarkable students. Ted Hoff was a postdoc for a number of years after completing his thesis. Then there was a new company getting started in Silicon Valley. The founder was a man named Robert Noyce. He was just getting a company started. The purpose of the company was to develop integrated circuit memory. The idea of storing one bit with a flip flop was radical. I suspect that when they were all working at Fairchild, they must have suggested this to management, and management said no, so they went and formed their own company that they called Intel.

Ted Hoff joined Intel. I knew that this was the right thing, that being a research associate is not a permanent thing in a university. This was an opportunity for a young fellow to go ahead and get involved, so he joined Intel. He told me his badge number was number 12 at Intel.

He worked there for a little while, and he came up with the crazy idea of putting the entire computer—the CPU [central processing unit], all the logic, and the memory—on one chip. I think he must have been influenced by the computer that he learned on in my lab, an IBM 1620, an ancient machine now, but then it was quite a fine minicomputer. The machine worked in binary-coded decimal, BCD. Everything was done with decimal digits. It takes four bits to represent a single decimal digit, so the first Intel machines were all four-bit machines, and some of the instructions, I think, were similar. Ted called it a microprocessor. He was very successful. He's a fellow of the IEEE, and his Fellow citation reads something like, "For the invention of the microprocessor." *Note:* The Inamori Foundation has announced the laureates for the 1997 Kyoto Prizes (Japan's version of the Nobel Prize). For the invention of the microprocessor, along with Ted Hoff are his co-workers at Intel at the time, Dr. Federico Faggin, and Mr. Stan Mazor, and a colleague from Japan, Dr. Masatoshi Shima.

I've had about sixty students who have gotten doctorates under my supervision over all these years, and almost every one of them has worked on something adaptive. Now we're back to neural nets again, and I can't find a student who wants to work on adaptive filters. Everybody wants to work on neural nets. So neural nets it is.

We've been working on neural controls for a couple of years. We had a number of students who wanted to work on controls. The first one was Derrick Nguyen. He did the first broom balancer of the new era. [The "broom balancer" or "pole balancer" is a classic problem in control, where a system must learn to balance an inverted pendulum without having it fall over.] We were doing broom balancing way, way back, but the broom balancing we did back in the early '60s was a system where it was learning with a teacher. The teacher was a control system that knew how to do the balancing, so it was able to adaptively learn to emulate a system that knew how to do the balance. This was supervised learning.

Now we start out without having a system that knows how to balance the broom, and we ask the neural net to learn all by itself how to do the balancing.

After Nguyen did the broom balancing, he came to me and he said, "Well, I've got this working; you saw it."

I said, "Yes, I saw it. It's marvelous."

He says, "What should I do next?"

So I thought about it, and the first thing that came to mind was a double broom balancer; it's a broom on top of a broom. I thought, that will fix him. But I thought, "Wait. I've got another idea." I thought about the truck-backing problem.

I can tell you where the truck-backing problem came from. It came from my father's ice plant. One day when I was a little kid, a big truck came into the ice plant to pick up a load of ice. I didn't know the driver; he came from a different city, not a usual customer. He didn't know where to back the truck up to get the ice. I was standing on the side lines with a few men, and the driver got out of the truck, stepped down, and came over to us and said, "Where do I put this thing?" Meanwhile, he just left the brake on, and left the engine running.

And everybody said, "Well, over there is where you back up the truck."

He said to me, "Kid, you know how to drive?"

I said, "Sure." I think I was about fourteen.

So he said, "OK, back up my truck to the platform, will you?"

I said, "Sure.

I was a little kid. I just barely was able to climb up into this monster truck. So I got in, and I can see the little diagram on the dashboard that tells you how to set the gear shifter. So I got it into reverse, very carefully letting out the clutch, and putting my foot on the gas pedal, and the thing slowly starts to move. Yikes! It just wasn't going where I thought it would go. I had never had any experience backing up a trailer truck.

I can tell you, all the guys were standing on the sidelines. They were all laughing. They were having a great time, and I was so embarrassed. I finally gave up. Got out of the truck. I said, "I can't do it."

Everybody thought that was so funny. The driver just got in there and backed up the truck to the platform, no problem. I guess I never really forgot that experience.

So when Derrick came in, and he'd done the broom balancer, and he seemed to be pretty pleased with himself, I said to myself, "I'm going to fix him. I'm going to make him back up a truck." So I suggested the problem to him of getting the neural net to steer the truck while it's going backward.

The broom balancer, you know, is a classical problem in control. It's written up in control books for the last fifty years. When he did the work on the broom balancer, I could just refer him to a control book, and he could get all the equations from the book. So he said, "Where am I going to get the equations for the truck?" He went into a toy store, and he bought a little plastic truck with a trailer and took that back to his desk so he could play with it. He wrote out all the equations of the truck as a nonlinear plant. It didn't take him very long.

He came into my office one day. He said he's got something he thinks I ought to take a look at. So I went down to the lab with him, and he showed me the computer screen with a moving image of the simulated truck and trailer backing up under the control of a neural net. My jaw dropped. I knew about the broom balancing, but I had no feeling for the difficulty of the truck problem. It looked like a very difficult problem. The neural net learned all by itself to steer the truck, by backing up many, many times.

What he had it do is back up, but if it hit something, it stops. He's trying to back up to a platform in a precise spot. You look at the state of the truck when it stops and compare it with the desired final state. The difference between the two is the final error, and it's a vector because you have many parameters on the truck to describe its position. Utilizing a form of back-propagation, the error vector was used to adapt the weights of the neural controller. Every time the truck backed up, if it were set in the same initial position and let back up again, it would do it similarly, but the new back up would come to a stop, and the error vector in the least squares sense would be less as a result of learning. Now, you don't necessarily back it up from the same initial conditions every time. What you do is scramble them all up. The idea is that every time you back up, the thing learns something and adjusts the controller. So if it were to back up again, it doesn't learn while it's backing up; it backs up and then sees what the final error is.

Now that it's got an error, it uses backprop to adjust the weights of the controller. Nguyen was able to do this with backprop. He developed an algorithm that he didn't have a name for, but it turns out that Werbos had already developed that algorithm for some other purpose. Werbos had given it the name "backprop through time." And what Nguyen was using was backprop through time for this control problem.

When the truck backs up, it backs in increments. Let's say a big trailer truck backs up a small distance, like one meter. Every time it backs up, it backs up one meter, one meter, one meter—a whole series of steps until it hits something and then it stops. You see what the error is, and you go back and look over all the steps that you'd gone through, and you change the controller so that you go though another set of steps where the error would be smaller. So what Nguyen saw was that the transference of the state of the system from one state to the next, to the next, and to the next is analogous to the transmission of data, of signals, from one layer to the next of a neural net. He looked at each of these steps as analogous to a layered neural net. So the neural net that he's dealing with, that he's adapting, is not a two-layer net or a three-layer net. He's adapting a hundred layers, all with backprop. He succeeded with the truck backer, and demonstrated great visualization and ingenuity. [*Note:* It is with great regret that I report the death of Derrick Nguyen in the year 1995. He was 30 years old.]

We didn't know originally that the truck backer upper problem would be amenable to control theory at all. It looked like a very difficult nonlinear control problem. My first thought was that this was beyond control theory. Then I talked to some control people, and they indicated that there should be some way to do it analytically. Just recently, I received from Shankar Sastry, a colleague at Berkeley, a paper he wrote that shows analytically how to back up a truck and trailer with n trailers; n could be any number you like. He has an analytic solution. You don't have to learn to do it; you can do it analytically.

But I think the point is that we're not in the trucking business. We're in the business of demonstrating a learning capability, showing that something can learn to do something nontrivial and that it can learn it whether it's a problem that's amenable to analytical treatment or not.

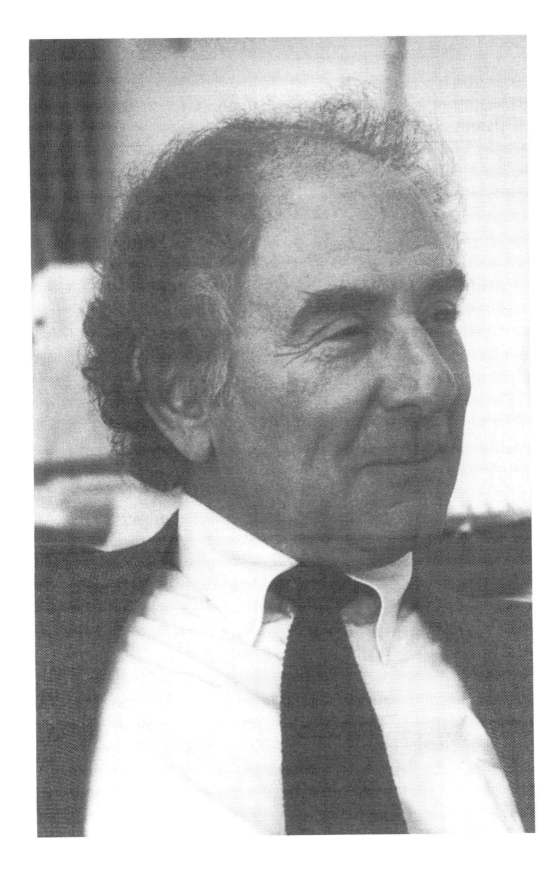

4   Leon N. Cooper

Leon Cooper is Thomas J. Watson, Sr., Professor of Science and Director of the Institute for Brain and Neural Systems at Brown University, Providence, Rhode Island. Professor Cooper was awarded a Nobel Prize in Physics in 1972, which he shared with John Bardeen and J. Robert Schrieffer, for developing a theory of superconductivity. A good reference for his work is a collection of his papers, How We Learn, How We Remember: Toward an Understanding of Brain and Neural Systems, *World Scientific, 1995.*

December 1994, Providence, Rhode Island

ER: Tell us something about your parents and early childhood.

LC: Now, you don't ask a person their date of birth. However, why don't we try February 28, 1930.

ER: We've asked everybody their date of birth, but we'll note your protest.

LC: I was born in New York City. I grew up in the Bronx and Mount Vernon and various places around there.

ER: What did your parents do?

LC: I don't think my mother worked after she was married, and my father at that time had a printing business. He was a typographer by profession.

ER: Did he stay with that business through your childhood?

LC: My childhood was complicated.

ER: What I'm really after in talking to people is to try to get some insight into what kinds of experiences have formed them so that they become the people they are.

LC: I wasn't prepared for deep psychoanalysis.

ER: It's not psychoanalysis, it's just ...

LC: Well, I lost my mother when I was about eight years old. My father sold everything he had trying to pay for the hospital bills—that's when he lost his business. A great illustration of what it means not to have generally available medical insurance. After that he worked in his profession. We were moved around for a while, and then he remarried. My father died a couple of years ago, and my new mother is living and very happy in Florida. The entire family celebrated her ninetieth birthday with a huge party last November.

ER: Do you have brothers and sisters?

LC: I have one younger sister, and I had a half brother, who died when he was about thirty.

ER: So when your mother died, this had a big impact on you?

LC: I think when an eight-year-old's mother dies it has a big impact on him.

ER: Did it affect your schooling?

LC: I was shifted around. I was pulled out of one place and sent to another, though I had some wonderful experiences at a foster home in Mount Vernon. The family took care of my sister and me for about two years or so. That was, I think, the first time I had a little laboratory. It was a private house, and they were nice enough to allow me the use of the basement, in which I immediately set up a chemistry laboratory, a photography laboratory, and a laboratory with all kinds of electrical things.

ER: How old were you when you had your first lab?

LC: Nine or ten years old.

ER: Where did this interest in science come from?

LC: That's a good question. I don't know. I don't really have an answer. My suspicion is that kids look for various things that intrigue them, and what gets them going is a little bit of success. You know, you do it, and you get a little something out of it. Then you do a little more, and you get a little something more out of it. I suppose I must have liked it.

ER: Most nine- or ten-year-olds are not even cognizant of electromagnetism.

LC: I can't say I was cognizant of electromagnetism. I had learned somewhere in magazines like *Popular Science* or *Popular Mechanics* that if you put a battery on an electromagnet, it attracted things. I liked to do that kind of thing. I think it pleases a child because he or she begins to know something that the other people around you don't know. It begins to make you feel a little special. I enjoyed it.

ER: Was there encouragement in school, or was this all on your own?

LC: This was long before I had any encouragement in school.

ER: So this was just your own interest.

LC: I don't remember too well the very early grades. I just remember isolated incidents. But later, when I was in junior high school, I remember getting a lot of encouragement from my science teacher. I won several science awards. By that time, I suppose I had an official interest as well as official encouragement.

ER: Where did you go to high school?

LC: The famous Bronx High School of Science.

ER: Was there a lot of encouragement there?

LC: There was encouragement. There were some wonderful teachers. There was also enormous encouragement because facilities were available. That's where I got interested in biology. The reason I got interested in biology was a great biology teacher and a wonderful biology lab. You could grow bacteria; you could do all kinds of things like that. I remember no corresponding opportunity in the other sciences. I used to work there all afternoon, everyday. A wonderful woman who was in charge would have to throw me out to close up. You had to wash your own test tubes, make your own culture media. Everything.

ER: So in high school at least you had made the transition from chemistry to biology?

LC: Well, no, I did well in all sciences.

ER: But you seemed to have had a very strong interest in chemistry as a younger child.

LC: I think it's because chemistry is easiest to do when you're little. You can buy a chemistry set and mix things together, and something happens—like things explode in the closet, which happened to me once. The reason I did biology in high school was because the lab was there, and I could put experiments together.

ER: Were you interested in physics?

LC: I was interested in all sciences. I didn't like physics especially. I liked it, and I didn't like it. I liked the deep ideas, but I didn't like the problems they gave. So boring. Biology was more interesting. First of all, I had a wonderful biology teacher. I could do more with my hands and really design experiments. I won the Westinghouse Science Talent Search with an experiment that I designed in that laboratory.

ER: Do you remember what it was?

LC: Of course I do. I was trying to develop a variant of *bacillus subtilis* that was more resistant to penicillin. I designed a dilution series to grow the bacteria in varying concentrations of penicillin. I would take the bacteria that grew in the highest concentration and then put them through a new dilution series and keep doing it. By the time I was finished, I had a strain of bacteria that would grow in higher concentrations of penicillin than the original wild type. The next part of the project I never got to do because I graduated, and they threw me out. I wanted to find out why it was resistant. Was it secreting something? It was not easy to do because even if you kept the more resistant type in the refrigerator, it reverted very quickly to the wild type. What I wanted to do was to see if I could filter out something. One possibility was that the bacteria was secreting something that destroyed the penicillin. I remember giving a talk on it and listing the various possibilities, so the next thing to do was to try to track them down. I don't know exactly what the story is now, but it was exciting to be able to do experiments like that.

ER: Obviously, you were motivated and driven.

LC: I really was passionately interested in science.

ER: Were you a good student?

LC: That's another story. In science I'd get 99s or 100s in various exams such as the Regents Exams. In science I was very good. I had a terrible time with French. This was what dragged me down from being first in the class to being only in the first ten percent. I did abysmally in French. I ask myself why, because I have a good ear. When I hear a phrase, I can repeat it. Just by living in Paris a couple of months I learned to speak colloquially. I think the bottom line is that I have a poor retentive memory for the sequence of actual spelling and for little grammatical points. I was a disaster on exams. I used to make numerous spelling errors. People tell me that's just because I'm stubborn, but I don't think so. I have a hard time spelling well, even in English, and so what this means is that if you have any brains, use a dictionary or a spell checker. This really tells you something about the way you should educate children.

Should you judge a person with a lower average if he or she has a weakness some place, if they're very good in other things? Suppose a person's a gifted musician, has a superb ear, and composes as easily as breathing, but can just barely make it through the sciences. What difference does that make? The point is that you should expose them to the sciences. To me that is one of the great things about the Brown curriculum. You expose the person to everything, but you only judge them on what they're going to do professionally because that's all that really matters.

And the ironic thing is that I love French. I read French easily and speak fluently, but I just couldn't learn it to spell it for exams. I still can't. In fact, maybe I wasn't even learning it so badly; it's just that I couldn't reproduce that one aspect of it. There must be dozens of stories like that. It's really a shame that the educational system finds it so difficult to come to terms with that idea.

ER: Were you competitive as a student? You mention that you would have been first in the class had it not been for your French grades.

LC: Competitive? Me competitive? You've got to remember that when I graduated from the Bronx High School of Science February of '47, I didn't have too many options for colleges. It was very hard to get into college. My only shot at an Ivy League college was Columbia because I couldn't afford the others. Three people in my class got into Columbia in February—a very close friend of mine who was first or second in the class, the son of an alumni, and me. The only reason I got in was because I'd won the Westinghouse competition. In June of that year Columbia changed its policy. Some thirty people from the Bronx High School of Science were admitted. Colleges were not easy to get into at that time.

ER: Because everybody was coming back from the war?

LC: I won't speculate on what all the reasons were. It wasn't easy. At least, it wasn't easy for us. So we were competitive.

ER: And what did you study at Columbia?

LC: I had to make a decision as to which way to go. I decided to major in physics.

ER: Do you know what the elements of that decision were?

LC: A kind of arrogance. I said to myself that I can always learn biology. I can always learn all these other things, but if I don't study physics, I will never understand those deep ideas. I think I was right about that, actually.

ER: As a teenager, what was your notion of what the deep ideas were? You've used that phrase twice.

LC: Einstein, relativity, quantum theory—all those incredible ideas mentioned in books and articles. I wanted to know what they were. I'm really glad I did. However, it wasn't quite as easy to learn the other things as I thought. It's not because it's so hard; it's just that you have to get into it.

ER: When you were a teenager, when you were first fascinated by these deep ideas, did you have an understanding of what quantum mechanics was?

LC: No, I didn't understand at all; it's just that I'd heard about it, and I wanted to understand.

ER: So it was something beckoning you on the horizon.

LC: I wanted to understand. I wanted to understand what the theory of relativity really was. I've always played with quote, "deep philosophical ideas," unquote. However, I'm very pragmatic. One of the nicest compliments that has ever been paid to me was by an anonymous English reviewer of my textbook who said that this text book was written by a "no-nonsense physicist." I love that. That's what I am, I'm proud to say. I'm a no-nonsense scientist. Also, it was a time when physics was suddenly very fashionable. The nuclear bomb had just exploded. It was rough, however, because between the deep ideas and what they put you through in the Columbia physics department, it wasn't easy.

Columbia College was an unbelievably rewarding experience. I loved the humanities courses. I loved the classics courses. I had a wonderful humanities instructor, Gilbert Highet, four times a week. There was Mark Van Doren and Moses Hadas. One regret is that I wanted to sit in on a seminar course on *Hamlet*. I won't mention the instructor's name, but he wouldn't let me because, given that I was taking four physics courses, I couldn't agree to do all the readings. I suppose he was right.

There was another course called "Colloquium." We read a book a week, and then we'd meet one evening for about two hours and talk about it. There were two instructors. I remember getting into an argument with one of them about Pascal's wager. Do you know Pascal's wager? Pascal says that we don't know anything about whether God exists. Since we are in total ignorance, the chances are fifty-fifty. Thus, he argues, it is your finite lifetime against eternity on a fifty-fifty bet. Any rational gambler would take the bet. There are various ways of showing this argument doesn't work. But my argument was that just because you're in total ignorance doesn't mean that the probability is fifty-fifty. Because if it were, you could say I'm also in total ignorance as to whether Satan exists, etc. Anyway, the instructor would not accept that. I was stubborn and he was pretty stubborn, too. We spent an hour and a half arguing about it. Nobody else got a word in edgewise. Then they called another special session. The argument continued. Finally, somebody said, "Just shut up so we can talk about something else."

But it was great. It was an enormously stimulating experience. Some of the ideas I sketched for that course I've since developed in lectures. I guess college is a time when people grow if they're lucky. You remember that period as the time when you grew up and matured.

At Columbia I didn't keep my opinions to myself. I took a course with Polykarp Kusch—an absolute marvelous character. The course was electromagnetic theory. He had a booming voice and was, I think, deaf in one ear, so he was very disturbed by people talking in class because he said he couldn't localize the sound. He worked with I. I. Rabi, did some very famous measurements, and later won the Nobel prize. I complained bitterly during the course about how meaningless the problems were, what a waste of time, etc. I was rambunctious and not fond of work.

In the middle of my junior year he called me in to his office. He was chairman. I said, "Oh no, they're going to throw me out."

But he says, "Cooper, how'd you like to be a teaching assistant at Columbia?"

And I said, "What does that mean?"

He answers, "It means you get your tuition paid and $90 a month."

So I said, "Where do I sign?"

That's how I made the transition from the college to the graduate school. I never even looked at another graduate school. They recruited aggressively in those days.

So I entered the graduate school in February of my senior year. I became a TA. I remember one of the earliest courses that I taught as a TA. I was probably just twenty-one years old. It was to a group of pharmacists-to-be. They were much older. They were the most undisciplined, unruly class. I couldn't stand it, so I would throw them out, one after another. They finally shut up.

I thought it was disgusting. So I asked them, "Why are you here? You have no interest in the material whatsoever."

They said, "Well, this is a required course and we are looking to graduate, get a job, and make our $87 a week." That was a high salary at that time. That was the depth of their intellectual interest.

I was a TA at Columbia, went to graduate school, did my thesis. All those good things.

ER: What was your thesis?

LC: It was on an aspect of nuclear physics, mu meson atoms. A mu meson is like a heavy electron. It doesn't have a strong nuclear interaction, but because it's heavy, about two hundred times as heavy as the electron, its permitted orbits are much, much closer to the nucleus. When it makes transitions between two energy levels, it emits more energetic photons than an electron making the same transition. By measuring the photon energy of the $2p$ to $1s$ transition, you could deduce the radius of the nucleus.

Well, the energy of the emitted light was something like a half million electron volts, more than according to standard calculations using the then accepted radius of the nucleus. The question was, why? When I worked on this problem, I was very fortunate. My thesis advisor was Robert Serber. If you've seen the TV play *The Day after Trinity,* Serber was an important participant in building the bomb. He'd been a student of Oppenheimer and worked at Los Alamos. I found it a little difficult to communicate to him because he was on too high a level. Fortunately, Ernie Henley, who was just a few years older than me, was a postdoc. Serber put me to work on this problem, and Ernie was also working on it. That was fantastic because I could have a very close interaction with Ernie.

ER: And so that problem was selected for you, as opposed to something which you came to yourself?

LC: It was suggested as a possible problem. The experiments were going on at Columbia; they were being done by Jim Rainwater and Val Fitch. Ernie and I finished it too quickly, so Serber said that I'd have to do other things before I could get my degree. So I did some other things. I worked with Rainwater, and I worked a little bit with T. D. Lee. They finally let me out. Do you want to know what I did after that? It has nothing to do with neural networks.

ER: Sure.

LC: Well, Serber got in touch with Oppenheimer, who was then director of the Institute for Advanced Study, and so I went to the Institute and worked there for a year. Then serendipity. When I was at the Institute, things seemed to be a dead end in my branch of physics. It was just after Schwinger, Feynman, and Dyson had done quantum electrodynamics. The normalization ideas were worked out. It seemed as though people were spinning their wheels. It was at the Institute that I had a conversation with John Ward, very well known in quantum field theory. I said to him something like, "After I have finished physics, I would like to go back into biology." He was shocked. I guess it was a bit presumptuous.

I probably didn't say quite that, but I always had the idea. I may also have said that I would write a few operas along the way. I wanted to do everything. It was difficult for me to accept limits. About that time, John Bardeen wrote to C. N. (Frank) Yang, asking if there was someone who was familiar with the current field theoretic techniques because he thought maybe they could be applied to superconductivity. Frank asked me if I might be interested, and I replied, "Why not?" Later, Bardeen visited and talked a little bit about superconductivity. I didn't know anything about it. I didn't know anything about solid-state physics, but the thing that intrigued me was that superconductivity was a problem that had been around for fifty years, and no one had been able to solve it. Almost every famous physicist had tried, but nobody had been able to solve it. And so I said, "All right, that's something for me to do. I'm not getting anywhere doing the kind of stuff people are doing here." So I figured I'd give it a try.

ER: Where was Bardeen?

LC: He was at Illinois. I sometimes wonder why I accepted because I didn't know anything about the field; I didn't know anything about solid-state physics, but it turned out that it was well chosen as a problem for me because I didn't have to know anything about solid-state physics. All I really had to know were a few things, and Bardeen taught them to me in days.

The first thing I did was dutifully to jump into the problem with all the latest, fanciest field theoretic techniques. No point in listing all the different things I did. Then, contrary to what almost everyone else thought, I decided that, you know, this doesn't make any sense at all. I'm doing all of this razzle dazzle, and when you look at the simplest elements of the problem, you ask people what the solution is in ordinary English, and no one can answer.

I started asking people, "How do you solve a problem of this kind?"

They said, "I don't know. Look it up in a quantum mechanics book."

And I said, "I already know what's in the texts. How do you solve it in the form it takes here?" No one had the vaguest idea.

This is really where I separated from everyone else. I was asked, "What are you doing? Why aren't you doing what you're supposed to be doing?" I feel uncomfortable working with complex technical tools if I don't have a sense in ordinary words of what it is that I'm working on.

I've developed several precepts over the years based in part on this experience.

1. Don't attack a complicated problem if there is a much simpler version that you are unable to solve. Solve the simple one first.

2. Don't believe what you don't understand.

3. Beware of those who say that the solution is in the complexity—that there is no way to see what's going on. Of course, in some cases this may be true, but most of the time it's just a way of throwing in the towel.

So I went back to fundamentals.

In about one or two months, I thought of a solution to the problem. In fact, what I had was an idea that would eventually lead to the solution. But to convince people, to convert that idea into a solution, was the period of greatest anguish in my life. You have to experience it to understand how you feel in the wilderness when you are totally unknown.

You go to meetings and say, "I think I really have solved this problem." People look at you as though you are a raving lunatic. Most individuals who think they have solutions to big problems are raving lunatics, so statistically they're right. I've always had a certain sympathy for these itinerant vendors of new ideas, but one has to face up to the fact that it's statistically unlikely. Anyhow, I went through about a year in this wilderness.

I buttonholed everyone I could grab at every meeting I managed to go to, Feynman may have been among them, repeating the spectacle of the earnest young unknown claiming he had solved a fifty-year-old problem that had baffled a substantial number of the Great Ones.

Now I know what I should have done. At the time I did all the wrong things. At every seminar I gave, and I gave quite a few, people would pose questions. I would try to provide answers. They'd say, "But how do you know that this is the case?"

And I would spend three months proving this was the case. And they'd say, "How do you know something else is the case?" And I would spend three more months proving something else was the case.

I spent all my time proving one thing after another. What I should have done, although that wasn't so easy, was to embody the idea and then calculate, do something. But that was done by three ideally suited people ...

ER: The three being John Bardeen, you, and Bob Schrieffer ...

LC: It's remarkable how each of us contributed things that the other person didn't see, really astonishing. We were and remain very different personalities. Bob and I are almost the same age. We used to commiserate with one another a lot. Bob, a graduate student, would say, "I'm never going to get a Ph.D. on this problem." He did, however, and it was a reasonably substantial Ph.D.

It all came together about January of '57. We decided that this was it. We were going to go ahead and work it out. We calculated literally day and night. Raw calculation for about three or four months. It is simply amazing the way the results came out. Absolutely astonishing. The techniques we used were so cumbersome compared to what became available even a few years later. It is hard to believe we did it, but when you're in the middle of things like that, we did just literally work day and night. I also remember, there were places where we were really stuck. I remember getting a critical idea at a concert. I had been thinking about the problem uninterruptedly for a week or ten days. It was a very intense period. After you're finished with something like that, what do you do next? I kept working in the field for several years, but ...

ER: By finished with it, you mean the paper was published?

LC: Yes, the problem was solved. The solution was accepted. Then there were all kinds of new techniques that came along. I worked in the area for quite a few years afterward.

ER: In Illinois?

LC: Illinois, Ohio State, Brown. Actually, at Ohio State with Sessler and Mills we published the first paper suggesting that helium 3 might be a superfluid. At that point the idea had always been that helium was one kind of a superfluid, and the superconductor was another. Helium 4 is composed of what are called bosons, while superconductors are composed of fermions. Helium 3 is made of fermions, so in principle it could be a superconductor. It turns out it's a much more complicated superconductor.

Anyhow, I kept working. Results kept coming. I published papers and produced Ph.D.s, but it was more and more technical. It didn't please me anymore. I didn't feel like going on for the rest of my life, becoming a superguru.

It's a very foolish thing to give up, when you think about it, because when you're that established, you can get money just by sending in a proposal. It's very easy because you know everything that's going on. But it really didn't interest me any more, and when you stop being interested, your work becomes mechanical.

So I began to look for other things to do. Among other things, I began to toy with my old interest in biological problems. And because by then I was very far from any laboratory, I didn't particularly feel like going into things like molecular biology. Also, I'd always had an interest in deep philosophical ideas. Mind-body problems, that sort of thing, although I take a very pragmatic point of view of these problems. I think the difficulties are mostly self-constructed to amuse philosophers.

Anyhow, trying to understand what the nature of the thinking process was seemed to me an incredible challenge, one I'd always been interested in. Also, my transition was aided by an illusion I had at the time when I began this work. I was an expert on many-body problems and quantum mechanics. Superconductivity was a many-body problem: many electrons interacting via known interactions. If you looked at physiology texts at that time, they would say that the properties of single neurons are fairly well understood. On the other hand, no one has any notion as to how memory is stored, or how any thinking process happens. So I said, "That seems like an interesting challange, and it might be a many-neuron problem."

I guess the whole thing came together when a graduate student, the famous Menasche Nass, walked into my office and said he wanted to do a biological-type problem. I don't remember if I'd suggested it to him as a possibility or vice versa. I told him it was really risky. It was bad enough trying to be a physicist at that time because the job market was tight, but this was totally unknown. You didn't know if you'd get a job; you didn't know anything. He still wanted to do a biological project.

At that time I had become aware of a paper by Longuet-Higgins proposing a distributed rather than local memory that seemed appealing. However, it didn't seem to be easily realizable in a physiological system, so I assigned

Menasche the task, a summer project, of coming up with a version that was more plausible. At the end of the summer, when I next met Menasche, I asked him to show me his results. It turned out he had found an easier way.

Menasche's family lived in New York. On one of his visits, Menasche went to visit Jim Anderson at Rockefeller University, who was supposed to know something about memory. Jim was a postdoc at Rockefeller at the time. Jim had developed an associative neural network model that was based on a simple learning rule, of the type that has become known as Hebbian. It learned using only local information available at the synaptic junctions between neurons. It did not give very accurate recall, but it did work and operated as a simple kind of associative memory. It was this solution Menasche presented.

When we developed this a bit, it became clear that with few assumptions you could get a lot. It wasn't the grand solution, but in the roughest sense you could see how associations could be built and put together.

Such things had been talked about for years. People regarded this as among the deep mysteries. And there it was, coming right out of the simplest assumptions. That, I thought, was very powerful.

At that time few people believed that understanding the brain was possible. They would say, "Well, it's an interesting problem, but it's not going to be done in our lifetime." The situation has changed dramatically in twenty years. I guess that's a reasonable part of a lifetime. But I don't think anyone feels that way now.

To understand the evolution of my own thinking you have to understand a bit the way I think and the way I work. To a certain extent I'm oblivious of the rest of the world. It's one of the best traits you can have, and one of the worst. As a marketer, as a person who can sell something, I'm terrible because I don't pay enough attention to anyone else. But when I'm satisfied in my own mind that something is understood, I don't care what anyone else thinks. At that point I said, "Those so-called deep problems about memory and association are just possibly understood in principle."

Of course, I was aware that a bit of additional work was needed. For example, the company I work with, Nestor, has been laboring for twenty years to try to sharpen things up so as to get commercially viable products. I wasn't oblivious to that, but I thought that on a deep level we might be beginning to understand.

The problem was that when I spoke to biologists, their reaction was, "a talented amateur, in never-never land." So I said, "You know, these guys are right in a way. I am in never-never land. What is required to take this from fantasy and make it absolutely convincing? What does it require to turn everyone around?" And as I saw it, what was required was to take the theoretical fantasy, make it absolutely concrete, and then show that you could make concrete connections between experiments that were being done and explain them.

It's my opinion that this was Galileo's greatest contribution to science. He was the first one who built a mathematical structure that could be put into correspondence in a detailed and quantitative way with what was observed. That's a very powerful idea. And that's what I thought was necessary.

At that time our theoretical models assumed modifiable synapses. Although that had been suggested in biology, there were very few biologists who took the idea seriously. Let me tell you, things have really changed. Now it is not uncommon to hear biologists talk about modifiable synapses and neural networks to explain their experiments.

In order to make this area serious science, to find a way to build a theoretical structure sufficiently concrete to be put into detailed correspondence with experiment, I began what now seems like an incredibly long detour into visual cortex. I was looking for a place where experiments could be done that indicated that some kind of learning was occurring.

The early experiments that seemed to show learning in visual cortex were controversial, ferociously controversial. I won't go through that whole sorry history, but this is what science is. If you looked at the situation with an unbiased eye, you'd say, "OK, maybe those guys aren't seeing exactly what they think they're seeing, but they're seeing something, and that something is very interesting."

Someone asked Einstein what he thought about flying saucers. He said, "Well, these people are seeing something, but don't ask me what."

So, these people who were studying visual cortex were seeing something. It was pretty clear that experience was modifying the response of the cortical cells. That's what I call learning, on a cellular level. And so some kind of synaptic modification ideas should be able to explain what was happening.

At that point, my own personal work branched. On the one hand, we tried very hard to make contact with experiments, and on the other hand, we in effect said, "Let's take it and build something with it." Just throw off all constraints and build something real. One way led to the commercial applications like Nestor, and the other went to see what was really going on in the biological system. In an interesting and curious way, they interact again because the learning rules that we proposed for the visual cortex, now known as the BCM theory, have turned out to be powerful statistically for dimensionality reduction. [BCM theory is named for a well-known paper by Elie Bienenstock, Leon Cooper, and Paul Munro, where it was first proposed: "Theory for Development of Neuron Selectivity: Orientation Specificity and Binocular Interaction in Visual Cortex." *Journal of Neuroscience* 2: 32–48 (1982). Reprinted in *Neurocomputing*.]

We and others have been applying these rules to feature extraction, dimensionality reduction. You start with let us say five hundred dimensions, and you can extract a few powerful features from them. So our initial idea that biology could teach us something is, I think, valid.

Anyhow, we worked on two tracks. On the biological track, we first tried to come up with some means of understanding what was going on in visual

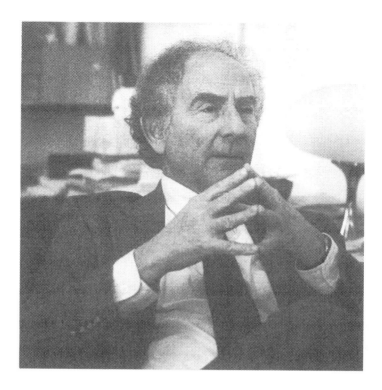

cortex. There was my paper with Nass. Other people were also working on this problem: Leon Glass, Perez Christoph von der Malsburg. There's a lot of work that's been done recently.

A key idea came to me in Paris. I was a professor of the Fondation de France. (I had by then conquered my high school aversion to French.) Michel Imbert called me to say, "We are trying to start something in the area of research involving neural networks. You come to France. You can be associated with the Institute Pasteur, the College de France. You name it, we'll get you space. Start a laboratory, and we'll give you a five-year appointment." And I said, "What happens after five years?"

Well, they said, "That's five years ahead."

I did a rapid calculation and said, "I'm not even going to be out of my forties in five years." I didn't really want to retire, and I didn't want to leave the whole group here at Brown. So I said, "Why don't we arrange something so that we can go back and forth?" We can join two laboratories. They accepted that. And that worked very well.

The first thing they showed me in Michel's laboratory in the College de France were their experiments with kittens raised in the dark. These kittens did not show the Hubel-Wiesel-type cell behavior seen in normal kittens, where cells in visual cortex respond selectively to particular orientations of lines. Cells in dark-reared kittens generally respond weakly and are very broad in their response to orientated lines. But if dark rearing was followed by just a few hours of patterned experience, the sharp tuning came out right away. That seemed to me a striking result that cried for explanation. Could one find a synaptic modification mechanism that could explain it?

According to our arrangement, I lectured in December. What made it really hard was I was lecturing in French. As I said, I'm pretty good using street French, but my technical French was almost nonexistent. It drove me crazy because I would mispronounce all the words. Finally I just gave up. One incident I remember was to try to say "action potential" in French. I'd say something like "potential d'action," and all my buddies in the audience would shout, "We don't say that. We just say 'spiking' the way you do in English." In French, that should be pronounced "speek." So I made it into a verb, and I said, "ça va speeker," meaning "that one's going to spike," and everyone began to laugh. They said, "We don't say that; we say 'ça va spiker.'"

I gave up. From then on I lectured in English. Or I mixed it up.

In the course of my lectures—I think it was December 1978—I really began to worry about Michel's results. The problem seemed extraordinarily simple. When neurons are in a patterned environment, they show sharp tuning. In a noisy environment, no sharp tuning. How do you get that? We should be able to understand that.

It was during those lectures that I thought of mixing an anti-Hebbian part with a Hebbian part. I was familiar with the work that Teuvo Kohonen had done with optimal mappings. While I was lecturing, it occurred to me that a selective cell is sort of an optimal mapping because what it's doing is mapping certain patterns to zero and others to a maximum. If the synapses were modified with a Hebbian rule, but with a minus sign, then cell response would eventually go to zero. Modifications with a positive rule would give a growing cell response. It then occurred to me that if the algorithm were such that all patterns but one resulted in negative modifications, then you would get the experimental results. That's how the idea was born.

Kay and I went to Finland every once in a while to visit Teuvo Kohonen. As a result of one of these visits, Erkki Oja from Kohonen's laboratory came to Brown. Fishel Liberman joined us, and we did a paper. It worked pretty well. But there was a rather amusing problem.

Fishel used to come into my office and say, "I'm losing cells."

I told him "Put the threshold in the right place. Fishel, you know you have to place the threshold so that the response to one pattern is above it, and the response to the others are below. If you put them all below, you're going to lose cells."

After some deep thinking, it occurred to me that it's hardly likely that every cell in the visual cortex has its own Fishel Liberman assigned to it to adjust its threshold. There must be some way that the threshold adjusts itself to achieve this effect. And so we began experimenting with thresholds that would move.

Now what is it going to be a function of? Well, the most obvious thing to do is to take something like cell activity or depolarization. That's when Elie

Bienenstock—who had asked me in Imbert's lab if he could come and complete his Ph.D. here—joined us. I won't go through all the stories about Elie. He had a rough time when he was here. We consumed quite a few glasses of Scotch in this office. He'd tell me about how awful Providence was, how the food was ghastly. You name it, it was awful. Everything was awful. Now he seems to be very content coming and spending lots of time in Providence, and he tells me how awful Paris is. I never stop teasing him about that.

Anyhow, soon after Elie joined us working with moving thresholds, we came up with an elegant possibility. Allowing the threshold to move as a nonlinear function of the activity also gives the whole system nice stability properties. Elie worked this out beautifully in his thesis, and we wrote the BCM paper. We've been playing with variations of that ever since. What we first did was somewhat of a skeleton, as always. Since that time I think we've made the theory more sophisticated and realistic. The real world is very complex, so one simplifies. One of the simplifications, for example, was the visual environment. We simplified the environment by saying that a normal environment could be represented by a certain number of patterns distorted by noise, as opposed to pure noise. Our justification was that if the receptive fields were small enough, and if you looked at actual images, probably the repetitive patterns would be edges of various orientations distorted by noise. That seemed to work well.

A real advance was made with Charlie Law and Harel Shouval, Brian Blaise, and others. We've been running the algorithms on real images (pictures taken by Harel). The retinal field is shifted over the images, and we get receptive fields coming out just the way they should. A little circle goes over the image at random. These are no longer patterns distorted by noise, so we feel we've made much more realistic contact with the external world.

We have also been working with Mark Bear and his experimental group. There seems now to have been confirmation of the phenomenon known as long-term depression [LTD]. For a long time we have known about long-term potentiation [LTP]. By stimulating a cell properly, you can enhance the responsiveness of the cell. This has been attributed to changes at the synaptic junctions of the cell and was seen first in the hippocampus. If the BCM algorithm is correct, by stimulating insufficiently you could decrease the response of the cell. People may have seen long-term depression, but no one was really sure. Depression might be obscured because you could kill a cell or ruin the synapse.

As Mark says, "Seeing is believing, but in this case it was necessary to believe in order to see."

For the BCM algorithm to work, in addition to potentiation we need the negative part, depression. Serena Dudek and Mark Bear did the experiment to look for it. I won't go through the design, but it's ingenious and maps the change in responsiveness of the cell as a function of its depolarization. For insufficient depolarization, learning is negative and then goes into the positive region. Long-term depression, then long-term potentiation. This has now been demonstrated in many areas of the brain, in young and old animals and in many species—including humans. There may still be a few skeptics, but I believe that most people are convinced.

The theory also requires that the crossover point between LTD and LTP move with cell activity, the sliding threshold. It is particularly evident in the experiment known as reverse suture in which you begin as with monocular deprivation, then open the previously closed eye, and close the other. The response of the cortical cells connected to the closed eye is driven to zero. But then if you reverse the suturing, the previously closed eye recovers. If the threshold weren't moving, the eye would never recover, so we know it has to move. Very recent work in Bear's lab by Kirkrood and Bear shows that the threshold does move, as expected.

Now no one talks now about whether synaptic modification occurs or not. What is talked about now is what specific receptor protein is altered. Within a few years, we're going to have an important story describing which receptor is modified, what it is that happens when memory is stored, and where it's stored. And we're also going to know the sites of short-term and long-term memory. The universe has changed. It really is a tremendous change. The consequences are difficult to predict, but you would think that if you know exactly what is being altered when memory is stored, there should be many important consequences.

My feeling is that one thing you can be sure of is Murphy's Law. If it can go wrong, it will go wrong. Every step in the sequences of events that leads to memory storage goes wrong sometimes. When it does, it's known by a Latin name. It's a disease of some kind. Of course, just because you know it went wrong doesn't mean you can do anything about it, but it gives one a chance.

ER: Want to talk a little bit about Nestor, your company?

LC: Sure. I'm always happy to talk about Nestor. That's the other branch. At Nestor we say, "Let's do something with it." We have produced useful commercial products incorporating what are now called artificial neural networks.

ER: Had you ever been involved with a commercial enterprise before Nestor?

LC: In fact, I have. With an old, old friend of mine, Conrad Taff, who was a venture capitalist, we started a company known as Science Resources. Then I drifted from that to the board of directors of other little companies and association with venture-capital people. The idea of forming a company was not unknown to me. Making it a neural network company, that just came together.

ER: When was Nestor started and under what circumstances?

LC: I remember writing to Charles Elbaum from Paris when I was there in '73 on sabbatical and saying to him, "I think it would be a good idea to start a company." And then when I came back, I got in touch with some of the people I knew in New York. They thought it was such a great idea they were here in Providence the next morning. We started as a limited partnership, back around '75 or so, raising a grand total of about $400,000, and we lived on that $400,000 for about ten years, which gives you some indication of our level of activity.

ER: So what were you trying to do in those early years with the company? To create a demonstration of the technology, to create a product?

LC: Well, I hate to be quoted on this, although I am aware you will quote me, but I don't think we knew what a product was. We were academics. We just had this idea that conceptually was very powerful. I guess we were trying to create a demonstration. The first thing we worked on was to try to create a demonstration of how you could recognize handwriting. Things were primitive then. Ironically, one of the things that made the company go wasn't an advance in software, or algorithms, but advances in hardware. If we wanted to recognize handwriting, way back, what we would do was write on a magnetic tablet and that was put on a tape. Then the tape was carried by hand to the mainframe, two days later we'd come back, and it would say that you wrote a "3." This wasn't the most impressive demonstration in the world. When machines developed to the stage where you could attach a magnetic tablet to an early workstation like a Terak [a small PDP 11–based workstation] and have someone write a numeral and have it recognized right away, then people said, "Hey!"

It was primitive by current standards. Still, it was all there in one place. It had impact. After fooling around this way, people said, "You guys ought to get serious. First of all, why don't you form a corporation, why don't you go public, why don't you hire a few people and try to do something?"

I think our first contract was with DEC [Digital Equipment Corporation]. They wanted to produce a Kanji recognition system. That's when we had our place on Governor Street and our first two people.

ER: How did that come about?

LC: As I recall, Terry Potter from DEC walked into my office one day. He said he had talked to John Hopfield and that John had suggested he talk to me. This eventually resulted in a project to recognize two thousand Kanji characters and to do it at the rate of several characters a second, using the tiny machines that were then available. Let me tell you, that was not easy. There was another reason why we thought a commercial company was the way to go. As soon as we began to use neural network–type systems to solve real-world problems, the problems didn't seem to be academic anymore. You had to use real data, in real situations. If you really wanted to develop such systems, it was no longer an academic project.

We've always been very conscious of potential conflicts of interest. We just wanted to get things to work and to separate commercial from academic. There is always the potential of conflict of interest, but I think we handled it. There are two ways: one way is to say there's potential for conflict of interest, so don't do it. The other is to accept the potential and handle it properly. We've always been very open with the presidents of Brown and let them know what we're doing. We've been scrupulous about making sure no Brown money was used for Nestor and vice versa, to the point of ridiculousness.

[Brown President] Howard Swearer said, "Go and make a fortune and make sure you contribute a lot to Brown." It's also been positive because it enables our students, when they want, to have practical experience. On the whole, I think it's been a good interaction.

Anyhow, we had this project with DEC. Charles Elbaum, Doug Reilly, Chris Scofield, and I worked together. We actually got to do the recognition, and then of course it wasn't fast enough. I got into all kinds of problems I'd never dealt with before, such as how to speed things up. I was fascinated because every day there would be new and very practical problems. It was really fun. By the time we were finished, we had two thousand characters being recognized with high accuracy, in real time, two to three a second, on the little DEC Pro series computers. One of the big problems was getting the characters, getting the training set. DEC did that in Japan. They got a training set for us. We trained on a DEC VAX 730, an old creaky VAX 730 that they lent us or perhaps was part of the contract. By the time the contract was finished, it wasn't even worth carting away.

We would train on two thousand Kanji characters, twenty to one hundred samples of each. The 730 would run all weekend. Our neural networks trained very fast, but it still took about a weekend. When we came in on Monday morning, there's the system, recognizing Kanji. That was pretty impressive. So DEC had the system, and they put it on their Pro. Then a guy from DEC named George Cassidy built it into a beautiful piece of software. I saw it running, and it was gorgeous. You'd write the Kanji. It would be recognized and put on the screen in a font of your choice. You could make it bigger, smaller, any color; you could do desktop publishing with Kanji. But then, after all that, the Pro series computers just weren't selling in Japan. How they expected a machine without any software to sell I don't know, but they expected to sell about ten thousand. They sold a few hundred, so they pulled the machines off the market.

Our project was pulled with it. Then we floundered for a while. We floundered because we kept wanting to do things with on-line handwriting recognition. It's a great idea, except the hardware wasn't there. Writing on a Bitpad wasn't going to work. We always keep thinking that someday this market is going to develop, and we're going to get into this again, but our feeling at the moment is that we're on hold as far as on-line written character recognition is concerned. Well, in the interim we raised money, and then we raised more money, and then we brought a president in. Presently, we have a great CEO, Dave Fox. He has tremendous business experience. After all these years we now have some solid products. We eventually made the conversion from a pure technology-driven company to a company that is driven by the market.

ER: So the products you are talking about are the off-line character recognition, intelligent character recognition, the one that detects fraud after credit card transactions, the chip with Intel ...

LC: Yes. We decided not to be a contract engineering company because we learned you don't make money that way. Our fraud detection system, for example, really is a risk analyzer that gives you probability ratings for events. It can rate risk and look for anomalies. It can be applied in many situations, but if you want to develop products for the financial market, you should have people who understand banks, how banks work—understand what they're doing, understand what kind of organizational change they will accept and what kind of change they won't accept.

If a product is something they would love to have, it usually must not disturb the system they have. Then if they buy it, they can grow with it. Once they have confidence in one system, they often want neural network technology to do other things for them. Our character recognizer, the Nestor Reader, is in use at other banks. It's cut their data entry costs enormously. [*note:* Since this interview, the Nestor OCR system has been exclusively licensed to National Computer Systems Inc.]

ER: What is your involvement in the company now?

LC: Officially, I'm a consultant. But, in fact, I'm an appendage, a fifth wheel. Since I know the people, I talk to them. I'm on the board, of course, and as a board member I'm involved in decisions at board level. My real technical involvement is that if Chris or Doug or any of the others want to talk to me about something, they are free to talk.

ER: Is there a flow to them from some of the ideas that you work on here in terms of algorithms or concepts?

LC: Sometimes. For example, if they have problems, they may ask one of my graduate students to come down and consult with them, but they are product oriented. If we were big enough, we would have a more research-oriented branch at Nestor, but we don't have the money for that. If the company evolves in the future, we'll have that. But at the moment, they're focused.

ER: What do you think of the neural net business? Do you think it's a field people should consider as a commercial opportunity?

LC: I think you have to make a distinction between the companies and the technology. The technology is just going to become part of the engineering toolbox. Which companies will make it commercially is difficult to predict. I think Nestor very likely will, but that's a bet on an individual company. As far as the technology is concerned, I think it is going to be incorporated in systems of the future. I think too much fuss has been made about neural networks as a separate mystery. These networks are part of the solution. They will work along with other technology. The brain is a perfect example. We have no example in nature of a neural network sitting on a table doing something. Take a piece of cerebral cortex, put it on a table—it doesn't do very much. It only does something when, for example, it's linked to some of the most magnificent optics ever built.

So we expect that the neural networks will be built into systems, working with conventional components and employing rules also. The dichotomy between rule-based systems and learning systems is a foolish one, like many academic dichotomies. Why learn what you already know? Why try to formulate a rule that is so complex that it's almost impossible to put it down, other than as a set of examples?

That's really where neural networks contribute. Our attitude always has been that if you know the rules, you might as well put them in. It's ridiculous not to. It shortens the learning process.

For character recognition, most of our competitors use some form of neural network. It's not anymore an issue of whether you use neural networks. The issue is more *which* networks are most efficient. The various algorithms have areas where they do best. What you should do is to use them in combination.

When we do what we call ICR, intelligent character recognition, we use neural networks for recognition, and then we might add sophisticated contextual checks to try to do connected or cursive writing recognition. As human beings we use context when we try to recognize things. Sometimes we use context with conventional means; sometimes we use recursive neural networks. It is less and less a matter of deep new principle.

ER: What would you advise someone who is just considering the field of neural networks?

LC: Well, the first thing I would say is, "Don't think of it as neural networks. Just make that a part of what you learn. Try to learn the underlying mathematics and statistics, neural network methods, and all the usual things that must be done to try to understand systems. If you want to go into the biological end, then you need a very good grip on the biology, the underlying ideas, what's possible experimentally, and what is going on now."

At this moment, we don't seem to have any trouble placing our students in good jobs. The students that are doing practical applications, at least as they come out of my group, have a variety of techniques in both neural networks and statistical methods and how to program computers. They're a very valuable commodity.

I suppose my advice is, "Train yourself in something that's useful, that you like, and that has possibilities." I think engineering applications are more interesting than academic problems. Some of the things that are worked on academically don't turn me on especially. I think some of the real-world applications are absolutely intriguing. They become engineering problems, putting systems together that function, but they may lead to some very deep ideas that we don't yet understand.

How do you take systems of this kind and put them together to arrive at something that associates—that reasons? And then the deep, deep question: how do you build something that feels, that's conscious, that is aware of itself? In my opinion, no one has the foggiest idea, not a clue. To me that's the great remaining deep mystery in this field.

ER: I noticed you used the term "has feelings," whereas most people talk about intelligent machines in terms of their reasoning ability.

LC: I think the problem of intelligent machines is already solved conceptually. That's arrogant, I know, but there are already machines that can do logic a million times faster than we can. I think we know how to begin to put them together. But a machine that reasons is not a machine that's aware of itself. In this field, that is the major unsolved problem.

The typical reaction to the problem of consciousness reminds me of Yogi Berra: "It's deja vu all over again." The typical reaction to really difficult scientific problems.

First, try to solve a difficult problem, you don't get any place. Then you prove that it can't be solved. Or you invoke a new law of nature. Or you solve one mystery by invoking another. Or you say, "For some reason or another, a solution is irrelevant." Or you do all of the above.

I remember that's what people did with superconductivity. They proved you couldn't solve it. "It's probably a new law of nature," they said. And one famous physicist whom I will not identify wrote afterward that it was somewhat of a disappointment that this beautiful phenomenon of superconductivity turned out to be due to small interactions between electrons, thus missing the point in operatic style.

How has this gone with consciousness? First of all you have the homunculus solutions—that is to say, you pour the conscious substance into the material substance. OK, that's one type of solution. Another kind of solution is to explain one mystery by invoking another. For example, consciousness arises in the interaction with the measurement process of the quantum theory. This is a subject I happen to know something about, and it doesn't arise there. Or in quantum gravity, where gravitation meets quantum theory. What they're really saying is that we don't understand the latter, and so maybe it can be used to explain the former. Another way is to say that consciousness arises quote, "somehow," unquote, when you execute algorithmic processes of a certain complexity. It's the "somehow" that I like. That's what I'm trying to find out: how does that "somehow" come about?

Or, another evasion under the cover of positivism is to say, "How do you know it's conscious?" I don't care whether I know it or not; I would just like to explain it if it is conscious. The Turing test is another way of evading this problem. All of these things have been said.

To me, it's all beside the point. I'm really, as this guy described me, a no-nonsense physicist. I just want to have a little machine, maybe a mental machine, that becomes conscious. I want to see the atoms going back and forth, and I want to see the thing becoming conscious, due to either the average velocity or whatever it is. That's what we don't know. I want to get it the way we get temperature—with primitive mechanical entities such as the average kinetic energy that you can identify with what we call temperature.

The way consciousness has to be explained from my point of view is that we have to find some combination of material objects about which you say, "That's just what we call consciousness because it has all the properties."

Either that can be done or it can't be done. I don't know. I haven't done it. I think it can be done, but it hasn't been done, and no one has a clue, in my opinion, as to how to do it. We can contemplate the possibility that it can't be done, but we certainly shouldn't begin by assuming that it can't be done. And if it turns out that it couldn't be done, that would be one of the profoundest things we have learned about ourselves in the history of human thought. I don't think it's going to turn out that way. It is a profound question, one that's really worth a little thought.

ER: I wanted to talk about government funding. You had mentioned that ...

LC: What do you want me to do, start complaining? I've been so cheerful all afternoon.

ER: Well, I just wanted to get your opinion on whether you thought that government funding was important to the field and your thoughts on the way it's changed.

LC: Government funding is important in all fundamental science.

ER: I know that your academic work has been supported by the U.S. Navy and many other funding organizations.

LC: ONR [Office of Naval Research] has been visionary and generous in their funding. They've been interested in the underlying biology, and they're also interested in the transitions between the underlying biology and various applications of interest. They feel as though the particular transitions that we've made in, for example, the Nestor-Intel chip or the use of the BCM algorithm for the separation of reflected acoustic or radar signals is the sort of thing they're looking for and are willing to fund.

ER: So do you see a continuation of government funding?

LC: Well, it's been very tight. If you look more broadly than neural networks, if you think about funding in fundamental science, I think the profound problem we have is people's desire for quick fixes or quick results. I'm not against quick results; I love them. It's just that you can't always get them. And in the area of fundamental science, you can show over and over again that if you had focused money on an attempt to get the solution of a social or medical problem with the technology of that time, you would not have funded what turned out to give you the solution.

I'll give you a few examples. Suppose that in the early '50s you had said that you'd like to find a new method for dense information storage and improved methods of, let's say, retinal surgery. Would you have funded Charles Townes's work on the interaction of molecular beams with microwave radiation? I don't think so.

Suppose you had been interested in these things in the '20s, would you have funded Heisenberg, who was working on some far-out idea called an uncertainty principle? Suppose you were looking for a solid-state device to replace the vacuum tube. You surely wouldn't have funded Heisenberg. You probably wouldn't even have funded Bardeen. Would you have funded Fleming, who in the course of an investigation on the color of bacterial colonies happened to discover the antibacterial properties of the penicillium mold?

Let me give the one example that to me is the archetype. At the end of the nineteenth century, Edward Bellamy wrote a book called *Looking Backward*. It was a utopian view, from the end of the twentieth century. One thing about that future world that particularly delights him is that everyone can have music in their homes at will. The way he did it is to have musicians playing in something like city hall connected to homes by acoustic ducts. Anyhow, he writes this marvelous paragraph that I'll paraphrase: "If in our time, we found a way to have music in our homes, in the quantity and quality that we wanted, whenever we wanted it, we would have felt ourselves as having achieved the limit of human felicity and would strive no more."

This is in approximately 1880. Now suppose that Her Majesty's Royal Marine Research Unit said, "He's right, what we have to do is to put all of our funding into getting music into people's homes." Translate music into your most horrible disease or anything; throw all your funding at it. Would they have funded Maxwell? Would they have funded Lorenz or Einstein or any of these other people? No, of course not. We would now have large Swiss music boxes. We would have automated piano players.

Two things are obvious. One is that sometimes it's clear that a precise development project is in order because you already know the underlying science. You just have engineering hurdles to solve, and with a little luck you can solve them. Pour money into it, and you'll do it. And you should certainly do that.

But for a cure to some diseases you're going to find that there are things that are unknown. We don't know how to discover those unknown things. So to take money from the National Science Foundation, pour it into various directed-research projects, away from what they call "curiosity"-driven research, is counterproductive.

ER: Could you give us your view of the neural network field in five years or perhaps even twenty years out?

LC: I think as far as the biological underpinning, that's now going to evolve in an almost predictable way. I think we're on the way to finding where short-term memory is stored, where long-term memory is stored, and what initiates the transfer between one and the other. I've always held that long-term and short-term memory are stored at the same sites. It's the simplest mathematical theory you can write. What you have are components that decay quickly, components that decay slowly, or not at all, and the question is whether you go from the quick decay to the slow decay guided by some global signal. I think that will be found.

Among the big problems are: How is the processing done? How is visual processing done? How is it all put together? It's going to be almost an engineering problem because you have the interaction of very complex systems, one with the other.

On the other side, as far as the practical applications of neural networks, I think they will grow, a little bit the way our cortex did it. First, you will have a little neural network inside a computer. Then it will be a slightly bigger one. Then it will be an even bigger one, and soon you'll find that what we call computers have processors asking neural networks what to do next.

I do have a concrete prediction. The twentieth century is the century of computers, telephones, cars, and airplanes. I think the twenty-first century will be the century of what we call intelligent machines—machines that combine the rapid processing power of the current machines with the ability to associate, to reason, to do sensible things. And I think these machines will just evolve. We'll have simple ones at first, and finally we're going to have reasoning machines.

Then you might ask, "What are human beings to do?"

The answer, I think, is really simple. It's what we've always done with machines that enhance our abilities. We are comfortable with machines that enhance the power of our arms or our legs. You see them all over the place. We're comfortable with computers that enhance our logic, our memory, and we'll be comfortable with reasoning machines. We'll interact with them. I think they will come just in time because the kinds of problems we have to solve, these very complex problems that are beyond the capacity of our minds, probably will be solved in interaction with such machines. We always have to keep control over them, but that same thing is true of all machines. In fact, the worst machines we have ever created, much more dangerous to our health than any reasoning machines, are our bureaucracies.

People will have various levels of comfort with this prospect. But I suspect that as matters evolve, we will, in the next hundred years or so, be interacting with machines that do really reason and that can be applied to very complex systems.

Let me conclude with this. Human beings have always been self-centered. The universe is built around us. Think of the extent to which intellectual problems are self centered. Why, for example, do we regard tic tac toe as trivial? And two-dimensional chess very challenging? No one plays eight-dimensional chess.

The reason is the capacity of the human mind. With a smaller mind, we'd find tic tac toe very challenging. With a larger mind, we'd be playing eight-dimensional chess. Now, the size of the human mind, I believe, is somewhat of an evolutionary accident. It could be twice as large or half as large. The same thing is true of the problems that we solve. And one of the little miracles is that there exist scientific problems that we find very important and that are solvable by our size minds. If our mind had been a little bit smaller, perhaps we never could have solved any interesting problems. What you have to think about is that there is a whole range of scientific problems that are enormously interesting that are beyond the power of our unaided mind. I think one of the things that will evolve in the future is that with enhanced power we may be able to tackle problems that are too difficult for us now.

We always have had the mystique of the human alone against the elements. I can imagine that on the plains of Troy, before the topless towers of Illium, Achilles lamented to his comrades, "With these new chariots, they're not going to need us anymore."

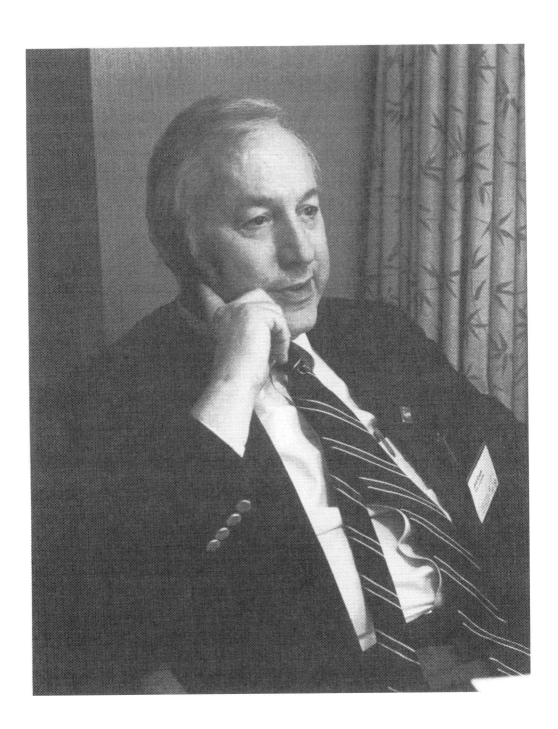

5 Jack D. Cowan

Jack Cowan is Professor of Applied Mathematics and Theoretical Biology, Department of Mathematics, University of Chicago, Chicago, Illinois. He is also Professor in the Department of Neurology in the Pritzker School of Medicine of the University of Chicago and an External Professor at the Santa Fe Institute, Santa Fe, New Mexico. A recent article on his work is "Neurodynamics and Brain Mechanisms" in Cognition, Computation, and Consciousness *edited by M. Ito, Y. Miyashita, and E. T. Rolls, Oxford University Press, 1997.*

December 1993, Denver, Colorado

ER: Maybe we could begin by talking a little bit about your personal background, where you grew up and your early education.

JC: I was born in Leeds in the north of England, but in 1939 my family moved to my father's hometown of Edinburgh. I grew up in Edinburgh and went to school there and went to Edinburgh University, where I did a physics degree, and then I joined Ferranti, an English electronics and computer company. My boss there had also been to the school I went to. He was very encouraging; his name was J. B. Smith. He and a colleague had designed a little machine that solved logic problems by trial and error. This was in 1954. I started work there in '55.

The Ferranti machine was sitting in a room full of dust, unused. I got it working again, and Smith asked me to take the machine to Imperial College and demonstrate it and talk to some of the people there. They got in contact with people in the electrical engineering department. Arthur Porter was the professor of light electrical engineering there and had worked on analog computing machines in the '30s, with Hartree. Hartree was a well-known physicist, numerical analyst, and computing person in the '30s and was famous for what's called the Hartree-Fock approximation in physics.

Anyway, I went there, and I hit it off with Arthur Porter. He introduced me to a very interesting man called Dennis Gabor. Not only was Gabor the inventor of holography, but he was one of the pioneers in communication and information theory. In fact, he wrote a paper in 1944, on "Theory of Communication," which is a very important paper in optics and was a precursor of his insights that led to holography. He also introduced what are now called Gabor functions, Gaussian weighted cosine waves, as a way to represent information in an optimal sense in optics.

He was also one of the first people, along with Norbert Wiener, to think about the problem of constructing learning filters—that is, filters with adjustable coefficients that could be used to predict the properties of time series and to filter signals. That's an activity that Norbert Wiener had been heavily engaged in during World War II and had written a very interesting little book on it. Anyway, Gabor introduced the method of using gradient descent to solve for the coefficients in a filter that was to be trained by comparing the input with the output. In fact, he essentially solved the problem of how you train such a machine in 1954 or '55. But in those days, life was very different from what it is now. There weren't many computers around. There were one or two in England, but they couldn't be used for this, so he and two or three of his graduate students spent seven years designing a fast analog multiplier, and they actually built a hardware version of the machine that finally got going in 1961. By then, Gabor had gotten interested in other things because lasers had been invented and laser holography burst on the scene. He was heavily involved in that.

When I was still at Ferranti in '56, they sent me to the first or the second International Congress on Cybernetics in Namur in Belgium. I met Gray Walter and Albert Uttley there. I heard some of the early stuff on conditional-probability computing in the nervous system that Uttley was doing, and I saw Gray Walter's striking demonstration of his little electronic mechanical turtle. This was after the first wave of cybernetics had been triggered in the late '40s by McCulloch and Norbert Wiener, and things were still going fairly strong in the mid-fifties. I guess that was one of the reasons I got interested in neural networks, that and reading von Neumann's article in *Automata Studies*.

Anyway, Gabor was interested in learning machines, and he was interested in the brain. I hit it off with him when I showed him how I had used many-valued logics to start looking at the problem of how you can do better than just simple trial-and-error learning in solving logic problems. One thing led to another, and I got a fellowship from what was then called the Hollerith Company, now called International Computers and Tabulators. I got a fellowship from them to go to MIT. I arrived at MIT in the fall of 1958 as a graduate student.

ER: Could we back up for just a minute? Because you went very quickly over your childhood. What's your date of birth?

JC: August 24, 1933.

ER: Could you tell us something about your parents, and how you got interested in ideas having to do with science and things like that?

JC: My grandparents on one side are Jews from near Vilna and on the other side from near Byalistock. My grandfather on one side was a tailor in Leeds, and my grandfather on the other side, I don't know what he did in the

Ukraine, but he had a cart; he peddled fruit around Scotland, just like a lot of other immigrant families did there. He died early. My father was a baker, and my mother helped my father. Both my father and mother were quite smart at school, but they had to leave to work. In those days, there wasn't anything else to do for first or second generation families.

My mother says I was a gifted child. I don't know why she said that, but she's a typical Jewish mother ... I was reading at some early age, and got scholarships to go to a very good Scottish equivalent of a public school, George Heriot's School. By the time I was about nine or ten, I was interested in science. It was all self-generated. I used to have arguments with my parents when I got to about twelve. They wanted me to be a doctor, the usual Jewish family dream. I kept saying, "No, I'm going to be a scientist." I decided that I was interested in physics, and I ended up winning all the medals at my school and getting a scholarship to go to Edinburgh University to do physics, but when I got there I found the style of teaching at Edinburgh University in the physics department was not to my taste. I got bored very rapidly. I went from being the top student in my school to just scraping along and doing physics courses that I wasn't interested in. I ended up going to Ferranti.

ER: Ok, now we can go back to MIT.

JC: I arrived in '58 at MIT. I had already had a thesis at Imperial College in which I introduced techniques of many-valued logic to start writing down parallel computer logic systems. I hit on the idea that you wanted to do things in parallel bundles. In '56 I got hold of the collection of papers by Shannon and McCarthy called *Automata Studies*. I got very interested in von Neumann's work on probabilistic logic and how you could synthesize reliable computers from unreliable elements. That was a big interest of mine when I arrived at MIT.

I didn't actually meet McCulloch then, but I met Walter Rosenblith, then the head of the Communications Biophysics Laboratory at MIT, and I became a member of the group. They were interested mainly in auditory psychophysics. I was there when Frank Rosenblatt arrived at MIT in the fall of '58 to give a public lecture on the perceptron. The year before, Marshall Yovits of the Office of Naval Research had publicized Rosenblatt's work and made a big splash about it. Here was a machine that could do pattern recognition in a humanlike way; it could recognize all kinds of things. Almost everyone at MIT was very skeptical.

The lecture was in the Research Laboratory of Electronics conference room. Everybody in the institute was there—Minsky, Shannon, Elias, Huffman, Fano—the whole group interested in information theory and in signal processing. I think Jerry Lettvin was there, but I can't be sure, but McCulloch was there.

Rosenblatt gave his lecture, and it was a terrible lecture. He kept saying, "Well, you can use information theory to do this, that, and the other." He made claims that you could tell a circle from a triangle with his early perceptron. It was all wrong; you couldn't do things like that. They went after him and really attacked him.

McCulloch didn't say anything. Shannon said, "It's worth looking at." Rosenblith's group had a little session after the talk, and there was definitely interest in the problem. Larry Roberts at MIT actually did a master's thesis in which he speeded up the way the perceptron behaved and got some nice results on it. But by and large it was clear that the perceptron wasn't doing the things that Frank claimed it could do.

JA: Did he know about the perceptron convergence theorem at that time?

JC: No, he didn't.

JA: He didn't mention it in his early papers, and I assumed that he didn't have the result because it's an important result.

JC: It appeared in two later papers in the *Reviews of Modern Physics.* Those papers contained an attempt at a formal proof of the convergence. In 1961–62 Al Novikoff recognized the essential similarity between linear threshold elements and the algorithm, and linear programming, and produced a very elementary but neat proof by contradiction that it converged in a finite number of trials. Novikoff's proof made clear what was going on and should have, actually, triggered a lot of work.

I think it was after that time that Marvin [Minsky] developed an antipathy to the perceptron and to everything that had to do with perceptrons. Ironically, he and Seymour [Papert] later worked out a beautiful treatment of perceptrons.

After about eighteen months in the Communications Biophysics Laboratory, where I wrote a master's thesis and where I extended the stuff on many-valued logics, I got to know McCulloch. He was a very interesting, generous and welcoming person. I took to him, and he took to me. I ended up switching groups, which was unheard of in those days. There was a lot of psychological tension between McCulloch's group, and the Rosenblith group and Norbert Wiener.

Norbert Wiener was a very interesting person. I sat in on his early lectures on nonlinear problems, stochastic theory, and random processes, and a strange thing happened, which I benefitted from. Norbert had used data taken by Margaret Freeman in the lab, to calculate the power-density spectrum of human EEG. She had made some mistakes in the calculation so there was a big peak in the power-density spectrum, and on either side there was a trough. So Norbert said, "Oh, maybe there's a clock there, a synchronization phenomenon."

Every afternoon, he would arrive at the front door of the Communications Biophysics Group in old Building 20, the building that had been the radar lab during the war, which is still there. Everybody in the entire group would disappear out the back door when Norbert arrived, except me. The reason was that Norbert would deliver a three-hour monologue on whatever he was working on at the time, and all he wanted was somebody to listen and say, "Yes, that's very good." So I stayed and listened. I got some private lectures from Norbert, which were fascinating.

Anyway, I ended up going over to McCulloch, and I met Lettvin and Walter Pitts for the first time. In '59, when I was still in Rosenblith's group, Rosenblith organized a very interesting meeting at MIT. There was a book published from it called *Sensory Communication*. Werner Reichardt presented there an early version of what is called the Reichardt motion-detector model. It's actually the Reichardt-Hassenstein motion-detector model. It was a great meeting for the graduate students who were there. Nevertheless, I decided my interests were more mathematical than the interests of the group, so I ended up going off to McCulloch and Pitts.

Pitts was very interesting to me, but let me talk about Warren McCulloch first. He and his wife had a house near Harvard Square. They would always have all kinds of interesting people staying with them. They were extremely gregarious, or he was. Rook wasn't quite as gregarious as Warren was, but she was very nice. And Warren was amazing; he would have cheerfully mortgaged his house to help one of his students, if need be. He did all kinds of very generous things for people. They had a big family farm, a 750-acre farm in Old Lyme, Connnecticut, where we used to go to in the summers.

He was definitely a link with a different kind of American culture from the one that was sitting around at MIT. He was unusual in many ways. He'd been trained as a neurologist and a psychiatrist at Yale and then at Illinois. He'd worked for two years in a psychiatric hospital and then decided that was enough; he'd learned enough about patients and psychiatry. He had gone in 1941 to the University of Illinois. I think he was at the Illinois State Psychiatric Institute. He met Pitts, and I can tell you something about that. Jerry Lettvin can give you a much more nonapocryphal picture of things, but I can tell you the stories I heard from McCulloch about it all. Whether or not they're true or not is a problem.

The wildest ones—the ones I can confirm—were true, and the plausible ones were false. But anyway, there they were in the basement of the Compton Lab, the early neurophysiology group—McCulloch, Pitts, Jerry Lettvin, and Pat Wall, who later went back to England. It was a really interesting group of eccentrics. That was the nice thing about MIT in those days; there were so many eccentrics floating around. There was Norbert Wiener, Warren McCulloch, Roman Jakobson, Emmanuel Sereno, and Claude Shannon. All kinds of strange and interesting people there. And Marvin [Minsky], too. I would say Marvin was in that category.

McCulloch at the time was interested in the reliability problem. He had gotten into that problem, he says, when he was talking with von Neumann. They had decided that it was an interesting question how humans managed to function, even when they were full of alcohol. Warren started to think, well, clearly the brain is reliable, but computers aren't all that reliable. What's the difference between brains and computers? How are they organized?

He started to design little neural networks, which would still give the same output, even though their thresholds were fluctuating back and forward. Earlier on, in the Macy Foundation meetings that McCulloch had organized with Wiener and the others, he was extremely influential in triggering von Neumann's interest in automata. And in computing, it was McCulloch and Pitts' formalism that von Neumann used in his first work on computers. They actually had a very important if indirect influence on the early development of computers in the U.S.

Turing actually met McCulloch at one time and thought he was a charlatan, but I think he simply underestimated McCulloch, in many ways. You could easily get the impression that McCulloch was a charlatan if you didn't know better.

ER: Because of his outgoingness?

JC: His outgoingness. He looked like Moses; he had this long beard and bushy eyebrows.

ER: There's this wonderful picture of him on the cover of *Embodiments of Mind,* [McCulloch's collected papers] and I figured that's what he looked like.

JC: That's right. He had a strange gleam in his eye. He really looked like he was crazy a lot of the time. He had grey eyes, and when they got really bright and glaring, he looked a spectacle.

Anyway, I started to work with him. I had done this stuff on parallel bundles and logic, so we actually applied that stuff to the reliability problem. We started to come up with improvements to some of von Neumann's schemes for multiplexing things. And then there was some work by Elias and Shannon and others on whether one could extend information theory to computing, rather than just to communication channels. I ended up recruiting to our group another graduate student by the name of Shmuel Winograd. Winograd is now one of the top mathematicians at IBM and is an IBM fellow. He has made all kinds of interesting discoveries on how you multiply and invert matrices using the Chinese remainder theorem and other fascinating mathematical theorems to cut down the number of operations that you need to use, thereby saving millions of dollars in computing time.

Anyway, in those days we got interested in this problem of the capacity of computing devices. We ended up extending Shannon's basic theorem of information theory, the noisy channel—coding theorem, to computers. We showed that von Neumann's solution to the problem of how you build reliable machines from unreliable elements could be thought of as one extreme, special case of this theorem. The other extreme was the Shannon theorem itself. In between, if some module had a certain complexity, you could calculate what the optimum design was for the network.

The information theorists didn't like our stuff because they said we hadn't properly taken account of the noise in the decoder, but in fact we *had* taken account of it. What we had discovered was one of the earliest constructions of a parallel distributed-computing device. We had set up a parallel machine in which any one thing to be computed is not computed in a single element, but in many places, and any one place does a mixture of many of the things.

We'd arrived at that by showing how you can embed error-correcting codes into the structure of a computing machine. It required devices that could compute functions of many, many inputs without being significantly more noisy than something that is a simple binary switch.

Such devices weren't available in those days, but nowadays it's possible to do things like that. In principle the architecture that we came up with is the kind of architecture you want for computing. Anyway, that work got us known. We wrote a monograph on it. We never published the complete theory, just part of it, because Shmuel by then was working at IBM. We never published the real guts of the thing. It's still sitting in my files. Shmuel and I agreed we would write it up one of these days.

It is quite interesting in the light of what's happened in computing. We basically had produced an optimal configuration for doing parallel distributed computing. It's immune to damage—if it's miswired, for example. It's taken care of by the redundancy in the network. If part of it gets hit by lightning, it will still work with fairly high reliability. In other words, it's got the same kind of error insensitivity that you would expect to see in something like a perceptron, which has a lot of parallel architecture.

ER: So the main reason this wasn't published was because Shmuel left to go to IBM?

JC: No. It was just that IBM felt it had a proprietary right to the particular thing we did at the time, so we wrote a monograph in which we did some of it, but the real stuff, which would have appealed to the information theory community, we never have published.

I went back to England after that, back to Imperial College with my own grant from the Office of Naval Research. And Shmuel went on to his work on matrices at IBM.

I think the main influence on my work was Walter Pitts. The first time I met him we had a general talk about neural networks. Warren kept talking about the relationship between neural networks and Turing machines and logic and things like that. And Walter kept saying, "Yes, but the really interesting thing is a continuous approach to neural networks." Norbert Wiener also used to say things along similar lines to me.

In '61, I took part in a symposium on information processing in the brain, in Holland. McCulloch was there, Norbert Wiener was there, Rashevsky was there, Gordon Pask was there, Albert Uttley was there. I gave a talk on this stuff, which went down very well.

Norbert Wiener was sitting there. Wiener and McCulloch had had a feud for years and wouldn't speak to each other. Norbert never let that interfere with his relationships with students and young people. He was very kind to everybody. One afternoon at the meeting we went off together into the town, and we sat in a little coffee house having coffee, and he sang vaudeville songs of the 1920s to me in a high falsetto voice. He was really quite funny; he wasn't what you might have thought he was. He always needed reassurance that what he was doing was great. And one time, in fact, he said to me, "You know, the reason I got all my results on what are now called the Wiener-Banach spaces and stochastic processes is because of my strong physical intuition." He said he got it from looking at all the ripples and anti-patterns in the Charles River. He had these thick glasses on, and he could hardly see where he was going. But it's actually true; he did have a strong intuition about these things.

Anyway, I gave my talk, and he was sitting in the front row, ostensibly sleeping. I gave my talk, and immediately he stood up and did his usual trick. He made a long comment on his own work, disguised as a question on my talk. I didn't really appreciate it at the time, but it was written up, and it's in the proceedings. It actually was a very, insightful comment about my work and his work and the way they might relate.

I was also very much impressed with Pitts and his insights. Walter was really the intelligence behind Lettvin and McCulloch. I think it was Walter who was the real driving intelligence there. Since 1921 Warren had had an idea of somehow writing down the logic of transitive verbs in a way that would connect with what might be going on in the nervous system, but he couldn't do it by himself. In 1942, he was introduced to Pitts, who was then about seventeen years old. Within a few months Walter had solved the problem of how to do it, using the Russell-Whitehead formalism of logic, which is not a transparently clear formalism. Nonetheless, they had actually solved an important problem and introduced a new notion, the notion of a finite-state automaton. So here was this eccentric but imaginative Warren and this very clever young Walter doing this stuff together.

ER: I was going to ask you to tell the story about how they met.

JC: This is where I have to rely on the stories I got from McCulloch about Walter.

The story goes as follows. Walter was born in Michigan, maybe Detroit or somewhere near there. According to Warren, he had run away from home. He was at the University of Chicago, sitting around and going to lectures. Anyway, he was on a park bench in Jackson Park near the campus. He was reading something by Rudolph Carnap, who was then in the philosophy department there. It so happened that Bertrand Russell was on sabbatical that year teaching at Chicago and happened to be there in the park and saw Pitts reading this stuff. So they got talking, and, as I heard the story, Russell took Pitts to meet Carnap, and through Carnap he met Rashevsky.

Nicholas Rashevsky had come from Russia after the revolution and had been at Rockefeller Institute; he had gotten a Rockefeller Fellowship, come to Chicago, and joined the physiology department there. Ajax Carlson, who was a very famous physiologist, threw him out after a year because he never did any experimental work. The story is that Carlson went into Rashevsky's office, and there was a desk and a chair and Rashovsky, sitting there with a pencil.

And Carlson said, "Where is your apparatus?"

And Rashovsky said in his Russian accent, "What apparatus? I am a mathematical biologist."

So he was thrown out.

The net effect was that Rashevsky set up a Committee on Mathematical Biophysics, as it was originally called, in 1938 in Chicago. He was the early pioneer in the field of mathematical modeling of neural networks, and his approach was to try to use differential equations rather than logic. Logic came along later in '43 with McCulloch and Pitts. Rashevsky had a flourishing group going with some very good people who later became distinguished in other fields. Alvin Weinberger, the former head of Oak Ridge, was a member of the group, so was Alston Householder, a distinguished numerical analyst.

Anyway, Pitts became a member of that group, and it was through his membership in that group that he got in touch with McCulloch, I think through Rashevsky. So if you believe the story, it was pure chance that led Pitts and McCulloch together.

ER: Pure chance and Russell and Carnap and Rashevsky. It's a wonderful trail.

JC: Whether it's true or not, I have no way of verifying. But that's what I heard from the lips of Warren Sturgis McCulloch one evening when he was in his cups. Where were we?

Pitts was at MIT as a research assistant with Wiener. Then McCulloch and Lettvin and Pat Wall formed the new group in the Research Laboratory of Electronics at MIT in 1951. But then Wiener and McCulloch had a falling out, and Pitts got caught in the middle and had a nervous breakdown and never really recovered from it. So there he was in the lab, but basically he wasn't doing anything. Lettvin looked after Pitts. Walter was sick. He was very shy. He was very easily startled by people. He would be somewhat hard to talk to or find. I managed to talk with him quite a bit, and always he kept driving home the idea that what one should really do is to look at continuous approaches to neural networks rather than the discrete approaches. There was far more mathematical machinery available, and it was more natural to try to look at the statistical mechanics of large populations than to look at just small network problems.

I already had some exposure to that idea because in 1956, while I was at Imperial College, I had gotten to know Raymond Beurle, who wrote one of the earliest papers on pattern formation in neural networks. Even though it turns out the mathematical details are wrong, nonetheless a lot of the basic ideas about the dynamical properties of networks of neurons are sitting in Raymond Beurle's work. I found what Beurle had done was really interesting mathematically. He had made a mistake in his calculations, so he thought that solitons were present in nervous activity. But they're not because refractory states in neural activity mean that any two waves that collide with each other will annihilate each other in a neural network, whereas in a network that supports solitons, the waves would just pass through each other.

Apart from that, the paper is full of very interesting things. In it is a description of associative memory; for example, a superposition of these waves leaves along the front a trace of both waves. If the waves affect threshold properties of cells, you can store information in those changes, so if you've got lots of waves, you can easily build up a store. Beurle showed that just giving part of a wave would regenerate the rest, for example, and he actually had a lot of properties of what we now know are associative memory in this paper. Actually, even earlier, Albert Uttley had already arrived at many of these properties in his own analysis of networks, using conditional probability ideas.

JA: There are many precursors. There's even some work from Lashley along the same lines.

JC: But Lashley's work was never expressed in a mathematical formal sense. McCulloch gave me a lot of Lashley's early papers.

But, anyway, I got this interest in a continuous approach, and I happened to run across some work by Ed Kerner, who had noticed that the Lotka-Volterra equations of population dynamics had a special mathematical structure to them that made them essentially equivalent to Hamilton's equations of motion and classical mechanics. I sat down, and I constructed a model neural network, which had similar equations in it. Then I modified the equations slightly so that they would be a little bit more stable, and I ended up with an analog neuron with the sigmoid function in it. So I had introduced a way to do the statistical mechanics of networks of analog neurons in the mid-sixties, about '64.

In 1963, I was over in Amsterdam giving some lectures, and Norbert was there, and we got together. We were going to work together on the statistical mechanics of neural networks. Unfortunately, before we got started, Norbert died. It was a big disappointment that I never got a chance to work with Wiener on this. I gave a talk at the Wiener Memorial meeting on it, at the same meeting at which Minsky and Papert presented their first work on the perceptron.

ER: That was in '65?

JC: '65, in Genoa. I was asked by Antonio Borsellino.

ER: How was your work received?

JC: Well, people were a little slow to see the point of an analog neural network, although Wilfred Taylor's work on associative memory was all done with analog neurons. He was perhaps the first person to explicitly produce an associative memory scheme. He didn't do it by theory, and he didn't do it on a computer. He actually built the hardware. In 1956, when I went with someone from Imperial College to University College London to meet him, there he was, and there was this huge bank of apparatus. There was the machine there doing its thing.

I tried to get him to explain to me how it worked. I couldn't. He didn't really understand himself what was going on, I think, and to this day in published papers you can't quite understand how it works. The learning rule he's got is not associative, and yet the performance is, so there's something fishy about it. It was all done with analog circuitry. It took him several years to build it and to play with it.

The idea of using nonlinear differential equations for neural networks was a little strange at that time. The Rashevsky group was trying to do things like that all along, but then the fashion was switching elements. I gave some lectures on it, but when I did it, it was ten years before the introduction of spin glasses.

In order to make the analogy with population dynamics, I studied the antisymmetric coupling case, where one neuron is an exciter that's coupled to an inhibitor, and then the inhibitor couples back to it, so the weights can be antisymmetrically related to each other. What I put aside to look at later was the symmetric case, which I didn't think was quite as veridical a model for a neural network as the antisymmetric case. Neither of them is actually a terribly good approximation.

ER: You had met and read Bernie Widrow?

JC: Right. In 1960, I went with McCulloch and Manuel Blum, who was a graduate student with McCulloch, to a Wright Patterson Air Force Base conference on bionics. I gave a talk on the reliability stuff. Then in '62 we went to Chicago, where there was a meeting on self-organizing systems arranged by Marshall Yovits, the supporter of Rosenblatt. Frank was there at the meeting and gave a talk on the perceptron. Bernie Widrow was there and gave one of the first talks on Adalines.

There was a certain skepticism from the MIT group toward Stanford engineering and what they were doing. I thought the Widrow stuff was quite interesting. When I looked at it carefully, I could see that it was essentially using the same methods that Gabor had introduced in the mid-fifties, the gradient-descent algorithm. I did not put it together with my own sigmoid work, even though I had alrady been getting preprints from Minsky and Papert about their perceptron studies. I knew from what we'd done with McCulloch that the exclusive-OR [X-OR] was the key to neural computing in many ways. But unfortunately, at the back of my mind I had the idea if I could work out the dynamics of analog neurons, later on I could start looking at learning and memory problems. I just put it aside.

That was a philosophical bias that I inherited from McCulloch. Warren always used to say that before you can study changes in neural networks, you should first of all study the behavior of systems where the connections aren't changing. "You have to get the anatomy before you can pervert it," he used to say. He was always philosophically biased toward the idea that if something is true, it works—rather than if something works, it's true. He was a great fan of Charles Peirce and pragmatism. Therefore, he always thought that it was the circuit first and then the behavior, rather than trying to use the environment to modulate the circuit to get the behavior.

All through the McCulloch group was this idea that there was an innate structure there. They believed in the Kantian notions of synthetic a priori. That's the kind of thinking that led Lettvin and Pitts to come up with "What the Frog's Eye Tells the Frog's Brain." They attributed much less importance to plasticity than to specificity in the nervous system. In retrospect, that was wrong. That was a mistake. That's the reason I never looked at the plasticity problems with the sigmoids early on because I had been biased to think about structural things and pattern formation first. That takes things up to about 1967.

ER: I'm curious about one thing. You said that Minsky and Papert first presented their notions about exclusive-OR in the Perceptron work.

JC: Well, they first presented their notions about the limitations of perceptrons and what they could and couldn't do.

ER: They hadn't gotten to exclusive-OR yet?

JC: They had, but that wasn't a central issue for them. The essential issue was, suppose you had diameter-limited receptive fields in a perceptron, what could it compute?

ER: How was that received at that first conference?

JC: Both of them were quite persuasive speakers, and it was well received. What came across was the fact that you had to put some structure into the perceptron to get it to do anything, but there weren't a lot of things it could do. The reason was that it didn't have hidden units. It was clear that without hidden units, nothing important could be done, and they claimed that the problem of programming the hidden units was not solvable. They discouraged a lot of research and that was wrong.

Everywhere there were people working on perceptrons, but they weren't working hard on them. Then along came Minsky and Papert's preprints that they sent out long before they published their book. There were preprints circulating in which they demolished Rosenblatt's claims for the early perceptrons. In those days, things really did damp down. There's no question that after '62 there was a quiet period in the field.

A thing that I didn't mention about Rosenblatt was that another person who was very perceptive about things was Mark Kac, a distinguished Polish mathematician who came to the Rockefeller University in the early '50s. He was the one who really promoted Rosenblatt. I think he had a very strong influence on Marshall Yovits at the Office of Naval Research. At the time, I think a lot of people felt that Mark Kac simply didn't know what he was doing, but they were wrong in retrospect. He knew. He had real insights into what was going on.

ER: It might be interesting to talk a little bit about funding at the time.

JC: Funding was in large part, from my recollection, the Air Force Office of Scientific Research, the Wright-Patterson Air Force Base people, and the Office of Naval Research [ONR], both the physics branch and the information systems branch. They were the main providers of funding for work in cybernetics and bionics and neural networks in those days.

JA: Was there any from NIH [National Institutes of Health] or NSF [National Science Foundation]?

JC: I don't think there was all that much. My recollection is that all the hardware and technological stuff and the modeling of the theory were all with DOD [Department of Defense] support.

ER: Robert Hecht-Nielsen has told me stories that long before Minsky and Papert ever committed anything to a paper that they delivered at a conference or published anywhere, they were going down to ARPA and saying, "You know, this is the wrong way to go. It shouldn't be a biological model; it should be a logical model."

JC: I think that's probably right. In those days they were really quite hostile to neural networks. I can remember having a discussion with Seymour, walking along the banks of the river Charles when I visited MIT. I think it was after I had gone, so it was in the '60s. We were talking about visual illusions. He felt that they were all higher-level effects that had nothing to do with neural networks as such. They needed a different, a top-down approach to understand. By then he had become a real, a true opponent of neural networks. I think Marvin had the same feelings as well. To some extent, David Marr had those feelings too. After he got to the AI lab, I think he got converted to that way of thinking. Then Tommy Poggio essentially persuaded him otherwise.

During the '60s there was a lot of pioneering thinking being done about continuous models of neural networks and pioneering thinking about associative memory. Associative memory really emerged in the '60s. As I said, Wilfred Taylor, Raymond Beurle, Steinbuch, and von Heerden had done work by about 1961 on associative memory. In '64 or '65, Christopher Longuet-Higgins got rolling, and by '68 there was Jim, Longuet-Higgins, Willshaw, and Buneman.

There was a wave of work after '43, when the McCulloch-Pitts paper came out, and then there was a wave of work after about 1954–55, with Uttley and Beurle's work, and then Rosenblatt's stuff came out, and von Neumann's work. There was a quietish period, and then there was another wave of work in the late '60s on associative memory.

ER: Were you at Imperial College during all this time, during the '60s?

JC: When I was at this meeting in '62 in Chicago, after my talk I was approached by two people from the ONR. The upshot was I ended up with my own personal grant from the U.S. Navy, by way of ONR, that I could hold back in Imperial College. I was there for four years. Then I spent a year at the National Physical Laboratory at Teddington, with Uttley. Then I got a job offer that I couldn't turn down as Rashevsky's successor at Chicago, where I've been ever since.

I can tell you a bit more about things in the '70s as well, and things that I've done with Hugh Wilson.

JA: That would be interesting because that was supposedly the dark ages of neural nets.

JC: I don't think it was the dark ages at all. There was a lot going on. The foundations were being laid or rediscovered for a lot of things. There was you and David Willshaw and Longuet-Higgins, also Gabor. Christopher got going with his version of associative memory and got furious with me when he first presented it at one of the Serbelloni meetings on theoretical biology that C. H. Waddington organized. I pointed out to him that what he had produced was virtually identical with Steinbuch's learning matrix. He got absolutely furious with me and wouldn't talk to me for quite a while. The funny thing was, Leon [Cooper] got interested in neural networks through our interactions at the Institute de la Vie meetings. Leon gave a very nice talk about the associative memory work at the Institute de la Vie meeting once, and Christopher stood up and very gently said, "You know, Leon, I published a paper virtually identical with this several years ago."

Leon smiled sweetly at Christopher, and he said, "Well, that's true, but you know, Christopher, you're famous for the statement, 'Reading rots the mind.'"

ER: Maybe we should talk a little bit about the '70s and about the period after you came back to America and decided to stay here.

JC: When I came back to the University of Chicago, the old Rashevsky Committee was moribund. The only person left was Peter Green. Peter Green was an interesting person. In 1960, he wrote a paper in which he tried to use an analogy between coupled oscillators, quantum mechanics and neural network behavior. It was full of suggestive things, but never got very far. In 1965, he wrote a paper which not many people know about, in Rashevsky's journal *The Bulletin of Mathematical Biology*, called "Random Superimposed Coding," in which he rediscovered and applied work by Calvin Mooers from the early days of information theory on the optimal storage of information in punch card systems. How do you code the inputs to associative memories in such a way that they are as unlike as possible, and yet you have as large a vocabulary as possible to work with. The Zator coding scheme as invented by Calvin Mooers solved this problem. Peter's paper is a complete description of how you go about producing a random superimposed coding scheme as an input to an associative memory, and then how you use the associative memory to store and retrieve the information in it. Interestingly, it's virtually identical with David Marr's cerebellum model, except it's not applied to the cerebellum.

ER: So it anticipated that work by ...

JC: By four years. It's an open question in my mind as to whether David knew about that work or not. David got into trouble with Longuet-Higgins for not referring to anybody in his thesis work. David had a very original mind, so it's easily credible that David just invented the whole thing himself. In fact, it's surprising how many people independently invented associative memories—all the way from Uttley and Beurle, Taylor, Steinbuch, Jim, Longuet-Higgins, Gabor, Kohonen, Marr ...

JA: It's a good idea.

JC: It's a very good idea. Anyway, I got involved in trying to build up the Committee on Mathematical Biology at the University of Chicago. I was fortunate because George Beadle was the president of the University of Chicago at the time. He helped me raise money from the Sloan Foundation and the National Institutes of Health. Very quickly we built up a good Department of Theoretical Biology. The first two appointments I made are now well-known MacArthur fellows. One is Stuart Kauffman. I met Stuart first in McCulloch's house. He was staying with McCulloch and working on neural networks with Warren. I hired Stuart right out of medical school. The other person I recruited out of graduate school was Arthur Winfrey. Both of them are distinguished theoretical biologists now. We built up a very good group and trained a lot of the current people in the field, like Leon Glass at McGill and John Tyson and others.

ER: What route did your work take after you came back to Chicago?

JC: What I started to do was to see if I could develop Beurle's work more. I had the good fortune to have a postdoc come to work with me—Hugh Wilson, who had done a Ph.D. in chemistry. Hugh and I worked on how we would actually clean up and extend Beurle's work so as to handle populations of interacting excitatory and inhibitory neurons, with or without refractory states. We ended up with a continuum theory for neural dynamics, which included the Beurle work as a special case, with the sigmoid function in it playing a key role. We basically showed that neural networks acted like transistor networks. They could produce attractors, or what are now called attractors. Switching and cycling and information storage could all be done within the framework of attractor dynamics. Those papers have become quite well known.

Later on I realized that we had created the neural analog of Turing's work on the chemical basis of morphogenesis. Now we know that neuron networks as pattern-formation systems are in fact typical of a universal pattern-forming system. You can use them as models for developmental processes, for hydrodynamics, and for all kinds of things. This is exactly in the spirit of the early McCulloch-Pitts work, which said that if you furnish a McCulloch-Pitts network with an infinite tape, it will act as a Turing machine, which we all know is a universal machine.

Jack D. Cowan

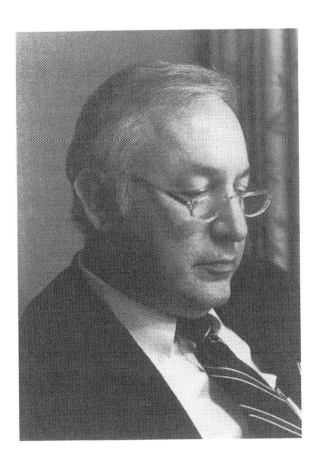

ER: A lot of people attribute the renaissance of the field to the spin glasses.

JC: In the mid-1970s I wrote a paper with Bard Ermentrout, the first of the set in which I actually looked at the symmetric case as well. It turns out a very old theorem in mathematical physics, called Maxwell's theorem, is relevant. Maxwell's theorem tells you that if you have a three-dimensional field —an electromagnetic field, for example—you can write it in terms of two potential functions. One is the gradient of a scalar potential function. The other is the curl of a vector function. Classical mechanics is basically the curl of a vector function. The mechanics, which has to do with attractors, comes from the other term, the gradient of the scalar. Classical mechanics equations are antisymmetric. The gradient of the scalar equations are symmetric. Any matrix can be split into the sum of the symmetric and an antisymmetric part.

So in general you can write any dynamical system as if it's built of a mixture of two parts. In n dimensions the theorem says that you have a gradient of a 1 form plus the generalization of the curl of an $n - 1$ form. I looked at the symmetric case, but again it was in a kind of continuum. Unfortunately, I didn't know anything about spin glasses, and I never followed that up either.

Actually, Erich Harth had seen in simulations that a neural network could act like a switch and show hysteresis. We essentially showed that with our continuum trick. But actually, that idea goes way way back to Neville Temperley's work. It was Temperley who first had the idea that a network of neurons in a sense could act like a network of spins. That was in the early or mid-fifties. He wrote a paper about the analogy between memory and hysteresis in networks of spins. So along came the spin glass idea in the mid-seventies. In the late seventies Hopfield and I ran a workshop in which we had various people interested in neural networks. In 1981 I spent the winter quarter at Caltech with John and gave a set of lectures on the stuff I had done. About six months later, John's first paper appeared on the symmetric case and the analogy with the spin glass. You know, I think that's neat stuff, but I still think it's an artificial system, as is the antisymmetric one. It may have nothing to do with the way things really work in the nervous system, but it's a very interesting idea.

ER: In terms of the sociology of science, what do you think happened with the Hopfield paper? It burst everything wide open. I suppose that's why people refer to the time prior to that paper as the dark ages.

JC: I think why is fairly clear. The theoretical physics community is like a swarm of locusts. There are far, far more theorists around than there are problems. There are only two or three problems, and whatever problem gets hot, a lot of them swarm onto it. That's what happened with the Hopfield paper. Here was this nice recognition by John that there was a close analogy between spin glasses and neuronlike networks with symmetric elements. So all the physicists landed on it. That created a lot of interest.

Independently of that, Geoff Hinton had been working first as Longuet-Higgins's graduate student and then later on at UCSD, and he was starting to get interested in neural computing, as was Dave Rumelhart. I think it was a sheer coincidence that the spin glass stuff occurred first. I think the other stuff would have occurred independently of the spin glass stuff.

JA: There was some other related work in the '70s. I was thinking of Shaw and Little.

JC: Right. Bill Little had noticed that if you took a one-dimensional network of neurons evolving in time and set out time as a second space dimension, then the equations you could write down—the update equations he came up with—were formally analogous to the Ising spin Hamiltonian network. His equations were very similar to my sigmoid differential form, except a discrete version of it. Again, he showed that in the symmetric case you could get long-range temporal-order effects and that you could store things in the attractors.

JA: That work never seemed to catch on the way Hopfield's did.

JC: No, it didn't. The reason was that there wasn't this population of physicists who knew about spin glasses. That didn't occur until after 1975. It was all a matter of timing with the spin glass model. I think all the time there was an evolution in the minds of people like Rumelhart and Hinton and also Terry Sejnowski. What Terry and Geoff noticed was that if you look at the spin glass Hamiltonian itself and think of it as an energy function, as in standard statistical mechanics, you could do things a little more flexibly than in the way Hopfield did it. So they came up with the Boltzmann machine. At the same time that they did the Boltzmann machine, they solved the credit assignment problem within the framework of the Boltzmann machine. They actually solved the credit assignment problem first. As far as I can see, they were the first people to publish a solution of the credit assignment problem.

Their scheme is very interesting. I think it's more biologically plausible in some ways than backpropagation, at least partly because what they did was look at the weight patterns in a network where you clamp the input and the output. Then they compared the weight patterns in that case with the weight patterns when you don't clamp the output. You just stimulate the net and look at the output. You don't try to force the system to do anything. Then they compared the two weight patterns and adjusted the weight patterns in the clamped case. They adjusted the network weights so that the free-running case would become more like the clamped case.

They didn't need any elaborate backpropagation scheme for changing weights, just a comparison between free-running and clamped networks. That's a bit more brainlike because you have an attentional mechanism that you're getting feedback from and error feedback, but it's done in a different way. Of course, it's much slower than backpropagation.

I guess it wasn't long before Rumelhart and Hinton and Williams noticed that you could solve the hidden-unit problem by a use of the sigmoid function. In retrospect, the extension to the hidden-layer problem is embarrassingly trivial. I mean, all you have to do is take a threshold logic neuron, as Bernie Widrow did, and just make the slope of that step finite, and then you can solve the whole thing by the gradient descent method using the chain rule of calculus. So, just going from something that has an infinite slope to a finite slope—that's the whole problem. It's so trivial it's embarrassing.

ER: What about the early '70s?

JC: In the early '70s there was quite a bit done. In the mid-1960s I did statistical mechanics with the sigmoids, but then in the early '70s I worked with Wilson on the continuum approach to neural tissue. That triggered a lot of interest.

There was a tremendous amount of excitement created by David Marr's papers; the 1969 cerebellum paper created a sensation. David's '69, '70, and '71 papers—the cerebellum, the hippocampus, and the neocortex papers—created a tremendous amount of interest among neurobiologists. Here for the first time was an attempt to actually give a role to individual cell types in a bit of brain tissue. McCulloch and Pitts had tried that with their '47 paper, "How We Know Universals." That wasn't a success, but this stuff of Marr's was very exciting, and it produced a lot of interest. Interestingly, a lot of the theoretical biologists felt that it was so speculative that it couldn't possibly be right and weren't impressed with it, but a lot of other people thought it was very exciting.

In the mid-seventies Tommy Poggio got going, working with Antonio Borsellino, on associative memory. He started working with David Marr. They produced a very nice cooperative model for stereopsis using the sigmoid elements and coupling them in natural ways, with lateral inhibition and excitation—a bit like what Wilson and I had done, but now applied to a specific problem, the problem of understanding Julesz patterns and what they were saying. That triggered lots of work. Then Kohonen's book on associative memory arrived with his methods for doing things. There was steady progress in the '70s, and also Steve Grossberg was publishing a lot of stuff as well.

I think there was a lot of activity in the '70s, but it was slightly unfocused. It wasn't as dramatic as the later work. Then along came the spin glass analogy and this large mass of physicists, and also along came personal computers and workstations. I think it was the workstations, the ability to do things that you couldn't do quickly before, that changed the landscape. That's when people like Sejnowski and Hinton and Rumelhart and company emerged and cracked the perceptron-training problem.

ER: Terry Sejnowski told us that he spent three years not touching a computer. When he left computers, it was batch processing, and when he got back, he had to learn UNIX and was on a workstation. It made all the difference in the world. Suddenly, computers became a part of the equation, rather than something distant and difficult.

JC: That's right. Backpropagation was the key to it, I think, though. If you read Rosenblatt's book [*Principles of Neurodynamics*], he talks about backpropagation in there—the architecture for solving the problem and everything, even including the term "backpropagation." The only thing that's not there is the actual algorithm, the details of it, but the structure and everything else is there. Poor old Frank was vastly undervalued in his day.

ER: In essence, aside from a couple of tricks and turns, Rosenblatt had the idea for backpropagation?

JC: He had the architecture, everything. He knew he had to backpropagate the signal. He just didn't know how to do it. He had a machine, too. He built a perceptron at Cornell, outside of Cornell Aeronautical Labs, and he would have had all the hidden units in there, chunking away.

There was a very heated discussion between Dave Block and Marvin Minsky. Block reviewed Minsky and Papert's book. [Block was a physicist at Cornell who worked with Rosenblatt in the early 1960s.] The review was critical, and then there was a rejoinder. Block claimed that the multilayer perceptron could do everything that Minsky and Papert claimed couldn't be done by a perceptron. With hindsight, Dave was correct, although he didn't know how to do it. He was right that the multilayered perceptron is capable of doing all the things that they said couldn't be done.

ER: Did you hear any stories about Rosenblatt's demise?

JC: Simon Levin at Cornell told me exactly what happened. He was out boating one day. The boat capsized. The bow hit him and knocked him unconscious. He drowned under the boat. It was accident.

ER: Can we talk a little bit about the '80s and what you were doing in the '80s?

JC: In the '80s I worked on stuff I'm still working on. In the late '70s I had an idea that I'm still working on. It's way, way out in left field, but I like to work on things there. I reformulated what I had done on the sigmoids as a probabilistic problem. You see, one of the things that I think is still lacking in the whole field of neural networks is some understanding of the higher-order correlations and fluctuations in nervous activity. All the equations, for example, the ones that I formulated, are basically the canonical equations, and everybody arrives at something like them. They are all expressions for the mean firing rate of a neuron. It's clear that neurons don't fire at a constant rate; they're fluctuating all the time. There's higher-order statistics in there. Neurophysiologists stick microelectrodes in, and they measure correlations. In the study of many-body problems in condensed matter physics, it's clear that the higher-order statistics are very important. They, in part, produce the physical phenomenon, the collective effects that determine whether you've got a solid or a gas or what have you. They're determined in part by the pairwise correlation functions of higher-order things that are there. In information processing, it's correlation functions that are really important. It's not mean firing rates, but it's correlations.

There is no decent theory of the dynamics of the creation and flow of correlations in neural networks. Anyway, in 1978 I decided I'd take a real stab at that problem, so I reformulated what I had done as a master equation of the kind that you see in chemical physics and physics. Instead of looking at the mean rate of firing of each neuronal population, I said, "Here we have neurons; they can be in one of several states. They can be quiescent, waiting to be stimulated, or they can stimulated, or they can be in refractory state after they've been stimulated. So let's roughly say there are three states to a neuron. And if you have n neurons, you've got 3^n possible configurations. What we really want is some way of writing down an equation that describes the evolution in space and time of those configurations and the statistics of that evolution. If we could do that, we would have a complete picture of the dynamics of correlations and how it flows back and forward. Now what is that like?" And the answer is that it's very like quantum mechanics, quantum field theory.

It's taken me since '78 to formulate the thing properly. What I've been able to do is to show that the mathematical problems are exactly the same as the mathematical problems that turn up in quantum field theory. Take, for example, the simpler case of neurons that are only either quiescent or activated. Now you introduce what's called a vector space representation of neurons. The vector with components 1 and 0 represents the active state, and the vector with the components 0 and 1 represents the quiescent state. Now you need things that flip from one state to the other. Those are two-by-two matrices. Those matrices that flip between the state 1 to 0 and the state 0 to 1. They're what are called "Pauli spin matrices," and they turn up in the theory of angular momentum in quantum mechanics. They're the thing that flip the spins back and forward. You can actually write down a description of the evolution of the configurations of a set of neurons—each with two states, 2^n configurations—which uses nothing but some combination of the Pauli spin matrices.

It turns out for three-state neurons in exactly the same way. You've got the vectors (1, 0, 0), (0, 1, 0), (0, 0, 1) as your basis, so you need three-by-three matrices to flip them back and forward into their different states and describe what's going on. And what are those matrices? They're nothing more than a subset of what are called the Gell-Mann matrices. They're exactly the matrices that turn up in the theory of quarks. So it turns out that the algebra of state transitions in a neural network, whatever its anatomy—it doesn't have to be antisymmetric, symmetric, or anything—are described by the same kind of mathematics that goes into particle physics. It turns out you can reformulate the entire structure of the flow of correlations in everything in terms of the language of what's called "second-quantized quantum field theory," where you have annihilation and creation operators which move states back and forward. All the machinery that physicists have worked out since Feynman is sitting there waiting to be used for neural network calculations. A student and I are calculating using Feynman diagrams in neural networks to see if we can say something about these fluctuations in activity and how information might be flowing back and forward in the form of long-range correlations in the network.

Anyway, that's one of the technical things I work on. Another thing that I did in the late '70s which attracted quite a bit of attention, but was a bit too mathematical for most people, is my favorite subject. That's the study of altered brain states. Among those are migraine states, epileptic seizures, and hallucinations—particularly geometric visual hallucinations triggered by things like hallucinogens.

At the University of Chicago there was a famous psychologist neurologist named Heinrich Klüver, who worked on mescalin and mechanisms of hallucinations. There are fabulous stories about Klüver in Chicago. He experimented in the grand physiological tradition on himself, so he used to take peyote. The story is that he told one of his colleagues in the medical school to come and check on him to make sure he hadn't taken too much peyote. So in comes this colleague, and there's Heinrich stretched out on the floor, completely unconscious; he had overdosed on this stuff.

Jack D. Cowan

Finally, he refined the dose; he'd take just enough so that he would stay awake, and after the initial period of vomiting, he would start to hallucinate. He described all of these hallucinations, and he classified them. It turns out there are four classes of hallucinations—patterns called "form constants" by Kluver. These form constants are ubiquitous. They're found in everybody who takes drugs or meditates or, like many people, hallucinates either when falling asleep or when waking up. I'm actually writing a popular book on all this stuff. There's evidence that many cave paintings are of hallucinogenic origins; Roger Lewin has written a little piece on that. There's all kind of evidence that the Mimbres Indians of New Mexico a thousand years ago used hallucinogens, and you can see it in the way they decorate their pottery.

So what are these pictures? Why this imagery? What's producing it? The Jungian mandala figures have a lot of the same kind of imagery. Jung claimed there was a kind of collective archetype to be found. Anyway, if you look at the form constants, you can do the following thing. In the mid-seventies, Eric Schwartz, among other people, and I independently worked out the coordinate transformation from the eye to the brain. So here's the visual field out there; we see the world with our retinas, but our retinas are hardwired to our cortices through the geniculate. The packing density of the retinal ganglion cells isn't uniform. In our fovea we have a lot of retinal ganglion cells, looking at the world, but out in the periphery of our field, we have only a few. That means there must be much bigger representation in the visual cortex of the center of our visual field than out in the periphery.

You can write down the equations that allow you to calculate what polar coordinates in the retina transform into in the cortex. You can take all the patterns that people see in visual field coordinates and transform them into what they look like in brain coordinates, in the coordinates of the visual brain, area 17 [the primary cortical visual area, now usually called V1]. When you do that, all the patterns turn out to be nothing more than stripe or blob patterns.

So it turns out that there's a very close relationship between the work that Turing and others have done on animal coat markings—and the fact that animal coats are either in the form of stripes or periodic blob patterns—and what's sitting in the brain. Bard Ermentrout and I worked out, using the techniques of nonlinear stability theory as applied to these sigmoid equations, what must be the architecture that spontaneously produces such patterns. The normal unpatterned resting state is destabilized by the actions of hallucinogenic drugs on the brain stem, which controls the thresholds of cells in the cortex. We came up with very plausible circuitry consistent with the neuroanatomy that had been discovered by Hubel and Weisel and others.

It turns out we've only solved half the problem. There are several kinds of form constants; there are checkerboard patterns, lozenge patterns, and bicycle spoke patterns. Many people see bicycle spoke patterns. They correspond to horizontal stripes in the cortex. Many people see concentric circles.

They correspond to vertical stripes in the cortex. But the most common hallucination of all is spirals; they correspond to oblique stripes in the cortex. And the spirals—the falling down a tunnel, with light at the end of it—that's just a pattern of stripes being produced in the cortex. But that's only two out of the four possible form constants—tunnels and funnels, and checkerboard patterns.

The other two are lattice patterns—thin-line lattice patterns that are even described in the Egyptian Book of the Dead as lattices of lights that people see when they're in trance states. Or cobwebs, spidery cobweb patterns. You can calculate the cortical projection of those spiderylike patterns. It is a hundred microns. You can also work out the cortical projection of the checkerboard patterns since one knows the details of the anatomy. It is a millimeter in human cortex. So what Bard Ermentrout and I had worked out was a theory of one-millimeter waves in the cortex. That corresponds in human cortex to turning on everything in a hypercolumn, in a Hubel-Wiesel hypercolumn. So basically you're turning on and off all the ocular dominance columns associated with one eye, for example, and that's why you start to see these patterns in the visual field.

But cobwebs and lattice patterns don't correspond to hypercolumn dimensions. The reason we know that that figure is correct is the following. If you measure the number of stripes in the patterns on the average that people report seeing, there are about seventeen stripes in a hemicircle, in 180 degrees. But that patch, that 180 degrees, maps to something that is 35 millimeters wide in the cortex; that's the width of the human area 17. So that means seventeen stripes in 35 millimeters—that's two-millimeter wave lengths in the brain. That's exactly the width of the Hubel-Weisel hypercolumns in humans, twice what it is in monkeys. But now this hundred-micron thing—it's got to be the width of an orientation patch. In other words, when you see a lattice pattern or a cobweb pattern, what you're seeing are, iso-orientation patches switching on spontaneously when driven by noise in a pattern that's reflective of the way they're coupled together. It's a kind of spectroscopy because we're studying the resonances of the brain as they're produced by a hallucinogen. What you see is your own anatomy basically.

Bernard Hassenstein and I did a study, which we never published, on visual migraines. I happen to get them every so often; every six months I get a visual migraine. I get all the fortification illusions. Bernard at the time had them every month. He got his assistant to make a fixation mark on a blackboard, and then she would plot where he told her the leading edge of the disturbance was and time it. You can get a plot of visual angle versus time in minutes. It's a curve. If you transform it with the retinal cortical transformation equations that I worked out, it turns out to be a beautiful straight line on the cortex. The slope is 1.5 millimeters per minute. Now that's much, much slower than the propagation velocity along axons that comes out of any of our network models. We know that hallucinations explode in the visual field and take about three seconds to cover the whole of the visual field.

Well, that's about a centimeter per second. That's like in epilepsy. Hallucinations really are a form of epilepsy, an epileptic seizure that's stabilizing into patterns.

A migraine is different. It turns out that it's a propagating wave produced by the diffusion of extracellular potassium or glutamate. You get a slow depolarization wave that moves along, exciting all the iso-orientation patches, and because of the way their circuits are set up to interact, if one turns on, others with neighboring orientations cannot. So you can see, in the angles that people actually see, evidence for what the weight patterns must be like in the cortex.

I'm not the first person to see this connection. Eric Schwartz actually wrote about it, but never calculated anything. He did the transformation, and he saw that these things corresponded to plane waves. I'm hoping to be able to deduce out of this hallucination study the details of the rolling and twisting of the actual zigzag patterns and all that. It turns out that you can also approach epileptic seizures from very similar points of view. I work now with neurologists on epileptic patients. You have to map out the locus of where the seizure is before surgery can be done on many patients. One of the things that's come out of that study is that most epileptic seizures that turn up are not propagating; they're not giving rise to traveling disturbance. They're just localized patches of oscillation in the cortex. That's something that Hugh Wilson and I described in our continuum model in '73. It means there's lateral inhibition at work in the cortex. There's still enough instability to produce an oscillation pattern, but it's not moving. But if it was strong enough, it would then break out, move, and start to give rise to traveling and rotating wave patterns. I'm sure that's exactly what's going on in seizures, except it could be patterned as well. There's all kinds of possibilities.

That's the kind of stuff that I'm interested in, rather than trying to train machines to learn to do things. I'm interested in altered brain states because I believe they can tell you a lot about the circuitry.

The same kinds of pattern formation tendencies are present in map formation as are present in hallucinations. You can start out with two sheets of brain tissue and randomly connected wires from one to the other, but with Hebb synaptic learning and winner-take-all, for example, the map organizes into a topologically ordered map. The reason is that the Hebb synapse acts like a recurrent excitation. The competition that's present in the winner-take-all mechanism acts like lateral inhibition. Again, you've got this mechanism that likes to make stripes or blobs.

In the space of weights, rather than the space of activity, making stripes corresponds to forming a topological map. In the late 1970s, Christoph von der Malsberg and I worked together on the formation of orientation detectors. I had the idea that maybe this idea of a natural tendency to form stripes and blobs was the key to understanding it, and all you needed was a two-layer network stimulated by noise, and it would automatically make the correct feature detectors.

Christoph didn't believe me; he said, "That's magic."

I said, "No, it's just spontaneous symmetry breaking."

It turns out I was right. We never did it, and I have been kicking myself ever since because Ralph Linsker did it. That's exactly what Linsker discovered: that stripes and blobs will spontaneously form in a map. That's the origin of center-surround orientation detectors in the visual cortex. The same epigenetic mechanism for pattern formation, the tendency to make stripes and blobs, is ubiquitous in nature. Cloud patterns, animal coat markings, hallucination patterns, maps—all that is sitting there. The brain is no different in many respects from any other physical organization. There's a tendency for pattern formation to occur because it's got all the same kinds of machinery in it.

Now I'm getting back to the philosophical bias that I guess I got from McCulloch. Here's the idea. There's an innate tendency to produce patterns of a certain kind. It's on those patterns that one should build theories of learning and memory, but that actually doesn't happen very much in the field as it is at the moment. They start with a tabula rasa, and they build in the structure completely with training. But we know that there's an enormous specificity in the nervous system. That's not the result of training; it's the result of genes. In my work on map formation, I've been studying the effects of gene products in the form of adhesion molecules, which tell fibers they've got to go to certain places. There's abundant evidence in frogs and fish that there have to be such chemical markers in the brain to specify which gets connected to what. That's totally absent in a lot of the theoretical work on learning and memory. Somehow they've all got to be put together. The architecture, a lot of it, is specified.

ER: You've talked about how you feel that a lot of the ideas having to do with brain states are more important for you in terms of your work than the ideas about learning.

JC: One should actually try to work on both. One of the things I'm trying to do as well is to study the dynamics of learning with the same mathematical methods that I've used to study the dynamics of activity. I'm convinced that there are instabilities in the dynamics of learning, just as there are instabilities to using activity. Jay McClelland, for example, one of the founders of connectionism, said something really interesting at a meeting a couple of years ago. He said, in his experience, when he does backpropagation, he can tell when the network is ready to learn from when it's not ready to learn. You can tell when it's not ready to learn because the differences between the biggest and the smallest weights in the network are small. Only when there are sufficiently big differences in the weights does it start to learn rapidly.

ER: That's the instability.

JC: That's the instability. I think in weight space there's the same kind of dynamics at work. It's nonlinear. Every nonlinear system looks the same to someone who studies instability theory. They can all be treated by exactly the same machinery. It's called bifurcation theory. That's what I do. That's my mathematical tool.

ER: What do you think about some of the other algorithms, like radial-basis functions?

JC: The radial basis function's an interesting idea. I'm actually interested in it for technical reasons. It turns out that radial-basis functions are closely related to wavelets. Interestingly, the first use of wavelets was Gabor's. Gabor functions are close to wavelets.

It turns out that in some of the machinery of quantum field theory that I use for neural networks are what are called coherent states. They're also very close to wavelets. Now Tommy Poggio has a view of the brain as a table look-up system using radial basis functions with some redundancy. It's actually quite an attractive idea. It's the ultimate expression of the grandmother cell. With the distributed features that it's got, it's a compromise between Lashley's equipotential networks and grandmother cells.

There's obviously a good bit in it. Of course, he's only been able to do it for feedforward networks. It's clear the brain is not a feedforward network; it's a recurrent network. I haven't seen any real developments of its use in connection with recurrent networks, whereas the recurrent backpropagation alogrithm as developed by Pineda and by Zipser and Williams is a very, very powerful tool. That's the tool that's going to allow brain researchers to understand the function of a block of brain tissue.

Zipser and Richard Andersen have already started to demonstrate that with their work on parietal and frontal cortex based on Joachim Fuster's and Andersen's data you can train monkeys to do delayed-response tasks, and they've clearly got to store the information about the task for a while before they do it. Hugh Wilson and I in '73 had a paper where we conjectured that the memory was in the form of reverberatory circuits that had the form of a bistable flip-flop, which didn't propagate, like the localized limit cycle in epilepsy.

We said, "Well, what's happening is a little bit of brain tissue is flipped on, and it stays on for a while before it's flipped off." It turns out that's probably right, but we didn't have the machinery for doing the flipping on and off. With a recurrent backpropagation network Dave Zipser simulated the monkey behavior and found in his hidden units two kinds—the ones that did the flipping on and the others that caused the flipping to go on and off. That corresponds exactly to what's found in the data. There are memory cells and gating cells in the frontal cortex that actually are doing the things that need to be done for the monkey to do the task. And you can discover what must be in there by using recurrent backpropagation models. I think that's actually the most interesting use of neural models for real brain research yet.

ER: Could you comment on what you think some of the most important trends are in contemporary neural modeling.

JC: One of the most important trends is the fact that more and more detailed modeling is going on. Experimentalists are finding more and more out about all the different kinds of gating currents and neurotransmitters that are present. On one side there's this push toward more and more accuracy in the description of what is actually there, trying to be more inclusive in modeling what's there. Rather than using these very simple toy models, they are actually trying to be realistic.

That's both a good thing and a bad thing. It's a good thing in the sense that for those people who are interested in the details, it's good to try to put them all into the model and see what they actually do. From my point of view of trying to understand higher-order things, it may be a bad thing because the forest gets lost in the trees.

Manfred Eigen, a friend of mine, is very smart about that. For years I went to a winter seminar that he ran in Klosters in January. In them he had people like David Hubel and Tommy Poggio and Werner Reichardt and myself. All kinds of people, a mix of theorists and experimentalists. Sometimes a distinguished experimentalist like David Hubel would get up and say things like, "What's the point in all this modeling? We don't know enough about the details."

He would say something like that, and Manfred would laugh and say, "Yes, but you have to have some good ideas before you can get the right facts."

Another thing Hubel used to say to me before we got to like each other was, "You know, Jack, all this modeling stuff you do is for the birds, but you tell really good jokes." But finally he said, "You know, I think modeling might be useful after all." He said that after about two or three years. He mellowed.

Another thing Manfred would say is, "A good physicist knows that the purpose of making models and doing theory is to provide insight and understanding of what's going on. It's not necessary to put in the kitchen sink to get insight." You have to abstract from reality, not face it, which was a gibe at Eccles's book, *Facing Reality.*

You have to abstract. If you're good at abstracting the essence of something, then you'll get real insights. That's what good theorists do. I think that just to simulate the hell out of populations of neurons with everything in the model is mindless. You've got to pick out of it the things that your taste tells you might be important and study those in some simplified context, where you can actually learn something. Otherwise, you're just mimicking what's there without necessarily understanding anything.

ER: Well, is there specific work going on now that impresses you?

JC: I think that Geoff Hinton's work is terrific. I think that almost everything that he does, right or wrong, is interesting. I think that a lot of the things that Terry Sejnowski and his students do is very good stuff too. I think Dave Rumelhart has got real insight into what you can do with backpropagation and how it's related to statistical things. One of the most interesting things that's coming out is that the statisticians are now starting to realize the power of backpropagation and the use of nonlinear functions of linear combinations in doing predictions. For reasons that aren't yet understood, these function approximations by systems of sigmoids are extremely powerful function approximators compared with almost everything that the statisticians have been using. There's something quite important in there from a theoretical point of view, from the point of view of prediction and filtering. The old Gabor idea of prediction and filtering with gradient descent is holding up well—except it's not with polynomials; it's with sigmoids.

ER: If you were starting out in the field, or if you were advising, as you do, people who are just starting in the field, what would you suggest to a newcomer?

JC: Well, what I would tell them is to go and try to work with Geoff Hinton. I think the best way to get into the field is to find somebody really good and go work with them. I was very lucky to get going with Gabor and then with McCulloch and Pitts and to interact a bit with Shannon and Wiener. I think that's by far the best way to do anything.

I took part in one of the Einstein Centennial meetings a few years ago at Illinois, organized by a philospher down there. Dirac was at the meeting.

Dirac gave a lecture on relativity and Einstein, a wonderful lecture after dinner. Then he answered some questions. He was asked three questions. None of them were very good questions, but his answers were gems.

The first question he was asked by a philospher: "What do you think of the philosophical significance of quantum mechanics?"

He said, "Well, I'm not interested in questions like that. I'm only interested in getting the right equations. If you get the right equations, everything else follows."

The second question he was asked, and this relates to your question, was by a physics student: "What would you advise a beginning physics student to work on?"

Dirac thought for a bit, and he said, "Whatever interests you most," which I thought was wonderful.

Then another student asked him, "How did you discover antimatter?"

Dirac said, "Oh, that was easy. In relativity, energy's the square of a quantity, so I just took the square root."

I mean, that's the real answer: just work on whatever it is that really interests you the most. But if you're really smart, you'll go and find somebody really distinguished and go and work on it with him or her.

ER: Where do you see the field going?

JC: Well, computer technology is increasing its power all the time. I can see that being a driving force behind ever less toy applications of the theory to real-world problems: the construction of artificial networks that will do more and more powerful things. At the moment these networks are still doing simple things, but later on they'll start to do things that will surprise people. I'm always interested to follow the debate between the cognitive psychologists and linguists, people like Pinker and others at MIT, who criticize the neural network approaches to language and say, "Well, you can't really handle this and that, or you can't do semantics, or you can't do this." A few months after some specific criticism is made, there appears a solution.

It's very like the content of the McCulloch-Pitts paper itself. The late Donald Mackay, whom I knew very well, characterized their theorem as follows: if you are arguing with someone about what a machine can or cannot do, and you can specify exactly what it is the machine cannot do, then their theorem guarantees that there exists at least one machine that can do exactly what you say it cannot do. If you can specify in enough detail what it is that you say a machine can't do, you've produced a solution. So the real question is, "Is everything out there describable?"

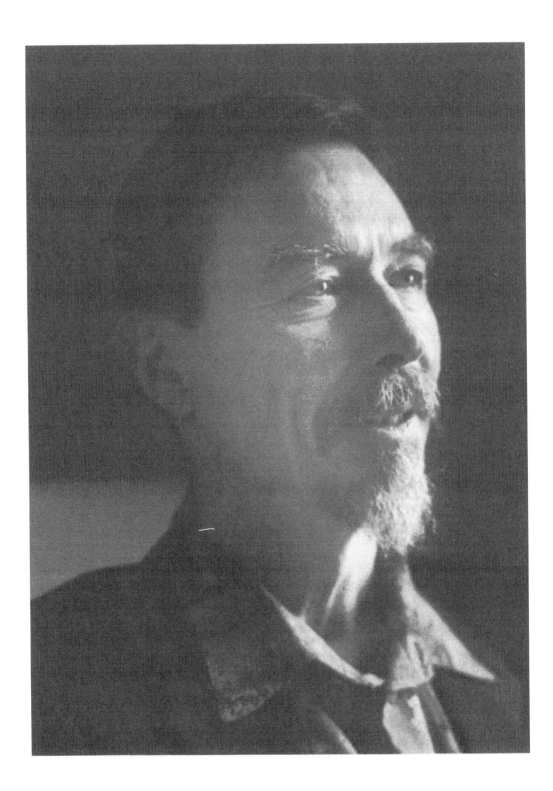

6   Carver Mead

Carver Mead is the Gordon and Betty Moore Professor of Engineering and Applied Science at the California Institute of Technology, Pasadena, California. Probably the best introduction to Professor Mead's ideas about the practical VLSI implementation of neurocomputing can be found in his 1989 book, Analog VLSI and Neural Systems *(Reading, Mass.: Addison-Wesley).*

March 1994, San Francisco, California

ER: I'd like to ask how you grew up and what your parents did.

CM: I was born in 1934 in Bakersfield, May 1, 1934. The reason it was Bakersfield was because my dad worked for the California Edison Company back up in the Kern River Valley. Bakersfield was the nearest place there was a hospital so that was where I was born.

I grew up up in the Sierra Nevada Mountains in a place called Bee Creek, east of Fresno, about thirty miles back in the woods. I went to a little school with twenty kids total for the first eight grades, one teacher. A wonderful, fun time.

ER: What did your father do?

CM: He was the guy in charge of the local power plant. I grew up around the power plant. He used to bring home electrical stuff, batteries and so on. I got hooked on electricity at a very early age, and I've been hooked on it ever since. It's never gone away. I never had any desire to do anything else.

When I was in sixth grade, a guy moved into camp. This was back in the mountains with a little group of houses around the power plant that we called the "camp." The guy who moved into camp was a radio ham. This was just as World War II was ending. He got to teaching me about this radio stuff, and I was just blown away. So I'd save all my hard earned money, and we'd go down to the big town of Fresno once a month. I'd go down to the surplus store and hunt for bargains. You could buy the most incredible pile of electronics for a dollar. I collected all this stuff so I could experiment with it. One thing led to another.

ER: Did you have brothers or sisters?

CM: I was the only child.

ER: Was your mother at home?

CM: She was at home. Once in a while she'd be secretary for the local school board or something.

ER: Did you build a ham radio station?

CM: I built all my own stuff. I couldn't afford to buy it. So you substituted labor for buying it. That was much better because you learned all about the stuff. I built receivers up until I could afford one of those little RME 69s. Remember them?

JA: I sure do. I had one of those.

CM: Did you? Well, that was the only thing I could afford.

JA: With the great big dial in the front?

CM: That was the one. Those were fun days. We didn't have test instruments really. I finally bought a Heathkit vacuum tube volt meter. That was as close as I could get to a real test instrument. You had to debug stuff blind as hell. You had no idea what was going on. That was excruciating, but it would also give you a sense for how to proceed when you didn't have but the tiniest bit of information coming back from the thing and no real instrumentation to find out. It reminds you of neural networks a whole lot, actually.

It was wonderful training. It gives you this confidence that if you muck around for a while, you'll figure it out even though you have no really sound fundamental basis for it. You just have hunches and you develop a feeling for it, and after a while it gets to working, and the more you work with it, the better it works. Then you can't remember why it was hard back in the beginning. It's an awful lot like research in that sense of being out there where you don't know what the hell's going on. There is no obvious reason to be able to succeed, and you just keep at it until you start developing a feel for it. It really tunes up your intuition.

ER: What was high school like?

CM: I moved away from home when I was fourteen. I went to the big town of Fresno where my grandmother lived, and I lived with her. I went to high school there. It was great because I didn't have to put energy into fighting with my parents. I got my commercial radio license. I ended up getting a job with the local radio station and the local two-way communication place. That was about all you could do in Fresno because that's all the electronics there was. But that was enough.

I rubbed against people who knew more than I did, and one of them said, "Well," he says, "you should take electrical engineering at college."

Of course, in Fresno, there was Fresno State College, but there wasn't any electrical engineering there. The closest you got was the physics department. There was one guy there who knew some electronics. I used to go over there when I was in high school. My buddies were all in college, and I'd go over there and sit in on their classes. We didn't have any of these AP [advanced placement] courses. You just made it up as you went along.

I knew this one guy up at the radio station who said, "You should either go to Caltech or to Stanford."

I'd heard of Stanford. Never heard of Caltech. I applied to both places, and I got admitted. I visited up here, and I visited down there. I struggled for a while. I finally went to Caltech because it was smaller. I've been there ever since.

I took a bachelor's and master's and a Ph.D. at Caltech. I had no idea I wanted to do a Ph.D. When I was doing my master's, I stopped by the office of a faculty member, and we got to chatting. He said, "Well, you know, a Ph.D's not much different from what you've been doing, except you make up your own problems instead of doing problems somebody else made up."

"Hey," I said, "That's what I've always been good at."

So I thought I could succeed in a Ph.D. program. It never had occurred to me before. Absolutely never had occurred to me. I had interviewed for jobs at places like Minneapolis Honeywell. I was thinking of going to work in a very standard industry job, and then this guy said what he said, and I went, "Hmmm."

ER: Was he an advisor or just somebody you knew?

CM: Just one of the guys on the faculty. I liked the way he taught his course, so I'd go up there once in a while and chat. Then I thought what the hell, so I applied.

I was one of these late bloomers. I had a miserable academic record from my undergraduate career, and I was just getting to be OK as I got into my master's program. So they made up a special exam to try to weed me out. This exam was what we now call a mini oral. We've since institutionalized it. We do it at the end of the master's year because it's such a graceful place to let somebody go because that way they don't look like they flunked their oral. It gets the faculty off the hook. I was the first one they gave it to because they figured, "This guy's got no business being a Ph.D." I'd done well enough on the master's that there wasn't any obvious way to keep me out, so they figured that an oral exam was going to make me fall all over myself.

It turned out that, of course, oral exams are more about understanding than they are about being brilliant mathematically. I've always been better at the intuitive side of figuring stuff out than grinding out long solutions to big complicated things, and so I did really well. They were blown away. They didn't think that that was going to happen, so I got to stay.

ER: And what problems did you choose?

CM: It was interesting. John Linvill at Stanford—ironically enough, the place I didn't go—had just come out with this thing he called the Linvill model for transistors. You basically did a lumped approximation for the linear behavior of the thermodynamic quantities in the transistor and then put the exponentials into the interface between that and the voltage switches —which is, of course, a brilliant way to look at the whole thing. I looked at it, and I said, "God, even I can cope with that."

Before that time there had been the Ebers-Moll equations, which were just these godawful nonlinear things. The nonlinearities were all mixed in with the other stuff, so you couldn't see the essential relationships because it wasn't factored in any nice way.

Linvill had factored in such a nice way that you could see what to do and where everything came from. So I said, "God, this is what I need to do transistor switching times and storage times." I went and worked all that out on my own. It was enough for a thesis.

In retrospect, it's kind of trivial, but at the time it was neat because I'd figured it out myself. You know when you turn a transistor off, it's a while before the minority carriers clear out and the thing goes off. You can predict all that. I had some fun with it, but mostly it was important to me because I'd figured it out myself. Nobody gave me the problem. It wasn't just one more homework problem. I had to figure out what the problem was.

ER: And you went directly from the doctorate into teaching?

CM: When I was a first-year graduate student, Dave Meadowbrook had just come down from Stanford. He was teaching a transistor course. I took his course as a first-year grad student, and I did well in it. The next year he was going to go off and write a book, but somebody had to teach the course. He came around and said, "How would you like to teach the course?"

Here I was, a second-year grad student supposed to teach a first-year graduate course. I had been teaching undergraduate courses all along since I'd been a senior. I'd be a lab TA and stuff like that because I liked teaching. This course was major because there were all these bright guys who were smarter than I was. But I figured it out, gradually. It really stretches the hell out of you when you've got to explain this stuff. You've got to really, really know it all the way down.

That experience was what got me in love with teaching. When I got done with it all, it turned out Caltech didn't have anybody else around doing this stuff. They were out recruiting young faculty, and in those days you couldn't find anybody in transistor physics because everybody had been slurped up by other universities. So they said, "How would you like to stay?" There wasn't anybody there to compete with, so I had the job to myself.

I went off doing tunneling and transport processes through thin insulators for about ten years. Then Max Delbruck came around and said, "Hey, these guys are saying that nerve membranes work like transistors. Is that right?"

And I said, "I don't know. Let me look at it."

He gave me a bunch of papers. People were copying Shockley's stuff and putting in ions instead of electrons, and it was all complete hogwash.

So I said to Max, "It's complete hogwash."

And he said, "Well, let's figure it out then."

Max was a gruff old guy. We started this little subterranean group. That was when work just started on bilayers [artificial monomolecular films that have certain similarities to cell membranes]. We did a bunch of bilayer stuff. I guess the only contribution we made there was that we were able to show that the channels were ohmic.

That was my only real biology. We did that with Max and a couple of students, one engineering postdoc and one grad student in biology. We called it our subterranean group because the bilayers would break if you shook them at all. We had one vibration-isolated darkroom way down in a sub-basement.

JA: No real animals?

CM: No, I have a hard time with surgeries.

ER: At this time were you aware of any of the the perceptron work or Widrow's work?

CM: I knew about the perceptron. I'd heard about Bernie's stuff, but just vaguely. I wasn't paying any attention to it at all. That was the time I was starting to get interested in VLSI. I had these long talks with Max about how, when you work with biological substances, you realize there's nothing precise. Everything has to be adaptive. I was getting the idea how that had to work and how it couldn't be that there were any precise parameters. How in the hell can you build a system like this? It has to find its own zero, find its own center, and tune itself up.

At the same time I was getting intrigued by large-scale MOS technology because I could see that if you're going to make big systems, that's the way you had to do it. That won.

In those days, digital systems were the easiest ones to conceptualize, so I did them for ten years. I figured out how to made software that would organize big systems and get them to work. I had in the back of my mind that what you really ought to do is to use all the physics of a device to do the computation, not just the on or off property. But you couldn't even imagine doing that unless you had ways of designing really complex things.

JA: You were always heading toward big analog circuits?

CM: They used all the physics. I was from the device side, so I wanted to use the physics. It was fascinating to me that you could get wonderful exponentials over orders and orders of magnitude. I had done a lot of that, taught courses on it. It always seemed to me a terrible waste to turn these devices into switches, but that was the only kind of system we knew how to imagine. It still isn't obvious.

ER: I think of the VLSI work as culminating with the Mead and Conway book. [A classic book on VLSI design. *Introduction to VLSI Systems.* Carver Mead and Lynn Conway. 1980. Reading, Mass.: Addison-Wesley.] I was wondering how that partnership came about?

CM: I had been doing VLSI. There was a talk around Caltech about having a computer science program. We didn't have one at the time. We were interviewing people for the job. They were all very traditional computer science. Nobody was really thrilled at having one more. We talked to everybody, and they'd say, "Yeah, you've got to have a guy on operating systems or this guy on languages." It didn't feel like the future exactly.

Then Ivan Sutherland came by and got all excited about VLSI. We ended up hiring him, and the two of us started the computer science operation at Caltech. Ivan introduced me to a lot of people he knew, like Dave Evans back in Utah and his brother, Bert Sutherland, who was running one of the labs at PARC [Xerox Palo Alto Research Center]. It turned out to be the lab where Alan Kay was doing the SmallTalk project, and right next door was Bob Sproul doing wonderful stuff that turned into Postscript eventually through a very circuitous route.

I went to give a talk up there and Bert said, "Why don't you come and consult with us?" So he stuck me next to Lynn Conway. She was at PARC. She worked for Bert. After my talk, she came up and said, "You know, Carver, you should really write a book about this."

Then Lynn went off, and the next week when I came back, she had every book on integrated circuits that was available on her desk. She had looked through all of them, and she said, "There isn't anything like it. Let's do it." So that was it. But that's typical. She did all the research, figured out what was out there.

ER: And how long did it take to write the book?

CM: Two years. In a year, we had a note version, and we distributed that to a number of universities that wanted to teach the course. We got feedback and finalized it the next year. That was great fun working with people, getting the courses started, giving them material, and getting MOSIS [the national chip fabrication facility] started so people could actually get chips made. That was a great partnership. We had really good times. God, it was stressful, trying to start this whole major thing, but it was fun too.

ER: You referred to it earlier as a ten-year detour. When did you start to get back on your main road?

CM: It was '82. I had been one of the people who had supported the move to get John Hopfield to come to Caltech because I'd known him from solid-state physics. I'd stopped by at Princeton a few times and got to chatting with him. So when they started a move to get Hopfield to come to Caltech, I said, "That's great. I like him."

When he got to Caltech, we started talking, and he said, "Let's do a course."

So Hopfield and I and Richard Feynman did a three-way course that we called the "Physics of Computation." We did that course for three years. Three more different stories you have never heard. You would never imagine the stories we told had anything to do with each other. We enjoyed it immensely because we could start making connections to each other's viewpoint. That was a three-year period when we were each evolving our own view of what it all meant. Then we went off and made three courses.

That period was when I learned about what is now traditional neural net stuff. I didn't know there had been any except for the perceptron, which everyone knew about. I didn't know there had been ongoing work.

I was frustrated because this work was all a very simplistic view of what was obviously a much more continuous, much richer, adaptive thing. So then I decided, "Hey, I've got to figure out how to make these adaptive circuits because that's the only way this is ever going to work."

I figured that in five years you could learn how to make adaptive circuits. I've been at it ten years, and we still don't how to do any but the beginnings of it. It's been much longer than I had anticipated. Meanwhile, it's interesting that simulations are getting more adaptive. Many of them are getting more like what you can actually build.

ER: I know that many of your students have gone into business and that you yourself have been involved with various companies through the years. Maybe you could talk just a little bit about how you've placed yourself within the commercial environment through the years.

CM: That was all started by Gordon Moore. When I was a first-year faculty, Gordon Moore came by, and he had one of these old briefcases that used to open up at the top. He came by with this briefcase, and he sat down in my office and said, "Hi, I'm Gordon Moore from Fairchild and I'm a Caltech alum, and I just stopped by to see what you're doing."

I told him about this device stuff I was doing, and he said, "Would you like some transistors?"

I said, "Yeah," because I was teaching labs, and transistors were expensive if they were any good, and if they weren't expensive, they were no good, and either way you were damned. So he opened up his briefcase. There was an old shirt and two old socks in there, and he looked up kind of sheepishly, and he said, "I travel light."

He pushed down his dirty clothes, and he pulled out these manila envelopes—you know, $8\frac{1}{2}$-by-11. Two of them. One was full of 2N706s, and one was full of 2N697s. I'd never seen so many transistors in my life. And he said, "Here's some rejects. I don't guarantee what they are, but some of them will be good. Come up and visit, and maybe you'd like to consult for us."

So two weeks later I went up to Fairchild. It was a little tiny place. There were probably twenty people in the whole company. I gave a talk about what I was doing, and then we all sat around a conference table. The whole group was there. We sat around and talked for an hour and had lunch. It was very laid-back. They were building these transistors in this little lab downstairs.

I started consulting for them. I'd come up every week and spend a day. I got hooked because I always learned something and I could get samples of different kinds of devices. I found out the things they didn't understand so

I could go back and work on them. That's kept up till the present day. It's been a source of an enormous wealth of research projects—the research part that you don't have time to follow up when you're in an industrial track. You've got to get a product out.

I've kept doing that. When a company got too big so I couldn't do that any more, I'd find a smaller one. A lot of my former students have started companies and asked me to get involved with them. I come up there every week. I've been doing this since the early '70s, more than twenty years. I keep track of what's going on. It's been wonderful having the best of both worlds.

JA: Do you have any interest in things like artificial intelligence [AI]?

CM: I never got involved. I guess I couldn't see a way to make a contribution there, is really the honest truth.

JA: Was there discussion about AI at Caltech in that era?

CM: A little bit. And, of course, at Xerox PARC there was a lot of it because PARC was crawling with AI people. But I never quite found how it fit with anything I know about. I'd have chats with those people and try to understand what they were doing, but I never quite got it. But with neural networks I felt right away that this was an analog thing. It's really a simulation of an analog property, and that made a lot of sense.

JA: The work you've done on analog VLSI has been largely in the direction of sensory processing.

CM: There's a reason for that. I started wanting to do learning systems. The very first chip we did was a learning chip. It was a feedforward net with outer product learning. It only had two bits of weight storage. That wasn't enough, but we didn't know that. We had no idea how many bits you needed for weight storage. It did its thing, and it incremented the weights and decremented the weights and so forth. We could never get it to do anything very interesting. Neither could anybody else. We didn't realize that if we had five levels, it probably would have been interesting.

But in the process of trying to make it do something, I realized that if this was going to be interesting, we needed real-time stuff coming in, and if we were going to have real-time stuff, we weren't going to get it out of a television camera. We ought to be doing something about the information coming in. That's been a ten-year detour. I really think of it as a way to get data that's worth learning. I'm sad to report that we still don't have data that's worth learning. It's been a much bigger detour than I had ever imagined to get sensory preprocessing to where it's in reasonable form to do anything. It's still not there.

JA: Most of the brain is preprocessing. That's really the most interesting problem.

CM: I think it is mostly. There's also a motor equivalent of that, which I don't even have a word for.

JA: I heard you give a talk a few years ago where you talked about the cognitive iceberg, which I always thought was a beautiful image. [Mead compared mental life to an iceberg: a little bit of cognition above the water-line and a huge amount of sensory preprocessing below the waterline, where most of the work gets done.]

CM: I think it was Wundt who came up with that image. When I first saw it, I thought, "That's my idea." It was a beautiful insight. I really believe it's true. We get these fully formed concepts and percepts that come floating up from below.

It's hard to do that, you know. I'm still trying to do it. I can't make an object. I can in trivial cases, but in the real world I can't make an object yet, and I've been working very hard. I want an object so I can learn stuff that is interesting. I haven't made phonemes yet or anything even remotely resembling a phoneme. I'm very frustrated because I feel like I should have made more progress, but this tells me that it's a lot harder than I thought.

ER: I was reading a section from a new book that says we must follow the rule of "microcosmic prophet, Carver Mead." The book quotes you as saying, "Listen to the technology and find out what it is telling us."

CM: Yes, I did say that.

ER: I wonder what you think neural nets are telling us.

CM: Adaptation. It's the whole game. I really believe that. It's not just because of the technology I work in; it's because of the nature of the real world. It's too variable to do anything absolute. You don't make a voice recognizer by looking at absolute frequency maps. You don't make vision systems by looking at intensities of pixels. You have to develop a higher level of abstraction than that, and you do that by comparing things and adapting to things. The nervous system figured that out a long time ago. But, boy, is that hard because nobody tells you what to adapt to what.

It's a problem, really, about the interface between the real world and computers. If you talk to anybody in computer vision, they'll tell you, "Yeah, you can make everything work, as long as you control the lighting really well." So they spend all their time going around controlling the lighting really well, and they get it all just right, and then you can go and do computer vision. It looks great, but nobody told you that they spent two hours getting the lights just right and if you change the light, it doesn't work anymore. You don't have that problem with your own vision system.

To me, that's the key. My own belief is that what started out as a dumb kind of adaptation has gradually turned into learning down through evolutionary time. This is wild speculation, but I just believe, deep down in my gut, that sooner or later that's what ended up as learning.

ER: It's a straight line between adapting and more complicated learning?

CM: A straight line on a log scale, yeah. What people do is take a given problem and set everything up for that. The brain couldn't do that. It had to

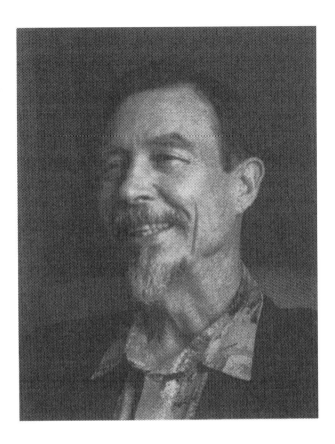

work with whatever came in, so that means it had to adapt much more than our technology has had to.

If new stuff comes along, it figures out what to do with it and just keeps going. I think the learning is really long-term adaptation. It's a way of adapting to things on a longer and longer timescale, and eventually that gets to be learning. I'm not clear in my own mind if there's a boundary between the rudimentary act of finding a level and the much more complicated act of getting rid of what I think of as the false entropy in the inputs—you know, getting rid of the junk that doesn't matter and pulling out the important things.

JA: There's not that many levels in the visual system to do it, either.

CM: And then all of a sudden here you are recognizing somebody's face. When you see your grandmother, there's a population that lights up that's different than when you see your grandfather.

JA: I remember a talk you gave in Washington. You had a lot of pictures illustrating the low selectivity of natural receptors. You pointed out that sensory receptors are mostly low Q. ["Q" in electronics describes selectivity of response. A low-Q receptor responds to a wide range of different stimuli; a high-Q receptor responds to a very narrow range.]

CM: Right. That was the thing that blew me away the most in the beginning. In color vision, I realized that you see yellows better than you see any other color because two broadly tuned filter functions are crossing at that point. That was a new idea to me—that you'd encode things using the cross-over, rather than by the selectivity of the receptors. Of course, if you're doing adaptive processing, it's the only way you can do it because all you can do is compare things. There are no absolute levels of anything. If you have a crossover, you can compare and you get a nice signal, so that made sense.

ER: You were talking about things that have surprised you. What have been the major surprises as you've pursued your work through the years?

CM: It was amazing to me how hard it is to have a new idea. I've always found that whenever I really understood something, somebody else had already figured it out a long time ago—like this thing about the cognitive iceberg. It's obvious once you've seen it, but then, of course, somebody figured it out a long time ago.

Adaptive circuits have been much harder to build robustly than I had any idea. I'd say that of ten circuits that get invented around our place, one will survive. For every winner there's ten that you think are going to be just as good, but there's something that isn't adaptive enough. You don't see it right away, and then later you realize, "Oh, it's because it wasn't really a rela-tive circuit; it wasn't working on the natural scale of the thing. It was work-ing on something absolute somewhere, and I just didn't see it." And then it isn't robust anymore. The difficulty getting to the solutions that are really clean and robust has been amazing.

ER: Are you surprised about the acceptance of your work?

CM: It's taken longer than I would have guessed to get people interested. I think part of that is that most people who know about analog stuff are electrical engineers [EEs], and they're still a little skeptical about the neural stuff. So I think as the neural stuff becomes more mainstream, then we'll get more EEs interested in the analog way of doing the neural stuff. I think there is still a lot of skepticism among the hard-core engineering community about whether this art form really is going to turn into anything, or if it is still fluff.

That's my constituency, the hard-core engineers. There was downright hostility in the beginning when I started talking about neural things. They'd bristle. Then when I started a little softer sell about adaptive analog and how people started out making digital filters and then they finally found out that they had to be adaptive filters. But if you're going to be adaptive, you don't need the precision, and so then you can be analog. Engineers understand that argument. But if you start from the neural perspective, they are still skeptical. I think it's turned from hostility into skepticism at this point.

ER: Could you comment a little bit on other people's work in the field that you think is important?

CM: I've learned a lot from everybody I've run into. I'm shameless about adopting ideas from people. I'm not sure I can even trace the important insights to any one person. I've learned a huge amount from Geoff Hinton. I think I learned more talking to Geoff than anyone because he thinks so differently from me. Just by struggling to cross that different way of conceptualizing I learn a tremendous amount.

My most intense learning experience—has been this thing called the Helmholtz Club. I don't know if you've heard of it. It's Francis Crick and Terry Sejnowski and V. S. Ramachandran and myself and John Allman and a group of other people. We meet once a month, and we invite two people. We spend a whole day, from noon on. We get two two-hour presentations and then discussion. There's maybe twenty people there. I never miss one. I have somebody take my class because it lands right on top of my class. I do it anyway because it's just too important to miss.

The reason it's named after Helmholtz is it's about the intersection of biology and harder-core physics and engineering. And it's exposed me to many different ways of thinking.

We had one talk on eye movements, and we had a guy talk about sleep and all the things that happen in sleep. I didn't know anything about sleep. It was wonderful hearing all that stuff from someone who was trying to think of a model. The last one we had was on the amygdala. We've had about three sessions now on attention.

JA: Attention is incredibly important behaviorally, and it's something people almost never build into a neural net.

CM: It seems to me it's a form of adaptation that's almost totally missing from our artificial models. It is extremely important because it gets the resources of the brain focused on things that belong together—not because they come through one sense, but because they're important to the animal for some reason. It's a way of aggregating the stuff that's in memory and the stuff that's patched together from all the senses and exploration—all pulled together into a context.

ER: What do you tell newcomers starting out in this field? How do you guide them or direct them? What do you tell them is important?

CM: When someone feels like they want to get involved, I try to find out what instinct base they have built for themselves. People with different backgrounds have different instincts about things. People who get really good at something develop a set of instincts around what makes sense and what doesn't. They can sort really rapidly through ideas. This field hasn't got to the point where you can just grind it out. You've got to have some instinct about what's important, or you just get lost.

I try to see a way in which that instinct base can be effective. Then I will usually try to steer them to someone where it feels to me like the things they have good sense for will fit in with the way that person works. I'll say, "You should go and talk to Terry Sejnowski" or "You should talk to Geoff Hinton" or "You should talk to John Allman," whoever might resonate with that person's native sense of where things are.

If people think really differently from me, it's hard for me. If I can't see a way to bridge into what they're doing, it's better they work with someone who has that bridge made already. That's happened quite a lot with people who have come to me, so I say, "Yeah, I think you fit really well here," and then I'll make an introduction because we're still not able to make big bridges yet in this field.

There's still pockets of stuff. You know that there are connections, but you can't always see them. Most of the time it's just hard work. We still haven't got the big blinding flashes yet.

JA: Occasional sparks.

CM: We do get occasional sparks. That's always fun. You believe there's a big lightning strike out there, someplace.

ER: Where do you see the field going?

CM: I've grossly underestimated the effort it's taken to get real-time data to the point where it was useful in learning systems. I would have told you five years ago that by now we would have real-time stuff that people would want to learn with—in other words, data that was good enough, with a good enough representation to feed into a learning system. We're not to that point yet. I still believe we're going to do it because it's just too important. It's in the real-time stuff that the richness of the network shows up. Networks will be doing things that you just can't do with AI. I don't know how long it's going to take. I'm getting gun-shy of making predictions.

We've got to be able to do it in real time with real-time stimuli and all adapted into some form where a lot of the invariance gets built in on the fly. That's my own personal goal. I want to provide the front end so people can build the learning system on the back end.

JA: Do you think we're still on an exponential learning curve in this area?

CM: I guess exponentials happen when one thing you do makes it easier to do the next thing. The places you get the big exponents are when you start getting crossings between areas of work so that something that happens in one place has effects elsewhere.

It feels to me kind of linear right now. We're riding on a computational paradigm that's getting better all the time, but in terms of the actual knowledge in the field it feels linear still. It doesn't feel like the insights from one way of looking at it play instantly into the other ways. That's what has to happen to make real exponential growth.

I think we still have the exciting period to go through in this field. It's beginning to happen. It feels like it's starting to tell us how it wants to be. We've been telling it how we want it to be, and it's just now starting to tell us the shape it wants to go into. When that happens, that will be the big exponential.

Part of what keeps me from being able to take immediate advantage of the rest of the community's work and vice versa is that the stuff I build is so hard to simulate. People don't have the computational resources to apply to things they are doing. There's so much energy put into getting networks to run well in the digital paradigm that all these issues of adaptation—how to have things be self-normalizing, how to have the levels find themselves, which are for me the really hard problems—those issues get swept under the rug.

ER: What about the commercial future of the field?

CM: It's beginning. There are two issues there. One is neural networks working on real problems. There's a lot of that now. Most of them are run on standard computers as simulations, and they're done in applications where it's not real time in any sense—like predicting the stock market. You don't need to have millisecond response, and you can wait till the market opens the next morning to get your prediction updated.

In the real-time area, first you use DSPs [digital signal-processing chips], and once you get a huge bunch of DSPs, then you need them to be in a little box. Then, as a last resort, you'll think about analog.

Analog is not the driving end of commercial neural networks. It can't be. There's too much momentum, too much knowledge, too much lore behind the software side and the digital side. Eventually some of that lore trickles down to applications where power and space are critical. Battery-powered things. At that point, somebody's going to be willing to invest in development of an analog system. Then we're going to gradually be able to grow the analog lore up to where it can start to be a real thing. Right now, it's a specialty item. By no means is it a commercial neural network thing. That's being done by the guys doing simulation software packages. And thank God for that because you need to develop a base of lore and credibility.

You really have to do a lot before you'll ever make an analog device because it takes so long to get it right. As time goes on, we'll get better at it, but at this point it is really important that we have the digital stuff out there commercially. Otherwise, as analog people, we wouldn't be able to keep the neural net paradigm alive long enough to learn the analog stuff well enough. As a field, we would be sunk if we didn't have the software that's running right now.

ER: Do you think that it's important that people are starting to make the transition from software simulations to making chips?

CM: It's a first step, right? It's beginning to make the point that there is a real thing here. It's very important that the neural paradigm is gradually seen as a thing that has its own structure, its own paradigms, its own way of being excellent, its own metrics or performance and value. What was scary for a while was that there were all of these announcements about stuff that was pretty clearly garbage and couldn't even compete with standard chips that were out there for other reasons. That gives the field a bad name, when people don't know that they could go and buy off the shelf something that would work better than what they just built. That was an awkward period. I think we're past that now. We're getting serious players who are going in and doing things in a serious way.

It's fortunate that there's enough awareness about the way things are done in a neural paradigm, enough different sets of requirements, that you can still do it in software, but much more optimally by building custom architectures.

ER: Your company [Synaptics, Inc.] is involved mostly with recognition problems. Do you think this is the foremost area where neural networks can make a commercial contribution?

CM: It's an area where it's very hard to do anything without a neural net. The AI people tried for years. With a neural network, you can do better in a week than people have done fooling around with AI programs for years. I'm particularly interested in the perception end of it because I'm working from that end.

With real-world data, where you don't know what the information is, neural network paradigms can pull out that information and make it useful. That is very, very clear. It wasn't clear five years ago. Then, it was a gleam in all of our eyes, but at that time it wasn't clear to anybody who was objective about it that it was going to be better than sitting down with a smart guy and writing a program. Now it's clear that there's no contest at all. That's been a big change.

You probably remember some of the early talks I gave which were, "Hey, let's not overhype this neural net thing because it could turn into another crash." We don't need another twenty-year famine like we had after the perceptron. I think we're well past that now. My own feeling is that it's not going to go away no matter what.

JA: It wasn't really a crash. Maybe a flat spot.

CM: I think we got through it. I think the group has been really statesmanlike in bringing in the old guys. It's like saying, "No, this isn't a community that pushes people out. Let's figure out how everything goes together, what the insights are, whereever they're coming from. Let's have a community that's open to new ideas and new ways of looking or old ways of looking, or whatever. Let's pull together and find what makes these big collective systems work."

To me, that's been the thing that got us through. There was a tendency for a while for people to break into groups. It feels to me like the statemanship won out over that, and that's really what caused the community to survive.

ER: Do you have any sense of what's going to happen in terms of the government's role? Traditionally, this field has been funded by the more defense-oriented needs of government, but now defense needs are changing.

CM: I can give you the jaded view, or I can give you the optimistic view. Maybe I ought to give you both. The jaded view is that the agencies will go after the hot new fields regardless of what their nominal role is. DARPA [the government's Defense Advanced Research Projects Agency] has been a great example of an agency that has figured out how to position itself to look like it's doing the current politically right thing. They've been skillful enough at it so that they haven't been bashed like a lot of other agencies have.

I don't think the basic forces in Washington—who does what to whom—are going to change very much. The fly wheel's too big. The names will just change around a little bit. The players will move around. They'll keep talking to each other, and they'll keep politicking the way they always have.

The problem of having something just defense related is it was always a sham, anyway, because with research you don't know what's really going to happen, so you have to make up something. The more you have to make up, the less relevance there is, and the less feedback there is between what works and what gets worked on. We've seen that played out over the last twenty years to the point where now there's very little feedback from what works to what's worked on. You see huge budgets going into things that have no relevance to anything that's ever going to be useful to anyone. You see things that are really very useful not getting any money.

In the military sector, it takes twenty years before anything gets fielded, and everybody forgets who did it anyway. There's no feedback. In the commercial sector, there's a lot more feedback because it's pretty clear what works and what doesn't. You're much more apt to get some sensible form of feedback.

I think, because of the fact that neural networks do useful things, there will be a net positive influence from actually looking at what they do rather than making up stories about what they might do. I mean, it took us twenty years to get completely disconnected from reality. It may take another twenty years of constant work to get back connected with reality.

JA: I asked about AI earlier. Do you have any interests in things like cognitive science?

CM: There are a whole bunch of cognitive people who come to the Helmholtz Club. We always try to pair them with a physiologist to try to get that bridge. I don't consider the whole cognitive psychology, perceptual psychology side, to be AI. I consider it central to everything.

JA: I'm glad to hear you say that.

CM: How would you work on a perception problem if you didn't know how you perceive?

JA: I think you have to know what the output is doing as well as what the input is doing. But there are a lot of people who don't think that, unfortunately.

CM: I think it's central. As a practical matter, we've actually gotten more from perceptual psychology than we have from physiology. Fortunately, physiologists are starting to use psychologically important stimuli.

JA: That's been a subtheme for a long time, but it hasn't gotten more respectable or popular until fairly recently.

CM: Now it's kind of expected that you'll do that because otherwise how the hell do you know what will happen? I find that the most important trend in neuroscience in recent years. Of course, there have been the occasional people who did it anyway, but it was an oddball thing, rather than mainstream. But now it's mainstream.

JA: It was always like: real scientists count photons.

CM: There was this terrible reductionist thing for years which was just deadly. If it wasn't reducible to that level of basic physics, then it wasn't real. And, of course, nothing could be further from the truth. I remember Feynman once gave a talk. Somebody asked him something about chemistry. He said, "There's a reason physicists are so successful with what they do, and that is they study the hydrogen atom and the helium ion and then they stop."

The chemists have to deal with real molecules that have more than one electron and more than one atom. Of course, there's no way to do that with physics. So then the chemists have to start making approximations. They have to start making constructs at a higher level, like the chemical bond. Well, what the hell is that? Yes, it has some quantum mechanics in it, but it's not something that you can just solve.

The more complicated the system, the higher level and the more approximate will be the concepts that you use. The good physicists knew that. They knew that the reason they were so successful was they didn't tackle the real problems. They made up a problem that was simple enough that they could actually solve it, and then they announced they were successful and left.

In our business there's no hope whatsoever of having that kind of reductionism work. We're more like the covalent and the ionic bonds. They're approximate ideas, but without them we couldn't make any progress at all.

But it is interesting that, having said it from that side, we can say it from the other side. There was a time when psychologists would argue vehemently over the meaning of some term. The philosophers were the same way, and they would yell and scream at each other. When you look back at those diatribes, you say, "What the hell were they thinking about?" It's like they were trying to be precise about something that was a very fuzzy concept anyway. It had very little to do with anything you could actually observe. Maybe what they should have been doing was more experimental. It feels bad arguing about the meaning of some word which doesn't really have a meaning yet because you couldn't operationalize it.

How many angels are dancing on the head of a pin? Maybe it was Aristotle or somebody who felt that you ought to be able to prove everything. It's been only twenty years that we've known that this was an oxymoron—since Gödel—and nonstandard analysis was worked out only fifteen years ago, so that it's OK to use infinitesimals again. Maybe Leibnitz had something after all. It was weird, the place we got into because of our Western upbringing that said you've got to be able to prove everything.

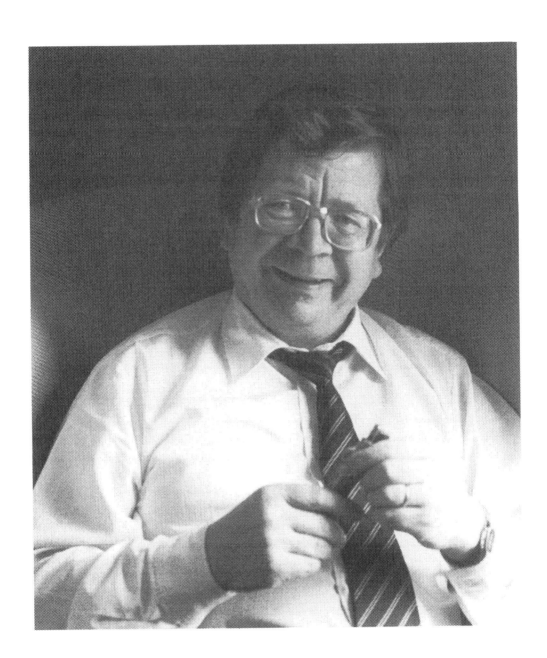

7   Teuvo Kohonen

Teuvo Kohonen is Academy Professor at the Helsinki University of Technology and of the Academy of Finland, as well as Head of the Neural Networks Research Center at the Helsinki University of Technology, Espoo, Finland. An introduction to his research can be found in his book Self-Organizing Maps, *second edition, Springer-Verlag, 1997.*

March 1993, San Francisco, California

ER: I'd like to begin with your date of birth, information about your growing up ...

TK: 11th of July, 1934. I was born in a small town in eastern Finland, in a lake area that has a link by a canal to Russia. The nature there is very beautiful; I think that it must have affected the people who are living there. My home town belongs to the western-most part of Karelia. There are eight or nine regions in Finland that are not bound to the countries, but to the cultures of people, and Karelia is one of them. The people there are said to be very lively, very, very friendly and talkative. But I don't know if I'm talkative at all. I'm rather a very silent type. Except sometimes.

I was raised in a family with two elder children. My brother is twelve years older than me, my sister is nine years older, and so I was just paid special attention, by my mother especially.

My father was a very busy man because he had many kinds of duties. He's a long time dead, but his hundredth birthday was in February 1993, and we collected his biography. Boy, I really heard interesting stories about him. As I was a child, my father was so much tied up with various duties. At that time he was a contractor in transportation. He ran first a one-truck business, but later he went into the construction area, making roads with tractors and excavators. He was all the time on the way to different places. I could actually very seldom talk to him.

My brother was involved with World War II, and after that he studied in Helsinki. I was still living in eastern Finland, and Helsinki is 240 kilometers away, so I also seldom saw him. My sister stayed home during my high school times. My mother sewed professionally. She learned that profession as a young girl. Although she did that in the country, she was almost like a salon keeper. People sometimes wanted to boast that they had a model dress.

Both my father and my mother were very practical people. They came from the countryside, so practical and very realistic, so there was no abstract kind of thinking. My father actually went to school very little because in the far countryside at that time, around 1900, the school system had not spread out very much in Finland, so he just attended what were called mobile schools, where the teachers came to the students. My mother went to regular school, but both had only grade school educations. My mother came from a country house to my father's family. She was also providing for the family with the sewing business all the time.

My father was also socially very active, and he belonged to the political life, to the leftist part of it, so he was asked to act in the town—what is it called, not government, but ...?

JA: The city council?

TK: City council, yes—sometimes either as a representative, like the congress, but sometimes in an office like the senate, and also as an alderman. He was also active serving on certain boards, like the social welfare board. He was chairman of the welfare board. I remember that when he came home from his far away business, and he was having his lunch, there was often a line of old women asking questions and complaining about things. He was a very open person, outward directed, who always wanted to help people, too much. I think that's roughly his character.

My father was ten years older than my mother, so there was also this age difference accounting for some polarization in the family. Mother was always taking care of all the practical things, and father was away, on the road, really, practically all the time. My elder brother is an engineer in telecommunications, and my sister has economical training, not the university training, but something which is professional economical training. She used to work for the truckers' union as the chief accountant.

In my school times, I went to school very early; usually children go to school at the age of seven, but I insisted on going to school at the age of six. I am biologically very young in regard to my chronological age, so I always felt like I was just a little boy among the others, which created a kind of tension perhaps. But my mother tells all sorts of stories about my childhood. For instance, I am supposed to have learned to spell at the age of two and a half, and to read at the age of three or so. I was a complete reader before I was four. Once my mother was telling me that she saw me skiing outside when she was sewing, and I was just standing there still and holding the poles, in this still position.

When I came home, she asked me, "What did you do?"

I said, "I was thinking."

Also I felt that many of the topics that were discussed at school were so naive that I would turn in better answers to them. But I was a nice guy all the way through until the university, so I never really objected to the teachers. In Finland, you had to be obedient, and that has affected Finnish people's lives, too.

We were asked to do much work at school, much homework, and so until the university, I really felt that that was a bore—not just a bore, but a nightmare. As a hobby I went to the Scouts. This lake area in Finland is so nice that also our family often went outside; we had a summer house. My father was fond of old motor boats, and he always assembled them himself, and I helped him, so I got some experience in how to deal with motors at an early age. And in school I had my favorite topics—mathematics, of course, physics and chemistry. Chemistry was not taught very much, but physics was very nice. As a special hobby I had psychology; I even bought books on gestalt psychology in high school and read them, so at that time I was really thinking about what is going on in the head. That must have been the first time when I was really working in this area of psychology.

ER: You were interested in gestalt psychology because you wanted to know ...

TK: ... how it works.

ER: ... how perception works?

TK: Yes, perception, yes. Perception and memory. That came to me at the age of sixteen, I guess.

I don't remember any other special hobbies, except the Scouts. At that time, I liked music, but the family could not afford fancy lessons. The only lessons that I got were a few violin lessons from a band player. We built radios; yes, of course, I have to say, radio building and electronics were also hobbies.

ER: This was when you were a teenager, or younger?

TK: Sometime after the age of fourteen or fifteen or so, I believe. I built a half a dozen radios, also the superheterodynes, and set up an electronic record player and things like that. I also experimented with chemistry. The neighborhood called it the "laboratory." I had this two-story board where I had the bottles and reagents. There was also the usual building of things. My brother was much more skilled; he built a kayak, fine model airplanes, and everything like that. I was not so skilled, but I was many sided, so I was trying this and that—optics, chemistry, electronics.

ER: You mentioned that the load of schoolwork was like a nightmare.

TK: Yes. They gave so much homework to us; the American people cannot believe how much homework we were given in school. I still remember all these exercises, like the declensions of the German language.

I think my memory for numbers has always been much better than my memory for names or faces. I forget faces; I forget the names of people. But once, as a school kid, I was trying to learn the decimals of pi. I took fifteen minutes, and then I could say pi to 108 decimal places. My brother was a witness. But of course such skills must be degrading all the time.

ER: And before you went to University, were there any teachers in elementary or high school who stirred you or interested you?

TK: Oh yes, my mathematics teacher, who also taught physics—he was extremely encouraging toward me. He supported my ideas. I think he was fond of my achievements, so he wanted me to study mathematical subjects or something, and so I went to the University of Technology, in applied physics. I have very warm memories of my mathematics teacher. He had practical advice all the time—"you must not be sloppy in your work," or whatever—and he gave us some extra advice and counseling when there were entrance examinations to the university. He gave us a course, for free, on special aspects of mathematics, but in university I didn't actually get a very good mathematics education. It was more like engineering mathematics. I still feel badly about it. I thought that at the same time I should start pure mathematics, but in our university there was at that time no abstract mathematical education. It was very practical. That was the University of Technology, where I still am, but nowadays everything is different.

ER: So when you went to university, you went to Helsinki?

TK: Yes.

ER: And were you living there?

TK: I was living at first in a dormitory, and then I moved to the home of a private family, but I was only a tenant. I was living in a rented room rather close to our university until I graduated. At that time, the Helsinki University of Technology was in a very antique building in the harbor of Helsinki city. Now it has moved to another city, which borders Helsinki, and we have grand new buildings, including modern architecture.

But at that time our university was situated in an empire-style, old building, which was in very bad shape. I was in the applied physics department, which was so small that the class had only eleven members and my professor, who is now a retired academician. He wanted us to go to the laboratory, so he said, "Classes must be kept at a minimum. You can always read the books later on, but just now you must go to the laboratories."

I did all sorts of reproductions of experiments. I myself constructed a continuous Wilson cloud chamber, Rutherford's and Millikan's experiments, and all sorts of things like that.

I liked my studies until graduation very much and also after that. I think that it is a very good idea to be in a laboratory and to have these experiences. I have always been very practical, I consider myself more like an inventor than a scholar. Scholastic studies are not my style. When I had almost finished my graduate studies for the doctor's degree—or a little bit earlier, in 1959—we moved to this new place, the new campus. I finished my doctor's thesis in 1962. I was among the first scientists who moved to our new campus, and I don't know for sure, but I might have had the first laboratory there, at least one of the very newest.

In Finland we have actually a succession of three degrees—a diploma engineer, which is very much like a master of science, then comes the licenciate.

In Russia, they have something similar which they call "candidate." Then comes a doctor's degree afterwards. It takes more time usually in many fields to take a doctorate degree in Finland than in other countries because the licenciate is in between.

We actually write three theses, one for each degree. For my first thesis, as a diploma engineer, I constructed, together with two other people, a simulator for the kinetic equations on nuclear reactors. For my licenciate thesis, I worked with nuclear electronics, constructing nanosecond time-measuring circuits, which were later used for positron lifetimes. So that was my hard experience with fast electronics, where you actually are working with waves and not signals, so you have to take them through coaxial cables, and you have to know exactly what to do. Your ground terminal is no longer a ground terminal; it's just a reflective plate.

I was not sure whether to write a theoretical thesis or a practical thesis, so I did work on both. I had theoretical work on quantum electrodynamical analysis of the scattering of polarized electrons and positrons. There I needed to use matrix algebra, which later was a good instrument. And as my practical work, I did the measurement of lifetimes of positrons. We were evaluating times in the subnanosecond region, with an accuracy approaching 10^{-11} seconds, and that included detectors, the scintillation detectors, too.

I was also doing work on tunnel diodes. That was a gadget which was popular then, but disappeared very soon. Even IBM made this big mistake, an odyssey to tunnel-diode computing circuits. Around 1965 they finally disappeared from the scene, but we still used the tunnel diodes in pulse-forming circuits. So many people thought that there's this nanosecond Kohonen.

I showed you the article in the *Journal of International Science and Technology*, written by four authors, which actually turned on my interest in neural networks in 1962. I was immediately caught by the idea. That article would be a very modern article, even today.

ER: That is the article about learning machines?

TK: Learning machines, yes. However, I couldn't work on neural networks because, although I had done my thesis in physics, I had to start teaching computers, because I was the only electronics expert in the department, in engineering physics and technical physics, whom they could use. It was against my real interests, using me for teaching computers.

Computer architecture teaching occupied my academic life for five years. Well, finally, it became interesting when I started to understand. When I was a professor, in my laboratory we built a computer which belonged to the second generation of computing. It was built with transistors, but it still used magnetic cores. So I am teasing the neural network people, "You are boasting these sixth-generation computers, but how many of you have done any of the earlier generations?" I started with analog computers, then went to digital computers, and finally to computing theory.

I was appointed associate professor in applied physics in 1963 and full professor in electronics in 1965. You must understand that there was a lack of people, and the competition was not as high as in the U.S.A., but I was a full professor when I was only thirty-one, and I had to develop the laboratory from scratch. There had never been any previous professor; the chair had just been founded. In Finland we have vacancies; we are not just looking for people, but we are filling vacancies, like in the U.S.A. civil servant system. So I was filling the vacancy and trying to develop a computer engineering education.

That occupied my life until I finally decided to go to the States. I got this possibility through an ex-Fulbright professor who was a dean at the University of Washington in Seattle. He invited me to come there during 1968–69. I had at that time an interest in neural networks, which I finally could continue, but even before that I had tried to create some algorithms which might nowadays be similar to genetic algorithms, systems that just learn by choices. Also, my idea of an associative memory was considered a little bit weird at that time. I had the idea that we must somehow implement an associative memory like the Fresnel holograms so that we are not really reconstructing pictures.

We see a virtual image through the hologram. That would explain, for instance, hallucinations and mental image scenes, our memorized image scenes, and almost anything. I still think that that would have been, and still could be, the highest achievement of my career—that I could explain these things. But, unfortunately, nobody understood it.

During the late '60s, I sent my paper to *Nature*, and it came back like a boomerang because people said, "Hey, you don't separate the key pattern from the recognized pattern," Later I was trying to make a more concrete model, like the correlation matrix model that Jim Anderson was doing at the same time. At that time I also submitted it to the *IEEE Transactions on Computers*, and again it first came back like a boomerang, so I decided to write an internal report after that. Remember that the internal report was after I had already done research, and that was 1970, so I could have had publications before that, but I didn't. But then there was a small conference in physiology from which I published "Principle of Virtual Images" in a Scandinavian series, *Acta Polytechnica Scandinavica*.

The principle of virtual images I documented also in a neural network article that started the journal *Neural Networks* and also published it in one of my early books, but I never saw any interest from people. I mean, people were not interested in that idea, although I think that it is a philosophically very important idea. We need not know who is looking at the hologram because we are not asking that question, even with a traditional Fresnel hologram; we take it for granted that we can understand it. Similarly we can separate the eternal question of soul from just practical conditions of associative memory.

As I was in the United States in 1968 and '69 I had the first possibility to think of the problem of associative memory. After that, I decided to start a new direction in our university, move it more toward the fundamental sciences and fundamental problems.

I was quite happy with this situation, but the political life was very disturbing in Finland in the 1970s. You said that you had your leftists here, but it created a very special aroma in Finland because of the Russian influence on our leftists. I don't know whether this is interesting at all, or whether I should even mention it, but I must say that the student political life was much more severe and grave than it ever was here.

Here it was considered as radical when the universities had courses on basket weaving and meditation, but these people in Finland—these student politicians—they later became important political leaders in our life, so they were almost professional politicians at that time, and they had great support by our state president. So in the 1970s the situation was very colorful. I had to fight for my scientific work, to get it published, and then there were the political problems and everything ...

Then I had a period in my life which very few people know because it is possible for professors in Finland to have extra business; they can take one day a week off or even other times to run a business. I was running a design office, an engineering office, together with my elder brother, for fourteen years. We started in 1964. In that office we designed digital control systems for Finnish industries. That was not a small activity in my life. We were actually delivering on the order of twenty rather large cabinets full of digital electronics to stabilize temperatures and the humidities in saw mill industries. They were drying boards. I abandoned this activity about 1975, but it was often parallel with my scientific activities.

JA: Did you find the practical work helped at all in your other work?

TK: Oh yes, yes. If you know that by your work you have to find the salaries for ten people, that creates a very practical view of life. I'm sorry, but I think that people here in our community, in the academia, just don't realize what it means if you have to do something which is so useful that it pays and that people want to pay for it. Maybe I have been doing too many things at the same time.

Still, my first journal article on the associative memories was published in *Transactions on Computers* in 1972, in addition to those I mentioned published in the Scandinavian series and in the internal reports. That article is now considered as one of the initial articles of distributed associative memory together with those by Kaoru Nakano and Jim Anderson. I became known. Then I started speech recognition research in 1975. Again we were asked to do something towards the "phonetic typewriter" so that one of the printing houses could have their raw material dictated. They said, "If you ever get 90 percent accuracy, that will be good enough." Now we have 95 percent, but I don't think that it is still useful for printing houses.

ER: What kind of approach were you using to speech recognition in the mid-seventies.

TK: In the mid-seventies we started first with the IBM type of approach. We had the analog filter bank and then did some kind of direction cosine comparisons with the correlation matrix formalism. I got these new ideas, two ideas in 1978. One was called the learning subspace method which is an early form of competitive learning, something which is similar to the map idea, except that every node was actually a subspace—that is, a set of codebook vectors which defined a geometric subspace in a high-dimensional space. And the learning subspace means that you are rotating these subspaces instead of making corrections on a single vector. It worked, but it is still not as good as the map or the learning vector quantization [LVQ] that I invented in 1986.

The other invention was a more symbolic method, which is called redundant hash addressing. Hash addressing means that you are storing strings of symbols at memory locations the addresses of which are computed as pseudorandom arithmetic functions of symbols, regarded as numbers, so you are mapping strings onto address space so that it randomly fills the address space. The mapping is deterministic, though, so you can find everything practically in one search operation. I just extended this method where by I created a multitude of mappings so that it was like a lens and rays—the address pointers—are converging onto the same location. This kind of redundant hash addressing would immediately find strings which were partly erroneous and it would be a very good method. We started the work in 1972.

James Albus has a somewhat similar idea called the CMAC. I had several doctors, at least two doctors, write their thesis on this method and some others who partly used it. We could encode networks of sentences, like one thousand sentences, and keep them in a packing storage on a disk, a separate disk unit, and find them on the basis of erroneous cues in real time. So this was a very interesting method, and we have written on it for some conferences. We call it something like "emulation of neural networks by software methods."

ER: Was it just a coincidence that you and your brother's business came to an end at the same time that this speech recognition work started?

TK: I can tell you a very good reason for that. It was because in 1975 I finally got this position of research professor at the Academy of Finland, and I had to stop all extra activities. Also, the worldwide economic depression at that time helped us make the decision.

ER: The other thing I was curious about is how did the printing company or publishing company know to come to you? I mean, were they aware of your work, and that's why they brought you this speech-recognition problem?

TK: We had at that time an associate professor who took part in so-called round table. I don't know if that is international, but they call it that there, like the round table knights or something like that. He was there together with the printing house director, so sometimes they talked science, too. Always these ideas and agreements come through some special way, so if you want to do something, you never get it, but you get much without knowing it, if you have some secret links, hidden units.

JA: That's the way the world tends to work, isn't it?

TK: But we were ready, we had all the infrastructure for that because we were interested in pattern recognition. We started with the recognition of characters, but we didn't continue for long because it was decided immediately that we would start with speech recognition. This started in 1975, but we were on our own in 1978. That could be described as a Mark 1 of our designs, and now we are working on Mark 7, which is the CNAPS computer-based system [special purpose hardware from Adaptive Solutions in Beaverton, Oregon]. What's in the journal *Computer* is the phonetic typewriter that was Mark 4.

JA: That's the article we put in our book, *Neurocomputing: Foundations of Research.*

TK: But at the time, when I actually presented this speech recognizer at the 1987 San Diego IEEE Neural Network meeting, I had this nice film. That was the first time I called it a neural typewriter or something because before this we didn't talk about "neural" anything.

I remember in 1987 Steve Grossberg calling me to ask whether I would like to join the INNS [International Neural Network Society] and be coeditor of the journal *Neural Networks,* and I said immediately, "Yes."

Then he started to talk about the term "neural." I said, "No, no, no, no." I said, "Why not learning machines or adaptive systems or whatsoever?"

So he said, "Yes, but we have so many opinions, and this seems to satisfy everybody." Still, I think that, well, much of the work could have been done in identical form under another name.

In 1975, I got a visit from the publisher Springer Verlag, and they were looking for authors, and one of my younger colleagues knew of my interests in associative memory. I said, "OK, I could write a book, a small book on associative memory," which I did. Yes, that was '75 when we made this agreement, and the book came out in 1977. I said to my colleagues, "Now I am putting my head into the ants' nest." I knew immediately how many reactions—not only positive, but negative ones—I would experience, and this was very true. But I was in the right place in the right time.

Writing that book was very good for my career. I could easily make new versions—like the self-organization of associative memory—based on material which I had already collected. I also collected maybe two thousand articles on content addressable memories. I still have this file in my room. It fills one wall. Then I published a book, *Content Addressable Memories,* because

I thought that there was some confusion in the context of associative memory and content addressable memory. People were mixing up these concepts all the time. This second book on neural networks was a strict literature study of the area of content addressable memories.

I had already started writing my first book while I was in the United States in 1968 and '69. There are these circulating agents of the press, and one came to the University of Washington electrical engineering department asking who would be willing to write a book on digital circuits, and I was caught. That was early, in 1969, when I started to collect material. I had notes already on which to base something, but practically I wrote the book after I returned home during 1969. The book was published in 1972. In 1974, it was noticed by IEEE because the *IEEE Spectrum* magazine made a study, a special series of reports, where they evaluated various areas, and they evaluated computer science and computer engineering books. I think that they went through hundreds of copies, and they collected something like twenty recommended books, and I got the highest points, mainly because the book had so much coverage.

Then the book was translated into Polish, the only language into which it was translated. That was before I started to write the neural network books. The book on content addressable memories came out in 1980, and both it and the books on self-organized associative memory, self-organization, and so on have come in many editions. The first associative memory book was translated into Japanese and Russian, and the content addressable memory book was translated into Russian, but so far I haven't heard of anything else unless there are pirate translations somewhere. The *Self-Organization and Associative Memory* book is an outgrowth of the old *Associative Memory* book, and now I have five books.

Starting in the middle '70s I also started to go to big conferences. In 1978, Professor K. S. Fu, who was a very well-known character in the pattern recognition field, asked me to establish the Finnish society for pattern recognition, which we did, and in 1978, in Kyoto, at an international pattern-recognition conference, we established the International Society of Pattern Recognition, where I have been active from the beginning in the same way as I have been active in neural networks. I was even the first vice president during 1982 to '84.

I think that the pattern recognition field contains so much material and basic insights into the recognition field that it should be taken into account much more in what the neural network people are doing. There's so much. I think that many of the articles that appear in our circles nowadays have ideas that were published earlier in pattern recognition.

In the 1970s sometime, starting 1974 or so, I often went to German conferences—small symposia on biological modeling on neural networks—where I met many famous people. I met German and American and many other scientists; I became acquainted with Fukushima and von der Malsburg and many others.

Germans love the type of symposia where they invite fifty people, of which half are giving speeches, and half of them are making comments, so the discussion is usually twenty to thirty minutes long. I've given some papers in those symposia. The German view into neural modeling was very scientific, what I characterize as scholastic, so that they would like to know everything about the details, all the biological details and functions. It was very difficult to get an engineer's point of view accepted, like I was doing, so I was actually a precursor of the developers of artificial neural networks because I characterized myself as an inventor. I said that we should actually be developing new paradigms for new technologies because if you are developing or inventing something, you must do the most with the least material. So I was making the first linear models of adaptive associative memory, correlation matrix and learning models, whatever, and they were not accepted until the 1980s.

I thought that the whole field was dead. I did not believe in it very much. I was just living the usual academic life in the late '70s and writing books until suddenly I was invited in 1985 to the annual meeting of the Optical Society of America. I was amazed they had accepted the idea of the linear associative memory. At that time they already had something like five experimental, optical associative memories. So that actually started my career. I was already known because I had books in the right place at the right time.

I don't know what my position otherwise would be. For some reason, perhaps because I had personal relations and the books, I was the guy who represented Europe in the first years. Then in 1988 I mentioned other Europeans who should have been drawn to the activities. I mentioned the names of Eduardo Caianiello, John Taylor, Igor Aleksander and some others, who then started to come to these conferences too. That was very interesting.

ER: Were you aware that neural networks had entered a period of quiescence in the United States in the 1970s?

TK: Yes, but I really didn't know about this reentrance of neural networks in the beginning of the 1980s. Of course, I knew about Hopfield's work, but because I knew that Jim [Anderson] had done similar work in 1978, I was completely confused. I didn't know what to think about the situation, but later I understood that where Hopfield started was in the physical community, and the physicists were so enthusiastic about the spin glass possibility. They thought that perhaps this was a new way to do physical information processing. And, you know, the Hopfield networks are still studied very much, but mainly among theoretical physicists.

I had also written something about a related idea in 1976 and in my 1977 book. I never had the positive feedback like Jim and Hopfield had, but I had feedback in another sense, on the correlation matrix memory. My feedback was adaptive and negative, while Hopfield's feedback was positive and non-adaptive.

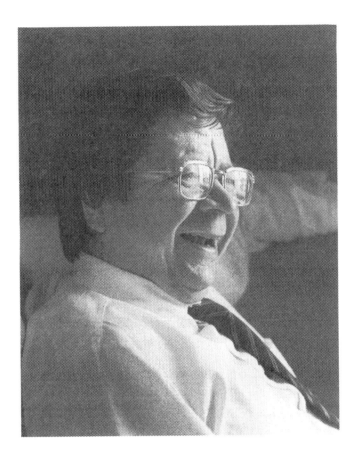

My correlation matrix feedback memory is called "novelty filter" because it creates this filter, which after exposure to a new pattern starts to become opaque to that pattern. The output fades out. For a new input pattern the output is the maximally new component in the new pattern, and then it fades out too. In this way you can train the network, really, to a set of new patterns, and as an associative memory it has the same capacity as the number of lines that is the dimensionality of the vector. I have mainly been able to publish these ideas both in the German journals and in my books, which are not refereed. But I had great difficulties in getting papers published in U.S. publications.

ER: Were you aware during the 1970s of the kind of switch from more biologically inspired models to the AI models—the more cognitively inspired models and the bruhaha surrounding Minsky and Papert's book?

TK: Yes, of course, I was one of the people suffering from Minsky and Papert's book [*Perceptrons*] because it went roughly this way: you start telling somebody about your work, and this visitor or whoever you talk to says, "Don't you know that this area is dead?"

It is something like what we experienced in the pattern recognition society when everything started to be structural and grammatical and semantic and so on. If somebody said, "I'm doing research on the statistical pattern recognition," then came this remark, "Hey, don't you know that is a dead idea already?"

Communities are very strange in the sense that some strong personality can lead it for a long time. He's going to dozens of conferences, and his opinions are cited and people ask each other, "What does he think about this? And what do you think that he thinks about this?" So it's like some kind of propaganda spreading in scientific communities.

ER: It cuts both ways because Hopfield influenced the community in a positive way about some of his ideas, irrespective of how innovative or original his thinking was. In part, it was the virtue of where it was published and the community that it managed to reach.

TK: I hoped that I could keep from mentioning anything negative about that work because it was Hopfield who put the neural network community on the bandwagon; but the truth is that Hopfield might have been the sixth or seventh who published the same idea. In some way, I think his work had a positive influence. You need some kind of support, and the support came from the physics community—especially in the area of, what should we say, statistical mechanics and certain people studying collective phenomena and people studying spin glasses because that seemed to be a very good theory for spin glasses. But there are also people like W. A. Little, who had actually written similar things on spin systems, so it is not too wrong to say that there were half a dozen articles along the same line as Hopfield's.

I have always found the lack of support the worst problem in my career. Finland is a small country; we are the dead end of the western world because behind us was only the Soviet Union, and nobody crossed that border very often except on the way to the conferences held in the Soviet Union. Finns are very apt to accept new ideas, but sometimes they also want to declare new ideas. It's either pure accepting or pure declaration. It's seldom transporting ideas from one country to another.

ER: When I met you in 1987, you had continued the speech recognition work. You were doing some of that work not just for Finnish language speech recognition, but also for the Japanese language under contract to Asahi Chemical Corp. Could you make a comment about how that came about?

TK: Sometime in 1983 or '84, there were very high expectations about the future of speech recognition. Some economics journals had published articles about the forecast; they had recognized the need in offices for dictating machines that automatically transcribe dictation, and they said that in the publishing business, speech recognition would have the potential to be a very, very good business. So the expectation of course went sky high.

At that time, Asahi was looking for partners; they were searching and visiting a lot of speech recognition laboratories, including MIT and Kurzweil Applied Intelligence and others. They came to my laboratory in 1984.

I had prepared a demonstration where I spoke Japanese words like "sakura" and so on, and they were most fascinated about the speed of the speech recognizer. The speed was so high that it was almost disturbing: when you saw the word appearing on the screen, it affected your pronunciation.

Asahi was immediately interested. They started research with us, and there was a contract for a two-year period of research, from 1985 to '87, something like two academic years. They sent one of their men over, who was with us all the time, and then there were two short-time visitors. Our objective was to transfer our technology into the Japanese typewriter. The motivation behind this objective was that the Finnish and the Japanese language are close phonetically. So I thought that our solution would be very good for the Japanese typewriter, and this guess was right.

In general I'm not willing to make guesses because like Einstein said, "I'm ninety-nine times wrong and one time right." If you ask me about the future of anything, or is it possible, I say, I don't know, but I will find out after I have tried it.

My algorithms include the self-organizing map, redundant hash coding, dynamically expanding context, the learning vector quantization and others. Each one I have simulated myself at least over a one-year period of time before publishing it. My computers run all the time until I have full comprehension of what is going on there. I have always said that you have to actually think like the process before you can make the process. You have to internalize all these ideas in your own brain so that you can imagine what is happening. After that, you can make the design.

But I haven't noticed that many people do it that way. They just take the algorithms, like some fast Fourier transformation, and they believe that if you put in some data, out comes a unique result—which is not true in learning machines and neural networks.

I once cited in 1987 the man who made artificial rocks for Disneyland and Disney World for twenty years. He said, "It is easy to make rocks when you think like a rock." You really have to live with it, and you have to imagine. So I think it is a common feature to all inventors that you must be able to visualize—not only visualize, but see inside. To visualize means that you must be able to internalize various kinds of things so that you are imagining what is going on.

This is the classical example. At Battelle Memorial Institute, one of their leaders said once that when he's testing new people, he gives them this problem: imagine Rubik's cube. Then you ask people the question, "How many of the little cubes have color on three sides, two sides, one side, and on no side?" The purpose is not to find the answer; the purpose is to watch what people are doing.

Most people are looking for a piece of paper and pencil, so either they draw figures or they start writing mathematical relationships to find it out. Real inventors see the cube like the eidetic image, and they put their fingers on the little cubes and they count them. So if you see a person just opening his eyes and start to look as if he saw the cube, then he's a real inventor. I could certainly say that I'm an inventor because the moment I read about this without yet knowing the answer, I was immediately sure that I had a cube in front of my eyes.

I spend more than a year with each major problem I study; that shows that you have to try many things. I have many notebooks full of ideas, wonderful ideas, elegant ideas, but maybe a fraction of them work well enough so that I can publish them. If I get an idea, I don't publish it right away.

I got my first shady ideas about the self-organizing map in 1975. I published them in 1981. It is usually several years before I'm ripe to publish, so I never publish anything right away. I have to be convinced. It must be credible, and to gain this credibility is some kind of growth process in my mind. I don't know if many people are that way. Many people say, "Oh, I must find a spot under the sun." They publish immediately, when they get something.

JA: When I get an idea, a great idea, it very often turns out to be wrong. I don't want to publish real fast.

TK: Exactly, yes. One of my colleagues in psychology says, "Oh, if I could visit all those places where they have my thesis on the shelves, I would go there and take it away!"

I just hate the idea of the so-called networking—what they have in the European Commission. The commission has now decided that it should establish centers of excellence and networks of centers of excellence, which are exchanging of people and ideas very fast by all possible means. Why should I tell my newest ideas to anybody? The biggest reason not to is, as Jim said, you are not quite sure whether they are right or wrong; you have to test them over a long time. Often, premature ideas cannot be told to other people. Or then, of course, if you want to publish something, you have to keep it to yourself at least until it is printed, so why tell all the ideas? Unfortunately there is so much competition, and many of us of the older generation have reached the stage where we are no longer so fast, so rapid, as is the younger generation. It takes more time for us to finish our paper.

ER: Besides speech recognition, are there other areas that you're focusing on?

TK: On the application side, I have left most of the work to some collaborators, students. For instance, there's this very promising work on texture analysis from images, which has been applied both in industry as well as in classification of various cloud types from satellite images. This is a good piece of work, and more than half of the work is included in the preprocessing analysis, where we have a very good person doing the work.

We have some directions in medicine where we are looking for new applications in medical engineering or analysis of medical data—like analysis of brain waves, analysis of lung sounds, diagnosis and clinical analysis of voice disorders, and so on. When people ask me what the three most important directions for neural network applications are, I usually say industrial applications, especially in instrumentation and robotics. Second are medical applications, and third, telecommunications. These are all areas for which neural networks are a complete fit. They all are dealing with difficult data and variable data—time-variable data for which you need the adaptive properties of networks. But speech recognition doesn't belong to that because it is more like an isolated problem area.

ER: Are there specific industrial, robotic and control applications that you're doing work on with your students?

TK: Well, actually some of the work has been initiated without my influence, but it directly comes from my ideas. Since 1985 there has been a professional installation that one of the Finnish papermill industries is using the texture analysis method for the analysis of fiber distribution in paper machines. It works in the production run, and it affects the control variables, which are set every week.

ER: It's an installed neural network application?

TK: It is, yes. I can be proud of it; it is the self-organizing map.

ER: What is the name of the company that's doing that?

TK: I cannot tell. It is a business secret. There's another Finnish company, a sawmill company, which is analyzing the quality of boards in such a way that when you make the first saw cuts onto it on four sides, by looking at the surface you can determine what quality of wood you have before you have to decide how you will optimize the sawing lines. This much I can say: both companies are in eastern Finland. But there are also other companies which use the maps.

It is my dream that the self-organizing mapper could be used as a monitoring panel for any machine where you have to monitor dynamic variables—or if not dynamic, then with lots of parallel variables. You could have that in every airplane, jet plane, or every nuclear power station, or every car. You could see immediately what condition the system is in. That would be something like what our nervous system is doing instinctively. There are now two small applications exactly like this.

In telecommunications there are also very good ideas—for example, our idea of developing detector systems for digital signals, discrete signals, that you might encounter in digital television and digital radio. This technology is just so new that if you want to use it, you must fit it to the existing standards.

JA: What are you doing in biology and medicine?

TK: I am no biologist, and the reason why I started with biological problems was that everybody thought neural networks are an explanation of the brain and cognitive processes. So during the 1960s and early 1970s I was actually desperately trying to relate these networks to biology. We did lots of literature searches and studies in order to find new experimental findings that would be helpful for us. But in this period, mid-1970s till the mid-1980s it was more like technological development along the pattern recognition lines, and it has been until quite recently.

Last summer I felt a real duty to relate the self-organizing map to some kind of biological process. I don't claim that it is exactly that, but if people understand, if people see the forest instead of trees, then they can see that there are plenty of avenues now if you start explaining biological things with the [wetware] models as well as with dry network models.

The techniques of distributing information by means of molecules is so simple; it is primordial in biology. Why shouldn't the brain be doing that? I think it is doing it all the time, especially in learning. Maybe not in a single transmission, but in learning you have to have some kind of sophisticated chemical processes in the brain. So this is my conviction now, and this is why I wrote that long article in *Neural Networks* ["Physiological Interpretation of the Self-Organizing Map Algorithm." *Neural Networks* 6: 895–905 1993], and I hope that it will be accepted by the community. I'm only afraid that I'm a spoiling their joy because so far everybody believes that we can do everything with networks of nodes and arcs.

As for medical applications, I mentioned the analysis of brain waves, where you can just map the various states of awakeness onto the map. In following experiments you especially need all sorts of monitors and indicators, and this might be very good, for instance, for the study of sleep or for the automatic study of epileptic people. It's time consuming and very straining to follow an experiment where you have to look at the EEG recorder and determine where it begins.

But if you can develop an automatic alarm method that says, "Please be alert now," and something interesting comes out, then the experimenter can do much better experimental work and clinical work. To aid medical experiments and studies clinically and in laboratories is one very important application area. I don't know about the prostheses and direct implants and so on. I don't want to speculate. We are not doing anything along those lines. But this monitoring business certainly is something which is very interesting and possible for us.

JA: Are you doing any projects yourself right now besides the EEG one?

TK: I don't say that I am doing these practical projects myself; there is always a group leader who is actually doing the research work and organizing everything. I'm more like a person who is keeping an eye on everything and trying to find out whether the work and what is done is sensible. I'm sort of a watchdog. What I'm doing personally is that I'm trying to develop these paradigms theoretically. The big question nowadays is what formalism I should use in order to prove the self-organizing map processor mathematically. We had a whole winter seminar last winter on the self-organizing maps; still, we are not so sure whether anybody has the right answer to it.

JA: How many people do you have working for you?

TK: It varies because they are from very different ages, starting from young undergraduates I have mainly three group leaders, but roughly fifteen people are paid from research money.

JA: Fifteen people, that's a big group.

TK: Yes, and of course there are separate subgroups. Also, people come and go.

JA: Do you get most of your funding from the Finnish government?

TK: Because I'm the research professor of the Academy of Finland, and I get my salary and my research from the academy, while I'm working at the university, according to the contract, the machines must be bought by the university, but all the other expenses come from the academy.

JA: Is that including the salaries of your coworkers?

TK: Yes, except if they are paid by the university, if they are laboratory technicians—I mean, academic laboratory technicians or perhaps permanent assistants. There are some lecturers who are permanent.

JA: Do you have to write grant proposals?

TK: Yes, well, to get to this position is of course very difficult because there are few positions and plenty of applicants, but I have been lucky. It is necessary to write a proposal only every four years, but I have done that every year just to be sure. In fact, the board has to accept every year's budget anyway, so I'm writing some kind of description every year.

JA: But it's not constant proposals, like the things you have to do in this country?

TK: Well, not at all in the same sense. If I count all the university salaries and the machines, then it is roughly fifty-fifty that my laboratory gets funds from the university and from the academy. But flexible research money comes from the academy. There are agencies in Finland that give out money, but there are also restrictions, much bureaucracy, and you have to find a partner from industry or something like that.

JA: It sounds wonderful.

TK: Yes.

ER: Years ago Bart Kosko said to me, "Don't you know, Teuvo is the Carl Sagan of Finland? He's the most well-known scientist in his own country." He also said that you have television shows?

TK: Television programs? There have been perhaps a dozen interviews on TV. There was one fifty-minute program. I had no talk show, but there was one fifty-minute program when they followed me during one week—my life, my home, and so on—and then they put it on the TV network. I think that there are dozens and dozens, maybe even more than a hundred, newspaper articles, interviews, and such that have been written.

ER: Is knowledge of your work in the neural network area widely known within your own country?

TK: At least the name of my research has been spread. I think so. I am not always so sure about the fare of my applications. Sometimes they are treated very well, but there are also some cases ... Although it is easier nowadays, life is never easy. You are living a dangerous life all the time. You cannot stop worrying. I'm sorry, but I'm of the worrying type, so that is how I feel.

ER: Is there work done by other people in the neural network field that you feel is particularly important or exciting to you?

TK: You mean theoretical or practical?

ER: Either.

TK: I could start answering about the practical. I think that some work which is done by the entrepreneurs is very good. I could mention Frederico Faggin [of Synaptics], whose work I really admire. Hecht-Nielsen has a view into the neural networks area. He has great virtues and profits in that direction.

In the area of theoretical research, I haven't been convinced of many breakthroughs. And by the way, like I said earlier, some algorithms could have been studied in mathematical statistics or statistical physics without any knowledge of neural networks.

ER: When you advise students, especially those who are just starting out in this field, what kind of studies do you suggest for them?

TK: Well, nowadays, if we have bright students, I say, "Don't forget mathematics." Then I advise them to read matrix vector formalisms and mathematical statistics, theory of pattern recognition and image analysis, optimal and adaptive control, and things like that. But computer science has never been very high on my list. The students have to know how to program computers and systems, but the problems of computer science are not important to this field at all. I had a background of being an experimental and partly theoretical physicist, a practicing engineer, and designer of electronic circuits; then I had to learn biology. You cannot become a neural network researcher without knowing at least the basics.

ER: I'm going to shift gears again. What do you believe are the questions in the field that you would personally like to see answered?

TK: Scientifically, again, on the psychological side, I would very much like to address this question of the virtual images, so that you are not working like a stimulus response machine, but you are creating some sort of understanding of what is going on. That doesn't necessarily need much mathematics, but it needs understanding.

I consider one of the greatest problems to be the preprocessing problem because if you look at various items, you can see how your field of attention is focusing narrower or wider, and so on. If you start doing this introspective experiment, you will be amazed about what is happening in our own system.

So the neural network or the neural system or some kind of cognitive system must build common case channels, which they first establish and then use.

People in research are doing it the wrong way. They are developing mappings that should be globally invariant. I think that is wrong. I have done and I let my students do a small experiment where we measure the reaction times to various sizes of letters, and I can certainly draw conclusions that there is first a set of channels established, and after that, these channels are used. I would like to have some kind of theory about this; that has been a dream. I think that locally invariant perception is the answer.

ER: I'd like to talk a little bit about the future. I wonder how you envision the field developing over the next three years, five years, ten years?

TK: I can only base my opinions on the results and progress that I have seen during the past five years and just recently. First of all, it will be realistic to say that like when microprocessors started, you could predict how they were developing. We can almost predict the development now of how the capacity of neural networks is growing. I would say that parallel processors or single processors are not what we need. We need some kind of circuits which have very flexible switching capabilities—partly analog, partly digital —and I see progress along these lines. And I think that this progress is visible in three years, in use in five years.

Ten years is a limit which is very, very fuzzy, so that it's difficult to say, but I think that the main incentive for building neural networks is that they will be cheap. The amount of information processed per dollar is orders of magnitude higher than by any other method.

But what else, I don't know. It's difficult to say. Maybe the dream about a really cognitive machine is too far away, not the least because it's difficult to define what these machines should be doing. We have made isolated demonstrations of abstraction and invariance formation and so on, but they work for rather clean experiments. If you take practical sensory signals, you might run into big difficulties.

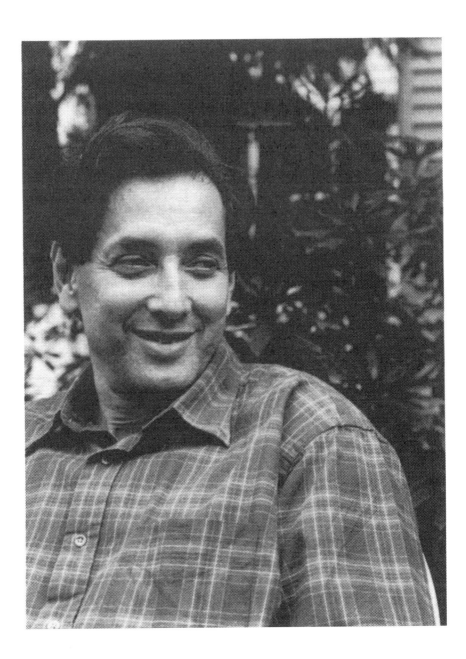

8   Stephen Grossberg

Stephen Grossberg is Wang Professor of Cognitive and Neural Systems; Professor of Mathematics, Psychology, and Biomedical Engineering; Chairman, Department of Cognitive and Neural Systems and Director, Center for Adaptive Systems, Boston University, Boston, Massachusetts. A good place to read further about Professor Grossberg's work is a 1995 paper, "The Attentive Brain," American Scientist 83: 438–449.

July 1993, Portland, Oregon

ER: What is your date of birth and where were you born?

SG: December 31, 1939, in New York City.

ER: Tell us something about your parents and what your early childhood was like.

SG: My grandparents were from Hungary, around Budapest, so I'm a second-generation American. My mother was a school teacher. My biological father died when I was one. My mother remarried when I was five, and I was adopted.

My new father was an accountant. My mother was a devoted teacher, and she got her Ph.D. equivalency at a time when it was hard for a woman even to go to college. She very much influenced my religious attitude toward learning. We grew up first in Woodside, and then when my mother remarried, we moved to Jackson Heights, Queens, to a lower-middle-class neighborhood filled with upwardly mobile Jewish boys who were fiercely competitive.

I was always very interested in art and music.

ER: Was that a natural inclination, or was that something that was fostered at home?

SG: It came from within. I was drawing from a very early age. I used to win a lot of art prizes, including study at the Museum of Modern Art when I was in high school. As for music, I went to the neighborhood library and discovered they had racks of records. I discovered all the major composers there. That made me want to play piano, so my parents started to save and eventually bought a piano. I learned very quickly. I actually did a lot of things well and was always first in my class.

ER: Before you were first in your class, what were your early childhood experiences like? Did you have a brother and sister?

SG: You'll have to prime me on this sort of thing because I don't usually talk about myself. I usually talk about work or other people. I'm a middle child. My older brother is two years older. My younger brother is the child of the second marriage. He's six years younger than me. This is a difficult position to be in if you want to be a scientist, apparently—to be the middle child and also not the child of the living father. How this worked out, I don't know. I guess it worked out just because I have certain talents, and I worked incredibly hard.

I knew I didn't want the life that seemed imminent. I looked around, and I saw a lot of very nice people who seemed unhappy with their lives. I wanted to find a higher form of life. I used to think about it almost in religious terms, although I'm not what you'd call a traditional religionist if only because I'm too much of a loner. I don't like believing things just because other people believe them. I try to find a path toward some higher form of existence. This is really fundamental to my whole point of view.

I was very aware of the fact that living things are either growing or they're dying. I had a strong sense of the dynamics of life—you know, blooming and decaying. It was already clear to me when I was very young that we have a short time on earth. It was also clear that society creates barriers to choice and that I had to find a way to keep my options open broadly so that I could eventually figure out how I could touch something that was more enduring. This, to me, was a deeply religious feeling: how to be in touch with the enduring beauty of the world, even though you can only personally be here for a very short time. It seemed the only way to do that at the time, given my limited options because my parents had no money, was to be incredibly good in school.

ER: What were your early childhood experiences like?

SG: How early do you want?

ER: As early as you can remember.

SG: Oh, I can remember when I was one.

ER: You can remember when you were one?

SG: Well, I have one memory, and that was when they took my dying father from the house to the hospital. The big black bag of the doctor was right in front of my face. That's my only memory from so early. Later, I was lonesome. I was very shy. In fact, one of the hallmarks of oh, the first twenty-odd years of my life was extreme shyness. I also didn't have much experience with how to be a man because I never knew my first father, and my second father was very distant.

My mother was marvelous—is still a remarkable woman—but being Hungarian was not good at showing or responding to affection.... I don't know if you know about Hungarians. They had the highest suicide rate in the world for many years, and one reason is that they wean you early from any show of affection. This isn't true of all Hungarians; for example, if you read the life of John von Neumann, you see that he had quite a different life because he formed a strong attachment to his father and was pampered by all the women in his extended family. One thing that made this possible was they had a great deal of money, and they led a privileged life.

We had little money. Although my parents were totally committed to their children and deeply loved us, there was a lot of stress, and little overt affection. My older brother was much more affected by my father's death than I was. That made him insecure and aggressive, and he used to beat me up regularly. That was frightening and made me feel vulnerable.

So I became shy and withdrawn, and—like a lot of people who are this way—became very creative, fantasized a lot, and tried to find another more appealing world. My world was the world of art and music at first and a world of trying to find approval. I found approval by trying to do very well in school, which also gave me great satisfaction because I was learning about things that often described other, more perfect, worlds.

In fact, many years later, when I read some of Einstein's essays, the phrase "the painful crudity and hopeless dreariness of daily life" stuck with me. Since that time, I've built a life with my family and friends that is happy, fulfilling, and full of meaning for me. But in my early childhood there was more painful crudity and hopeless dreariness because there were no examples of lives around me that I wanted to live. There were good people who were doing their best, but I viewed their lives as painfully crude and hopelessly dreary, so I had to find something that wouldn't feel that way to me, and from an early age I found it in learning more about the world. I also realized that I wanted to better understand why so many really nice people seemed unhappy, so I got very interested in people.

Also, you know, if you grow up in New York, there are only two major forms of life: people and dogs. You can't even see the sky half the time, so it wasn't as if you were in Nature and looking upon wonderful seasons and constellations. I therefore got very interested in the most interesting thing in New York, which was human life, and how people get on, how we come to know things about the world, and so on. From an early age I had a yearning to understand people, and I figured I would become a psychiatrist, as soon as I figured out what a psychiatrist was.

ER: And how early in your life did you start to draw?

SG: Oh, from the earliest years. I was drawing, oh, goodness, certainly well before I was five. First, I had all the usual coloring books, but then I started more active drawing, and I drew at a high level for my age. In fact, it became ridiculous when I was in public school and high school. I used to generate these large illustrated books that shocked my teachers because they were at a professional level.

The problem was that, even though I was in gifted classes, there was no one there to really help me build my confidence or move as fast as I could. Instead, it was a highly competitive environment. My public school, which was PS 69 in Queens, turned out to have kids with an unusually high overall cumulative IQ.

For example, we took standardized tests in the eighth grade, on which the highest you could go was the equivalent of having graduated from high school. It was called 12.0 plus, the twelfth grade plus, when you were in the eighth grade. The teacher foolishly read our scores out loud. It was 12.0 plus, 12.0 plus, 12.0 plus, until there was one poor kid with an 11.9—that kid was crushed. It was a sick environment. There was really little opportunity to enjoy being smart, apart from the fact that the satisfactions in learning were great, but the competitiveness was horrendous.

ER: You said you were also very involved with music, and I was wondering what form that took.

SG: Well, basically, my parents knew how much I wanted to play, and they were able to manage buying a little piano when I was in seventh grade. Within the year I was playing pretty advanced things—like Bach partitas, Gershwin's "Rhapsody in Blue," and lots of Chopin. My teacher called me a "genius," but I guess every music teacher tells parents that their child is a genius! One reason that I didn't go into music was I realized that, although I could play pretty well, I didn't have great hands; I also didn't have absolute pitch. I also tried composing some pieces for piano, and enjoyed this a lot but this still did not satisfy my yearning to contact enduring truths.

I wanted to do something where I could touch the eternal. I had this feeling that we're only here for a moment, and when we're not growing and helping others to grow, then we're dying. My hope was that the fruits of my mind might live longer than my body, and whatever understanding I could achieve would endure even as my body collapsed. So I very much needed to find something more enduring, more universal. These was this religious sense of needing to be in touch and commune with the world at an early age. This was my way of seeking a better future: to find a level of reality in life that could endure.

ER: Where did you go to high school?

SG: I went to Stuyvesant.

ER: Which is one of the New York schools for gifted children.

SG: It was either Stuyvesant or Bronx Science. Bronx Science was about an hour, an hour and a half away, and Stuyvesant was forty-five minutes, but in those days you could take the subway and feel safe. When I first attended Stuyvesant, it was a wonderful experience. I had some very good teachers, and I flourished in many ways there. But I was also aware of the terrifying statistics of the place. What do I mean by that? We had a class of maybe seven hundred kids. This was a time when there was still prejudice against

Jews in schools. There was a quota system. And only the top, a small segment of a place like Stuyvesant, would even get into college. Of course, you could go to CCNY [City College of New York] which brought out generations of great scientists. But I didn't even know about CCNY then.

Let me just give you an anecdote to set the stage. I remember going to a party after I graduated from Stuyvesant for kids from Bronx Science and Stuyvesant. One kid came up to me and said, "You're Grossberg, aren't you?" and I said, "Yeah," and he said, "I've hated you for four years."

I said, "But have we met?" and he said, "No, but I wished you would die."

I said, "Why?" and he said, "Because if you'd died, I'd be one higher in rank at the school."

I felt that all the time. There were several hundred kids who all had grade-point averages of around 92 percent—that's several hundred kids within fractions of a point from each other, which determined whether they got into college. I also knew kids who got three 800s on their college boards, but didn't get into any college to which they applied on the first round.

There were quite a few of us who had three 800s. I had three 800s on my boards, too, but I was also, fortunately, first in my class with 98-point-something average. So I succeeded within this system. I realized, though, that I couldn't stand this relentless competition much more. I needed out. I wasn't getting a chance to pursue my own goals, my own aspirations. My whole life was being spent on competing to escape, and I realized I had to find a way to get free from this relentless rat race fast. I didn't yet know what freedom meant, but I knew that I needed it to find out what I was going to do with my life.

Unfortunately, my family had no money with which to visit colleges. It was also a conceit of the time that, if you wanted to escape, you should try to go to an Ivy League school; that's where smart Jewish kids went. And so I started looking at Ivy League schools, and applied to several. Dartmouth had a senior fellowship program, which meant that if you were good enough in your classes, then in your senior year, you didn't have to take courses anymore. You'd have a free year to do research, whatever that was. That was one reason I applied to Dartmouth. Anyway, I got into a number of these schools with fellowships, including Harvard and Yale, but I got a bigger fellowship from Dartmouth, which was important because my parents needed the money.

In Dartmouth, my goal was to try to do so well that maybe I'd get a senior fellowship. I worked so hard at Dartmouth that many professors said that I was the best student that they ever had.

I was so highly motivated to find my way that, when I took Psychology 1, it unexpectedly created a storm of ideas in my mind. I got immensely engaged by human verbal learning data, animal discrimination learning data, and human attitude change learning. I was entranced by the implications of these data for how things are going on moment by moment in our minds— the kind of things that I still talk about: the real-time dynamics of individual minds. I could see that studying mind brought together several of my yearnings.

First, it was a good way to better understand people. Second, it gave me a way to better understand the processes of adaptive growth and development that were so much a part of my view of the world.

In fact, just anecdotally, I don't know if you know who Stuart Kauffman is? [A MacArthur Fellow, now at the Sante Fe Institute.] Well, Stu and I were classmates at Dartmouth, and we met just before school started at an overnight hike where new freshmen got a chance to know each other. Stu and I found each other that first day, and got into this long philosophical debate having to do with the mind: how do you know and how do you see, etc.

I can't remember the details, but I do remember being up in a loft one night, and we were still talking away while other kids who were trying to sleep were saying, "Shhh, shhh."

Even then, what would happen in our debates was, we would be discussing some topic during which I would say something, and Stu would say, "But that's not philosophy" because, you see, both of us were deeply interested in philosophy; we were high school philosophers! I had always thought of myself as being interested in philosophy and trying to define large issues and how to understand them.

Stu went on to become a philosophy major in college, and then he went to England on a Marshall scholarship in philosophy. It was only later that he came around to my view that philosophy doesn't have the methods that we need, and then made a big switch to medicine and from there to his present research in evolutionary biology.

But already, as freshmen we were having this battle. I'd say, "But I don't care if it's philosophy or not; this is what I want to know, and I want to find the right tools to know it." I was already searching for tools to understand better how our minds know the world, so when I read classical psychological learning data—the data of Hull, Guthrie, Pavlov, and all these other people —they really changed my life.

That year (1957–58) after Psychology 1, I went through a major intellectual struggle trying to figure out how to represent the real-time processes underlying these learning data. That is when I introduced the so-called Additive Model, which later in 1984 was called the Hopfield model by various people who didn't know the literature of our field. By then I had published at least fifty papers on it.

This misattribution. You know, when I introduced this model, indeed this modeling framework, it was really original, because there was nothing like it in the field. AI [artificial intelligence] was itself barely formed in 1957. There was just nothing to turn to for guidance. One had to find one's own way. I derived a lot of guidance from the bowed serial position curve of human verbal learning. The bow reflects the fact that the middle of a list is often harder to learn than its ends. Why does it bow? Why is learning asymmetric between a list's beginning and end? When you have rest periods between learning trials, why does the whole bowed distribution of errors change? Why do errors occur in the forward direction at the beginning of the list and the backward direction at the end of the list? To me, these data seemed extraordinary: first, that learning could go forward and backward in time; next, that silence between successive list presentations—the nonoccurrence of items in the future—could retroactively reorganize the entire distribution of learning. Events going backward in time excited me a lot and made me think about how to represent events in time.

I loved these data, and it was through studying them that I derived the Additive Model neural network with its short-term memory traces at network nodes, or cell populations, and its long-term memory traces in neural connections going forward and backward between these nodes, with the long-term memory traces at the synapses.

I think it's an interesting fact that I didn't know any neurophysiology when this model was derived. It was through quantitatively trying to understand the real-time dynamics of the serial position curve that I realized that there were short-term memory and long-term memory traces and competition among these distributed traces. I was also talking to my premed friends who told me about what they were learning about nerve cells, axons, synapses, transmitters, and the like when I realized that my model already had all of these properties.

I can hardly recapitulate my excitement when I realized this. It was such a passionate time. When it dawned on me that by trying to represent the real-time dynamics of behavior, you could derive brain mechanisms, I started reading neurophysiology with a vengeance. This first experience captures the story of my life as a thinker: To first try to understand behavior in a top-down way, always focusing on how behavior unfolds in real time, moment by moment, and trying to keep all homunculi out of the explanation. The model has to do it by itself, whatever its explanatory range. Such analyses have always made a link to neuroscience, and then computational and mathematical analysis showed how interactions among many neurons led to emergent properties that linked to behavior. Given the neural link, I'd then work bottom-up and top-down to further close the gap, pushing on both ends, between brain and behavior.

At that time, doing this work involved pretty extreme feelings of passion, terror, joy, and love. I was quite alone and pretty young—only 17 or 18—to be trying such a difficult path.

Anyway, to make a long story short, I did get a Senior Fellowship, and I spent my senior year continuing my research, including human verbal learning experiments. I knew that I had to make a difficult decision about what sort of career to follow. I loved psychology, and I view myself primarily as a psychologist and neuroscientist even today, rather than as a mathematician. I realized, though, that there were already many wonderful experimentalists but very few theorists. And I realized that, to be a good theorist, I needed mathematical techniques I didn't have, because from the first equations I wrote down as a Freshman, when I was the deriving the Additive Model, I needed systems of nonlinear differential equations. I hardly knew any appropriate math for analysing these equations.

Before I derived the Additive Model, I was stimulated by Bill Estes's papers on learning models that were just coming out then. He used Markov models to describe his Stimulus Sampling Theory. In my analyses of serial learning, I remember trying to express some of the distributions of learned traces and errors by using Stimulus Sampling Theory. I finally managed to compute a formula that went on for pages. I then realized that this couldn't be the correct method. The results were uninterpretable and meaningless. After struggling very hard, I began to understand that there were both fast rates and slow rates hidden in the data. In this way, I was able to start teasing out short-term memory and long-term memory traces, network nodes, and directed paths between them.

The dynamics of these short-term memory and long-term memory made me start to use differential equations. This was all exciting, but also terrifying because, at first, I couldn't prove anything about these equations. After going through the model derivation phenomenologically and being very clear about the steps that led to the equations and qualitatively being able to argue why they should be able to explain the data, I couldn't prove it. Computers weren't there to help, either. I can jump ahead and say that when I went to Stanford to do graduate work, one of the first things I tried to do was to work with one of the top programmers there to help me program the model so that I could compute the distribution of errors. He wasn't able to do it, for one reason or another. That created a major problem and source of anxiety, because how do you convince people of something that you can't prove mathematically and for which there aren't any other computational tools?

By this time, I had qualitatively derived a lot of results about human verbal learning and about animal discrimination learning. I also had related ideas about the dynamics of attitude change. I had replaced statistical psychological models with neural network models, and was aware of the importance of competitive normalization and contrast gain control to link the two types of description together.

As this was happening, I became the first joint major in psychology and mathematics at Dartmouth. It was also made clear to me that I couldn't hope for a career in a psychology department at that time as a full-time theorist. One had to function primarily as an experimentalist. Even Bill Estes, I was told, had a lot of trouble getting his modeling papers published at first, even though he was already a distinguished experimentalist.

My equations for short-term memory and long-term memory were nonlinear, many-body, fast-slow systems of differential equations. This was challenging mathematics. I needed a way to make it look simple. Although I was, at first, more interested in human verbal learning and animal discrimination learning, I then saw how to derive the equations from simple ideas about classical conditioning. That was exciting because both human and animal learning laws then had a similar form. These laws illustrated the type of universality that I was seeking.

Of course, none of these activities had anything to do with getting good grades. I became first in my class at Dartmouth for doing well in the standard curriculum. My research activities, in contrast, were not about getting grades; this had to do with how to be spiritually alive in the world. On the other hand, no one else was working to link brain to behavior with nonlinear neural networks. My intellectual work gave me a sense of purpose, but it also isolated me from my colleagues. Social acceptance and survival became a major issue, despite my intellectual success.

It was clear that I had to develop strong mathematical techniques in order to survive. I mean, how else could I prove anything? The computers weren't there. How else was I going to escape being considered a nut? At Dartmouth I was not considered a nut because I handed in one brilliant final exam after another, but I was still too shy to approach my professors personally. My own struggles to overcome my shyness have motivated me to set up an educational framework in our department that is designed to help students to be open and comfortable in their interactions with faculty.

It was not easy, while I was at Dartmouth, to figure out what to do with my life. One possibility was to become a mathematician because all science eventually becomes mathematics. If I could prove theorems about my neural models, then perhaps in that way I could continue my work.

But to become a mathematician when you really wanted to be a psychologist was no easy thing. I psyched myself into it with the following kinds of considerations. First, mathematics is a form of thinking, of cognitive processing. I tried to think of it as just one of the highest forms of cognition. This approach also helped me to better teach mathematics later on. Second, mathematics provided a way for me to learn large amounts of science fast, and I knew that I needed to learn a lot of science as part of my interdisciplinary training. I realized that if I opened a physics book on quantum mechanics, I'd either get stuck on trying to figure out how to read the equations, or I'd feel so comfortable with the language of mathematics that I could read the equations fluently and then be free to think about what the equations physically mean. Finally, I realized that I needed a virtuoso mathematical technique to express my own physical intuitions in an appropriate formalism, and then analyse the behavioral consequences of this formalism.

With these kind of intellectual rationalizations in mind, I decided to try to get a Ph.D. in mathematics. As you can imagine, I was pretty anxious about how all this would work out. Then the question arose as to where to go to graduate school. An advisor recommended that I go to Stanford because, at that time, Stanford had the strongest group in the world in mathematical psychology: Bill Estes was there, as were Gordon Bower, Dick Atkinson and Pat Suppes, among others. Stanford also had a strong department of applied mathematics.

So I figured I'd apply in mathematics at Stanford so I could also be close to the psychologists. Even if I got a degree in math, I wouldn't be out of touch with why I'm going into science, which was to understand the mind. And that's what I did. I went to Stanford.

Throughout all this, I can't overemphasize my sense of loneliness. I had a few wonderful professors, notably John Kemeny and Albert Hastorf, who were really very supportive, but there was always great anxiety because no one seemed to really understand what I was doing. I think they had the sense that because I was so "brilliant," unquote, I couldn't be a nut. I was doing what I as a young person was supposed to be doing: breaking new ground; and they tried to help me get to the people who could really evaluate what I was doing.

While this was going on, I wrote my senior fellowship undergraduate thesis at Dartmouth in 1960–61. It introduced the Additive Model and used it to analyse a lot of data about verbal learning. Because of this background, I don't believe that this model should be named after Hopfield. He simply didn't invent it. I did it when it was really a radical thing to do. My goal, to jump years later, was not to have any of these models named after anybody. I felt that models should have functional names—like Additive Model. Various power cliques do not seem to see things that way. They seek to aggrandize themselves even if, in so doing, they do violence to history.

When I went to Stanford I was sustained by my passion and love for science. My results enabled me to feel a little closer to the enduring beauty of the world, and gave my life a growing sense of focus and purpose. This was balanced against widespread indifference or skepticism about what I was doing. Without strong enough computational or mathematical tools, I realized that I had a limited amount of time to continue in this mode, because I was living off people's largess. I paid my dues by taking ninety credits of graduate mathematics, but there was no particular reason for established faculty to let me continue surviving as a scientist. Everyone else was planning to get a job in a well-established field, but there was no field that represented what I wanted to do.

Pat Suppes had been particularly active in getting me to come to Stanford. In fact, I was accepted in psychology and sociology in addition to mathematics. He was, however, incredibly busy. After I got there, I would hand him paper after paper that I was doing while I was taking my math courses —on human verbal learning, on animal discrimination learning, on competition, and so on. He never read any of them. When I would get up the courage to visit his office intermittently, he would ask what I was doing, and I'd give him a manuscript to read. I'd say, "I'd really appreciate if you'd look at it or maybe tell me what's wrong with it." I'd go back six months later, but he didn't have time to look at anything.

I greatly admired Bill Estes. I was unfortunately very shy, and Bill Estes was not exactly talkative. Whenever I visited him, I was always amazed by the fact that he was so quiet. He would sit there without changing his facial expression or saying a word and wait for you to talk. I very much wanted to communicate with him because I could see why Stimulus Sampling Theory worked when it did. I had stimulus sampling operations in my neural model. I could see how, in the neural model, if you changed variables, you'd get ratios of long-term memory traces that were just like stimulus-sampling probabilities. I could see why Estes' model worked and why it would fail. But I found it almost impossible to talk with him. I've never resented him for it because he's a marvelous man, and that's just the way he is. But it would have made my life much easier if he would have been able to draw me out a little more.

I realized later that Estes and his Stanford colleagues had a real struggle of their own to get Stimulus Sampling Theory accepted by experimental psychologists and to make it work. Then here comes this kid with neural networks. Well, what are they? Nonlinear differential equations, emergent properties. They didn't understand it well enough to want any of it. And I was too young to have the social skills with which to try to change their paradigm. It was also too soon—this was in 1961 to 1964. The failures of Stimulus Sampling Theory were not yet obvious enough for that paradigm to be abandoned. My experiences at Stanford were, by and large, a great disappointment because I only went there to try to get in touch with these people.

Since I couldn't sell any of my work, all I could do was to work even harder to try to understand more and to get closer to the communion with Nature that I desired. The good things that Stanford offered me were that I took ninety credits of graduate mathematics and read lots of physics, psychology, and neurophysiology, so I kept growing intellectually. I worked hard as a graduate student although I was a very unhappy one as I took course after course.

For the first year and a half or so, at Stanford, I didn't do any of the research that I did as an undergraduate. I didn't work on neural networks because I was trying to cope with the very real challenges of being a mathematics graduate student. I did love studying mathematics. I found the mathematics to be really beautiful. And I was able then to read a lot of physics quickly because I learned all the relevant mathematics. Socially, though, the first year at Stanford was so disappointing that I thought the second year had to be better, because I'm an incurable optimist. I figured, "This is so bad that next year has to be better." Well, the next year was equally bad. So then I tried to get out. An unfortunate accident then occurred. I was on an NSF [National Science Foundation] fellowship, and I realized that I hadn't yet heard about my fellowship renewal. When I went to the office in the mathematics department, they said that I probably should have heard something by then. They inquired for me because renewal was supposed to be automatic. As it turned out, the NSF had mailed my renewal notice to the wrong address. I just had to fill it out and send it back, and it would have been renewed, but because of the delay it was just past the renewal deadline. So suddenly not only was I unhappy, but I also didn't have any money.

Then Stanford did a very nice thing. They gave me a fellowship that supported me for another year. After that, I knew I couldn't stand it there any more. I got my Master's degree, and thought I'd try to go to MIT, in part to study under people like Norbert Weiner, and also because my girlfriend was then a graduate student at Harvard.

By this time, I had been reading a lot of papers by people at the Rockefeller Institute—papers by the neurophysiologists there and also papers by people like Mark Kac on statistical mechanics. So I wrote a letter to Rockefeller asking for information about its program too. This was a period when Rockefeller had a lot of money. They responded to my letter by checking up on me. I don't really know how they did it to this day, but the next thing I knew, they invited me to visit there.

I figured that I'd visit Rockefeller and then I'd also visit MIT and see if I could get an interview there too. My visit to Rockefeller seemed unreal. It had a gorgeous campus right in the heart of Manhattan. There was a guard at the front gate whose name was Angel. It was really like going to Heaven. You could go from Heaven to Manhattan and back every day if you were a student at Rockefeller!

So I transferred to Rockefeller instead of MIT, and that was a wonderful experience for me in many ways. On the other hand, I still had the usual problems there. My primary mentors were Mark Kac and Gian-Carlo Rota, who had just come from MIT. Rota had a sense of what I was doing because, in addition to being a mathematician of great breadth, he also was a professor of philosophy. He kindly became my "protector." At Rockefeller you really needed a protector! Rockefeller was then set up as a set of laboratories, and there were no required courses at the time. There were a number of lecture series. Still, various students went to Columbia or to NYU to take other courses.

Because Rockefeller was so unstructured, if you didn't affiliate yourself almost immediately with a laboratory and get a lab chief to claim you, you were vulnerable to the fluctuating winds of political change. My protector was Gian-Carlo Rota. During my years there (1964–1967) I continued to make lots of discoveries. Then I also had to write a Ph.D. thesis. What I did for a thesis was to develop methods to prove global limit and oscillation theorems for the Additive Model, treated as a content addressable memory [CAM]. They were, I think, the first global CAM theories.

Even then there were problems because—I don't want to go through the sordid details—there were some professors who did not believe the theorems. I had struggled very hard to find a way to demonstrate that my models worked as I claimed they did. And what could be more secure than a theorem? The shock was that they didn't believe the theorems! They thought that there must be a mistake. These people called me crazy before I proved them. Then they said that the theorems were crazy!

Fortunately, by that time Los Alamos had a big enough computer to run the equations, and this was done by Stan Ulam's group. They were interested in the theorems because they described a nonlinear collective phenomenon. At first they didn't believe the theorems either, but then they ran the networks on the computer, and the simulations did exactly what the theorems said they should. These CAM theorems analysed associative pattern learning in several critical cases: fully connected autoassociators, feedforward networks, and partially connected feedback nets. Given the difficulties I had in getting good scientists to believe my CAM theorems for Additive Model autoassociators in 1966, you can see why I am so annoyed that various people credit Hopfield for this model based on his work in 1984. I'll say more about this later.

Each graduate student at Rockefeller wrote up a first-year project. My first-year project in 1964–65 turned out to be a monograph of around five hundred pages, which synthesized my main results of the past ten years. It was called "The Theory of Embedding Fields With Applications to Psychology and Neurophysiology." It took me a long time to write it, and then the question was what to do with it. Several professors realized that students don't write five-hundred-page monographs every day. They wanted to get someone to evaluate it, so they arranged with me to mail it with a cover letter to 125 of the main psychology and neuroscience labs throughout the world. It went to David Hubel. It went to Steve Kuffler. It went to Eric Kandel. It went, actually, to most of the major neuroscientists and cognitive scientists in the world at that time. Unfortunately, no one seemed ready to understand it. But that monograph had the main results of my work of the past ten years and the seeds of my work for the next ten years. My published papers in the '60s and early '70s either published or worked out results that were in the monograph. It had a lot of results in it about reinforcement learning and human verbal learning. It also, among many other things, introduced a cerebellar learning model, which predicted that you'd have learning at the parallel fiber–Purkinje cell synapse. That was in 1964. David Marr made a similar prediction in 1969; Jim Albus in 1971. I published this model formally in 1969. Despite this background, the model is today often called the Marr-Albus model.

This has, all too often, been the story of my life. It's tragic really, and it's almost broken my heart several times. The problem is that, although I would often have an idea first, I usually had it too far ahead of its time. Or I would develop it too mathematically for most readers. Most of all, I've had too many ideas for me to be identified with all of them.

Please don't misunderstand my concerns about the so-called Marr-Albus or Hopfield models. My goal wasn't to get priority. Please understand that, first, shy people don't name things after themselves, and, second, I'm nothing. God is everything. I can't name after me something that is God's creation or God's proof. That's why I would try to give things functional names. But then many things that I discovered started getting named after other people! And I was not the only victim. Paul Werbos, David Parker, and, Shun-Ichi Amari should have gotten credit for the backpropagation model, instead of Rumelhart, Hinton, and Williams. Christoph von der Malsburg and I developed competitive learning and self-organizing feature maps between 1972 and 1976. In fact, Teuvo Kohonen's first version in 1982 wasn't the version that he used in 1984 and thereafter. At the meeting in Kyoto where he presented the first version, I was the chairman of the session. After his talk, I went through his model's properties as part of the general discussion, and I noted that my 1976–78 version of the model had certain advantages. That is the version that was used two years later in his 1984 book. And now the model is often named after Kohonen. Well, if it's named after anyone, the name should include Christoph and me. To leave out Christoph, who had a key 1973 *Kybernetik* paper, which adapted aspects of my 1972 *Kybernetik* paper, or me for my 1976 *Biological Cybernetics* papers which put the theory in its modern form, that's just historically wrong.

If you're doing a reputable history, you have to get right who really invented things. For example, for Amari and Werbos and Parker not to be given primary credit for backpropagation is wrong. How did this happen? In the early 1980s, a type of social autocatalytic wave broke that led to renewed acceptance of neural networks. This wave had been building since the 1970s; I could feel it building then. Some people who were in the mainstream of various related disciplines rode this wave, stoked the wave, and marketed the wave, and they deserve credit for that. Rumelhart has done a great service to cognitive science by promoting neural models, but he, Hinton, and Williams didn't invent backpropagation; he and Zipser didn't invent competitive learning; and all you have to do is to read the published literature in order to see that what I say is true.

Parts of my 1964 monograph were broken up and developed into ten research papers. While I was a graduate student at Rockefeller, I submitted all ten papers to *The Journal of Theoretical Biology*, including my verbal learning model and my derivation of the Additive Model. When the journal got these ten papers from this unknown scientist, they didn't know what to do with them. Bob Rosen, with whom I became friendly years later, was one of the receivers. He said, "If you had sent us one article we would probably have accepted it, but we didn't know how to handle ten." So they rejected them all. That was in 1964–65. This was, of course, a major disappointment for me.

Despite these problems, I got a job at MIT because my advisors at Rockefeller wrote strong letters on the strength of my Ph.D. thesis. When I visited MIT, I was interviewed by both the electrical engineering department and the applied mathematics department. Both departments offered me an assistant professorship because my thesis was considered to be very original. I had introduced a new class of models, these nonlinear short-term and long-term memory models, and I had proved a kind of theorem that was unfamiliar, these global CAM theorems. Then I did something which I think in retrospect was a mistake: I accepted the job in applied mathematics rather than in EE. I didn't realize that MIT was, at that time, really a big engineering department and that the power and influence of that department was overwhelming. I was influenced by the fact that Rota was returning to the MIT mathematics department when I arrived there.

Several of the math faculty were very kind to me. Norman Levinson was Norbert Wiener's greatest student, and he was one of the great mathematical analysts of our time. He and his wife Fagi took me under their wing as a kind of scientific godchild. They had two daughters about my age, but no sons. Fagi is, in fact, the Godgrandmother of our daughter. I wrote a large number of papers after I came to MIT in 1967, and Levinson, being a member of the National Academy, submitted a series of my notes in *PNAS* [*Proceedings of the National Academy of Sciences*]. There were three notes about neuro-biological and mathematical properties of the Additive Model and the more general Shunting (membrane equation) Model. Then I got a series of mathematical papers in the *Bulletin of the American Mathematical Society* and the *Journal of Differential Equations*.

MIT was a good experience in many ways. First, there was the challenge of teaching math to kids. I'd never taught before. My first assignments were to teach math courses in things I'd never even studied! I met the challenge by being so overprepared that I had the whole course totally polished before the first lecture began. Having never lectured, I would go into classrooms to practice my lectures to empty rooms. No one at MIT gave us any advice or help with our teaching. Now such skills are taught in our department to students in a one-on-one faculty-student setting as part of their Ph.D. training.

I remember the first day that I went into a classroom at MIT; the kids saw me, and they audibly groaned because I looked very young at the time. They figured they were getting yet another graduate student teacher. Anyway, I was so overprepared that it went OK, and my teaching was effective. My research also went very well. I published forty-odd papers on an ever expanding set of topics during my first few years there. Because of the range of this work, I'll have to skip it in this summary.

As a result, I was promoted after my first year at MIT from assistant professor to associate professor. I also won a Sloan faculty fellowship. Everything was finally going really well. I was verbally promised a professorship, but then when the time came, there was a major recession. I don't know if you remember in the early to mid-seventies there was a deep recession. A lot of schools got scared. It was the first one for a very long time in the postwar era. Essentially everyone who got a job at MIT after World War II got tenure, but then things crashed, and they started dumping us all. Traditionally at MIT, after you were an assistant professor, there was a critical decision point when you'd either be asked to leave or you were honored by being made an associate professor without tenure. The idea was that everyone who was chosen associate professor would eventually be a professor with tenure. You didn't have to worry about tenure, because you'd already gotten a verbal assurance of your future at MIT.

When the recession hit, I was not helped by the fact that some people considered me a "controversial" case. And no one advised me as to how you go about getting tenure. I was simply asked to give the department a representative list of people to write to for recommendation letters. I naively gave them a list of about fifty names of distinguished people across the fields of psychology, neuroscience, and mathematics. I got a very wide range of letters. A number of letters said I deserved a Nobel prize and I am a genius. I also had other letters that said, in effect: "Who the hell does he think he is trying to model the mind?"

At this point the department tried to break this deadlock by asking somebody whom everyone in mathematics would respect and who really knew what was going on. I don't know if you know who James Lighthill is? He was the Lucasian professor at that time in Cambridge University. That was Isaac Newton's chair. Lighthill had just written a scathing attack on AI. So they figured, first, he's a very substantial mathematician; he can understand all the math; and second, he has very strong attitudes about AI. Maybe some of them also thought that he'd therefore nail me and get it over with.

Anyway, he wrote a glowing three- or four-page letter which basically said that I was doing exactly what AI should have done. I've seen all these letters. I wasn't supposed to, but there were some people who were so upset that MIT didn't keep me that they wanted me to realize that the letters were, by and large, quite wonderful. They presented the type of case that an experienced reader expects to find when someone is doing something highly original, interdisciplinary, and technical.

I stayed an extra year at MIT. That's the year that Gail Carpenter came to the applied mathematics department at MIT. She's the best thing MIT ever did for me. It was because we overlapped that we could get together. Now we are very happily married and best friends. We have also done a lot of science together.

Then I went to BU [Boston University], and faced my next problem. I am telling you about these problems in order to reassure young people that you can hope to survive a lot of problems if you are true to your craft. A professorship of mathematics was created for me at BU through the President's office. I was told that my letters were the strongest that they had ever seen, but since President Silber was away in Europe, they couldn't offer me tenure until he read my case in the fall. A new dean then came in that fall, and said that he opposed creating professorships through the president's office. He said he would oppose me coming up for tenure in the fall, as promised by the previous dean, but would support me if I waited two years before going through the entire tenure process. Unfortunately, this man was no longer dean when I came up for tenure two years later. Who was? The man who had supported my tenure in his role as a Vice President two years earlier. No problem, right? Wrong.

This new Dean fired me. Why did he fire me? Because he claimed that the mathematics department was too big already. (It has since grown to more than twice its size then.) So I was fired from BU a few years after I got there, and I again lost the tenure that was verbally promised to me.

To make a long story short, the next six months were a very unhappy time. I appealed this decision to President Silber. It took quite a while before Silber considered the case. When he did, he also called up a lot of people to ask about me. Finally, he called me in to his office and said, "You're exactly what we want. I'm really sorry for the inconvenience." So I finally got tenure in 1975 after having been twice rejected for tenure. After 1975, for the first time I had some stability. It took me a few years to adjust to that. Now I hold an endowed Chair at BU and am one of its most respected faculty. My advice is: Never give up and don't hold grudges.

ER: You wanted to talk about Paul Werbos ...

SG: When I was at MIT, Dan Levine was one of my graduate students, and Dan was a friend of Paul Werbos who was then at Harvard. Dan told me about his very bright friend who was trying to do some work in neural networks, and he was having a lot of trouble with his Ph.D. thesis committee. So Paul came over and talked. The main thing I remember was that he seemed very bright and enthusiastic, but also talked a lot about all his troubles in getting people to understand and support what he was trying to do. This was a recurrent theme—that people who were making important discoveries about neural networks were hitting political brick walls.

The advice I gave him, which was the only thing I could do, was that he work out examples for people so they could see how his model worked. This he did, and he eventually got his Ph.D. thesis approved. You see, it was a period when I wasn't the only person experiencing brick walls right and left. I met a lot of very smart people who just vanished from the field. They just couldn't find a way to survive. Paul found a way. He deserves immense credit for that. The fact that, more than a decade later, people like Rumelhart, Hinton, and Williams were able to run with his ideas and further apply them when the scientific market was ready to receive them shouldn't deny the originators the credit that they deserve for introducing the ideas. I believe this both because it's the right thing to do, and also because that's why the field developed so fast in the 1980s. The foundations were already there; a lot of the main models were known. One can't believe that in 1982 suddenly everything was discovered. This just isn't the history of our or any other scientific field.

Around 1980, the Sloan Foundation started to give out grants in cognitive science. In college, I had gotten a Sloan predoctoral fellowship and at MIT I won a Sloan postdoctoral fellowship, so I figured I might get lucky again. I therefore called them up, and I asked, "If I submit a grant in cognitive science, would you consider it?" They said, "Well, you can't because you're not a center. We only make grants to centers." It was at that point that the concept of forming a center, a new administrative unit that could support people from many disciplines, firmly took hold in my mind. If I could only become a center, then I could work with people from many different disciplines without having to change departments.

I was at that time already working a lot with Gail Carpenter. I was also working with Michael Cohen, and more and more with Michael Kuperstein. Based on these and other projects, I was able to get a center grant, which allowed the Center for Adaptive Systems to get started in 1981.

The Center enabled me to start building up an interdisciplinary community of people interested in real-time modeling of mind and brain. I also wanted to help smart young scientists to have an easier time than I did. I almost didn't make it at multiple points, and I felt a commitment to making it easier for others to do so. After the Center succeeded, in 1988 I was able to get the university to start a graduate Ph.D. and M.A. granting program in Cognitive and Neural Systems. This program became a department two years later. It has developed an interdisciplinary curriculum so that graduate students can learn the field in a more systematic way. I also introduced the *Neural Networks* journal, and while introducing the journal, founded the International Neural Network Society [INNS], which began to bring together people from a lot of different disciplines.

One of the unfortunate facts about our field was that it was broken up into cliques that didn't cooperate. Physicists don't all love each other; in fact, I think they're probably one of the most competitive groups of scientists in the world. But they've learned how to cooperate to get more resources for all physicists. I hoped that INNS would help to fix this problem. So far, it has only achieved partial success because clique activities still tend to divide the field.

ER: Maybe you could say a little bit more about the more recent scientific work you've been doing.

SG: There've been a lot of streams of work in my life. The most pervasive stream has to do with parallel information processing and learning—the interactions between short-term and long-term memory. The earliest work was on human verbal learning—the problem of serial order in behavior and how you can get distributed patterns of errors that would evolve in a given context, like the bowed serial position curve, and why paired associate learning and serial learning were different.

I also did a long series of papers about global CAM and associative pattern learning. The problem was, how do you know it works as you would like? I spent years on proving that about what I call the Generalized Additive Model, which includes the so-called "Hopfield model," that I hope will not be called that for much longer.

I also did a lot of work about animal learning. If you think about conditioning—operant (or instrumental) and classical (or Pavlovian)—it forces you to also think about decision making, and associative learning between cognitive and emotional representations. Putting these concepts together leads you to think about the feedback between cognitive and emotional representations and how it focuses attention upon salient events. So, in thinking about this sort of decision making, I realized that I needed short-term memory nets that were self-normalizing. I had this insight first in my 1964 monograph and developed it for conditioning around 1969. My first paper on operant conditioning, per se, was in 1971. It has supported a lot of subsequent work.

My early learning theorems included outstar theorems, in which single cells can sample distributed patterns. I then realized that, once you have stimulus sampling, you need to ensure the selectivity of sampling in response to the proper combination of environmental cues. I then introduced instar theorems to ensure selective sampling to trigger outstar learning.

My 1970 paper on neural pattern discrimination used Additive Models with thresholding of signals to show how you could construct selective instar pattern discriminators. I realized around this time that you have to match what you can learn and what you can discriminate through information processing. This insight led to instars in 1970. These discriminators needed two layers of inhibition. In a 1972 article, I pointed out that these layers were reminiscent of retinas, where the first layer was like the horizontal cell layer and the second like an amacrine cell layer. This article also showed how an instar could adaptively change its selectivity to input patterns. This 1972 paper influenced Christoph von der Malsburg, who used the Additive Model but also introduced the key idea of tuning the adaptive filter with the weights in the filter, whereas I was using adaptive thresholds. His article came out in 1973.

In the interim, because of my interest in how short-term memory works during discrimination learning, I had mathematically attacked the problem of how you design short-term memory networks. It was a thrill to prove mathematically that properly designed networks had self-normalization and limited capacity properties as emergent properties of the net. Then I started classifying signal feedback functions, and I proved that sigmoid signals had very good properties; they suppressed noise, and also had had partial contrast enhancing properties.

I also proved how to design a winner-take-all net. That caused a little debate between Jim Anderson and me because I liked using the membrane equation, or shunting net, wherein I could suppress noise and still get self-normalizing contrast enhancement. His Brain State in a Box got contrast enhancement at the price of also amplifying noise.

I summarized all these results in a 1973 article, wherein properties of shunting competitive-feedback nets for short-term memory were classified in terms of how different signal functions altered the pattern stored in memory. I think that this was the first paper that mathematically proved why a sigmoid function is important. When I read Christoph's paper in 1973, which I thought was a remarkable paper, I was very gratified that he had used the Additive Model, but he also modified it. In my 1972 article, I had used a learning law that included both Hebbian and anti-Hebbian properties. I introduced that law in 1967 and 1968 in PNAS. It was also used in ART [Adaptive Resonance Theory] later on.

Stephen Grossberg

When I saw Christoph's 1973 article, I realized that it had several problems. One problem was that he had used a purely Hebbian learning law. Left to its own devices, this law would only allow adaptive weights, or long-term memory traces, to grow. To prevent this, he alternated learning intervals with trace normalization intervals. The model thus did not run in real time and it used nonlocal interactions. Based on some modeling and mathematical work that I'd done in the past few years, I saw how to design a real-time local model.

One step was to control the contrast enhancement and normalization of activity in the category node level of the network. The theorems from my 1973 article on recurrent on-center off-surround networks helped me here. In that paper, I described the first winner-take-all competitive network. More generally, I proved how a sigmoid feedback signal function could achieve self-normalizing, partial contrast enhancement, which Kohonen now calls "bubbles." I also realized that the input vector needed to be normalized, and discussed how to do this with an L1 norm in my 1976 article. Later, in my 1978 article on human memory, I generalized this to an arbitrary Lp norm, and singled out the L2 norm case for its unbiased properties. Kohonen used the unbiased L2 norm in his articles from 1982 onward.

With these innovations in place, I could then return to the use of the mixed Hebbian/anti-Hebbian learning law of my 1972 and earlier articles (it was introduced, actually, in 1958 when I started my work at Dartmouth). This learning law kept the adaptive weights bounded without violating real-time and locality constraints. I saw that this model was far more general than the application to which Malsburg had put it, which was the development of hypercolumns in striate visual cortex. For me, it became a general engine for classifying the widest possible range of input patterns. That is why I titled my 1976 *Biological Cybernetics* articles "Adaptive Pattern Classification and Universal Recoding."

The "Universal Recoding" part came from my observation that you could map the outputs from the classifier part of the network into the inputs of an outstar pattern learning network to learn an arbitrary map from m-dimensional to n-dimension space. This fact is of historical interest for two reasons. First, Hecht-Nielsen presented basically the same model again in the mid-1980s and called it counterpropagation. It has since achieved some popularity under that name. Second, when people popularized backpropagation in the mid-1980s, they often claimed that, whereas backpropagation could learn such a map, previous models could not. That, like so many other claims during that period, just wasn't so. In fact, my "universal recoding" map could learn such a map in an unsupervised way using purely local interactions, whereas backpropagation always required a teacher and used a nonlocal transport of adaptive weights.

Trying to live with so many false claims has been difficult for me, at times. If I try to get credit where it is due, then people who want the credit for themselves often mount a disinformation campaign in which they claim that all that I think about is priority. Because I have been a very productive pioneer, who innovated quite a few ideas and models, that can create quite a chorus of disinformation! If I don't try to get credit for my discoveries, then I am left with the feeling that eventually most of my ideas may become attributed to other people, especially if I have them too far ahead of my time.

Anyway, that's not why a person who has been scientifically active for as long as I have—now 40 years—keeps working. So, after designing the first self-organizing feature map of the type that is now used, I proved a theorem in a 1976 *Biological Cybernetics* article which says that such learning is stable in a sparse input environment; that is, an environment in which there aren't too many inputs or input clusters relative to the number of coding nodes. In fact, this learning has Bayesian properties, and I showed that the model's adaptive weights are self-normalizing and track the density of inputs coded by each recognition category. These properties were later exploited in the 1980s and thereafter in many applications by people like Kohonen.

My own interest was, however, primarily in how to classify arbitrary input environments, because no one controls the sparseness of inputs in the real world. I therefore also described examples in the 1976 article in which you could cause new learning to catastrophically erase old memories if the inputs were dense and distributed through time in a nonstationary way. This raised the urgent question of how the system could learn stably in a general input environment. I thought of this as a *stability-plasticity dilemma*, or how could a system continue to learn quickly in an arbitrary input environment without also forgetting what it earlier learned? Said in another way: Why doesn't fast learning force fast forgetting?

At this time, something exciting happened. I had published an article in 1975 in the *International Review of Neurobiology* on a neural model of attention, reinforcement, and discrimination learning. This model culminated almost two decades of work on classical and instrumental conditioning, which —as noted above—is the name given to those animal and human learning situations wherein rewards and punishments operate. In this article, I developed a model of cognitive-emotional interactions to explain how attention gets drawn to motivationally salient events. These phenomena included what is called attentional blocking and unblocking; or how do we learn what events predict rewards or punishments and focus attention upon them, while learning to ignore irrelevant events? This paper included my first adaptive resonances, which were feedback interactions that matched cognitive with emotional representations to focus attention in the desired way. I also needed to analyse what happened when a mismatch occurred, and this led me to introduce an orienting system that would search for and unblock previously unattended, but correct, cognitive representations, that could reliably predict the types of rewards or punishments that might be expected to occur.

One of the most exciting moments in my life occurred when I realized that the same dynamics of match/mismatch, search and learning that were needed to focus attention during adult cognitive-emotional interactions were also

Stephen Grossberg

needed to stabilize the development and learning of purely cognitive representations, from childhood on, including the learning of visual object recognition, speech, and other cognitive codes. This brought the reinforcement and cognitive literatures together in a truly radical way. Before that time, there had been bitter controversies between reinforcement and cognitive approaches to psychology. People like Skinner on the reinforcement side and Chomsky on the cognitive side were at each other's throats. In like manner, cognitive models in artificial intelligence were attacked for not being able to incorporate intentionality or feelings.

Part two of my 1976 *Biological Cybernetics* article introduced Adaptive Resonance Theory, or ART, to unify all of these apparent antagonisms. The key was to understand the central role of the stability-plasticity problem, or how to learn in real time throughout life without experiencing catastrophic forgetting. I showed that self-stabilizing learning required, among other things, the learning of top-down expectations, which focused attention on expected aspects of events. In other words, the stability of learning implies the intentionality of cognition and the fact that we pay attention. The universal status of the stability-plasticity problem helped to clarify why it could bridge between the cognitive and emotional domains. I also suggested that *all conscious states are resonant states*, and still have read no experiments that have led me to abandon this view.

I then did a lot of work on cognitive information processing, and I began realizing that I could only go so far until I knew what the functional units were that were being processed. These cognitive resonances were able to provide an intermodal binding of information from different sensory streams. But each of the sensory streams had its own heuristics. If you didn't know what the sensory units were, then you could go only so far. So I started working more and more on vision and language. I guess the most fundamental paper of that period was my 1978 human memory paper that was published in *Progress in Theoretical Biology*, because in that paper I offered a unified analysis which generated a lot of insights about perception, cognition, and motor control. That paper became a launching pad for the next ten years of work—just as my 1964 Rockefeller monograph had been a launching pad for the previous ten years of work.

Another stream of work tried to understand how to design neural net content-addressable memories. These networks always converge to one of a possibly very large number of equilibria in response to a fixed input pattern. That work greatly generalized my 1973 analysis of winner-take-all nets, sigmoids, and the like. Through it, I gradually identified in the mid-1970s a class of models which generalized recurrent on-center off-surround networks with additive or shunting dynamics, and which always approached equilibrium points. To prove convergence in all of these models, I introduced a Lyapunov functional method that made precise the idea that you can understand a competitive process by keeping track of who is winning the competition at any time. These results led me to conjecture that networks with symmetric coefficients always converge, as a special case of one of my general theorems. Mike Cohen and I then tried to prove this. We ultimately failed, but in the process, and because we were thinking about Lyapunov methods, we came up with a Lyapunov function in 1981 that helped us to prove the conjecture directly. We published this work in 1982 and 1983.

This work is now known as the Cohen-Grossberg model and theorem by a lot of people. We didn't name it that ourselves. The name came about because John Hopfield published a special case of our result—the case of the so-called Additive Model—in 1984, and it was called the Hopfield model by his colleagues. I had actually introduced that model almost 30 years before and Mike and I had published the Lyapunov function for it before, so quite a few people were not happy about naming it after Hopfield. They called our, more general, work the Cohen-Grossberg model to protect it from being misnamed later on. This sort of thing unfortunately happened all the time.

I also was very interested in understanding how a more complex form of content addressable memory was designed; namely, a working memory. This is the type of short-term memory whereby, say, you can remember a new telephone number for a short time after you first hear it, but can then forget it entirely if you are distracted before dialing it. A lot of data now points to the frontal cortex as a site of working memory. I realized that this problem of short-term memory was intimately linked to a problem of long-term memory, which is the type of more enduring memory whereby, say, you can remember you own name. (Presumably you don't forget your own name every time that you're distracted!) The main issue was that, as a novel list of items—like the numbers in a new telephone number, or letters in a new word—is presented to you, you don't want its storage in working memory to force you to forget familiar learned groupings of those items. For example, if you've never heard the word MYSELF, but have learned the words MY, SELF, and ELF that are subwords of MYSELF, you don't want the storage of MYSELF in working memory to erase the long-term memory that you have of its familiar subwords. If this were true, then we could never learn a language. This study thus identified a variant of the stability-plasticity dilemma that applies to temporally ordered memories.

I was happy to identify two postulates for such a working memory that would realize this goal. These postulates guaranteed that the familiar learned groupings would not be forgotten if they were coded by the type of bottom-up adaptive filter that occurs in a self-organizing map or an ART system. That enabled me to write down rules for generating all of the working memories of this type. Remarkably, these postulates could be realized by a specialized version of the recurrent on-center off-surround nets that I'd already studied! I was then able to prove something really surprising. Previously, it had often been thought that you could just have a recency gradient in working memory, in which more recent events were performed before earlier events. But just at around the time that I was working—in the mid 1970s—data began to appear suggesting that you could have an inverted U of short-term memory activity across items, with the earliest and most recent items performed before items in the middle of a list. In my model, larger activity of an item's representation translated into earlier performance. It turned out that I could characterize the conditions under which you'd get recency, primacy, or bowed (inverted U) gradients in working memory activity. I used this result to explain, for example, data about human free recall of recently presented lists of items. Here, items at the beginning and end of a list are recalled earlier, and with higher probability, than items in the middle. The main paradoxical result was this: The need to be able to store items in short-term working memory without destabilizing previously learned groupings in long-term memory sometimes implies that the *order* of storage is not veridical. It was veridical for short lists—a result which clarified concepts like the immediate memory span—but not for longer ones.

These results, combined with my earlier work from the 1960s on the long-term memory of temporally ordered lists, were both included in my 1978 human memory article, along with a lot of other stuff. They provided the foundation for more recent work about speech perception and motor planning. One of the most interesting things to me about results like this is that they showed how an adaptive property—like the stability of learned groupings—could lead to a maladaptive property—like the wrong order of storage—in certain environments. Many of my results are of this type, including results about mental disorders like schizophrenia, juvenile hyperactivity, and Parkinsonism, or about maladaptive partial reinforcement effects like persistent avoidance behavior, gambling, or self-punitive behavior.

ER: I wanted to discuss some of the other things that have gone on. You have patents, and I know that you've served on the science advisory board for Robert Hecht-Nielsen's company, HNC Software, and I was wondering if you could talk a little bit about some of the applications of your work.

SG: We've gotten patents on several of the ARTs—ART 1, ART 2, ART 3, ARTMAP. We've also gotten a patent on the BCS [Boundary Contour System, a computer vision algorithm] and on the Masking Field multiple-scale short-term memory and coding network. Our goal was not to interfere with research and development. We want to encourage that in every way possible. But if a company uses ART, say, to make a lot of money, then we would like to get some of it back to further energize the research that led to it. BU has been very good in helping us get patents under its university individual investigator agreement. I would say a lot of people are using ART, and more and more people are using our other models, but so far, most of this activity is still in the research and development phase.

ER: Do you have a relationship with any other company besides HNC?

SG: Well, I don't even have a relationship now with HNC; I was its first chief scientist, but am not any longer. To talk about more history, did you know that Robert Hecht-Nielsen entered the field in part because of me?

ER: He said that in his interview.

SG: My understanding is that Robert was reading the *Journal of Differential Equations* in the late 1960s where my early CAM theorems on the Generalized Additive Model were proved, and he got really interested in them. Robert then started to call me up every couple of years or so when he'd be in town on business, and we'd have lunch and talk about neural nets. I'd known Robert during years when one could only dream that neural net theory would be turned into a technology. When HNC started, Robert invited me to be its first chief scientist. It wasn't entirely clear to me what that would mean given that we were three thousand miles away from each other.

At the same time, Frederico Faggin and Carver Mead invited Gail and me to join their company, Synaptics. That created a serious conflict for me because I knew Gary Lynch was involved, and he's a really good neuroscientist. Carver and Frederico are, of course, top chip designers, and they promised to put some of our key algorithms into chips.

But I felt an old, even romantic, debt to Robert, and so I said yes to his offer. Apart from periodic meetings at HNC, not much happened. As the company faced the realities of trying to survive in a market where there weren't yet any niches, they needed very near-term products and business plans. My sense is that they changed direction several times before the company became a big success. I was too far away to be a large contributor to these strategies. So after our initial agreement wore off, it wasn't renewed.

ER: Do you hare other commercial relationships with other companies?

SG: We [the Center for Adaptive Systems] had a relationship with Hughes Co. on a joint DARPA grant. Gail has consulted for Boeing. A lot of our students have been getting good jobs at high tech companies. Several of our students were hired by MIT Lincoln Lab.

I feel that one really has to try to train people in the many interdisciplinary tools that the market needs. The nice thing about backpropagation is that it's easy to learn, so a lot of people use it. But backpropagation has a limited range. It's good for certain stationary problems where the variability in the data isn't too great, where there aren't too many inputs, and where you can run learning slowly and off-line. Fortunately, there are a lot of problems where these constraints hold. Backpropagation was there to help energize interest in the field, but there are at least as many problems where you want to learn in real time, on-line, with fast learning. Our students know backpropagation and ART, among many other skills.

ER: How many students at the Department?

SG: At this point there are fifty Ph.D. students and up to thirty M.A. students. The M.A. students are very interesting; all of them have full-time jobs in the area; for example, one of our M.A. students who recently graduated is an M.D.; he's at the Eye Research Institute. He's a clinical eye researcher, and he came to take courses to learn about neural models. Others are at Raytheon, MITRE, MIT Lincoln Labs, and so on. They're all already working professionals. We've had people come from the National Security Agency to get a masters, who now tell us that ART is being used to guard the nation's safety. The masters' students form a very interesting pool. They are one reason why we teach many of our courses once a week in the evening, so that qualified working people can set aside an evening each week to take a course each term, or possibly two courses.

ER: This leads me to my final question, which is to ask you to speculate about the future of neural nets. Where do you see the field going?

SG: I don't really feel comfortable talking about the future because I could never have predicted the present. I have hopes rather than predictions. I hope there will be more harmonious interaction among neural network colleagues.

ER: Well, I was going to give you a last opportunity to address nonorganizational and nonpolitical issues about the future of neural networks.

SG: I'll build my answer on some thoughts about why the brain is special. The following anecdote may help to make my point. Richard Feynman came into the field because he was interested in vision. When he realized that the retina is inverted, with the photodetectors behind all the other retinal layers, so that light has to go through all those layers before reaching them, he got out of the field. He couldn't figure out what kind of rational heuristics could be consistent with such a strange fact.

So here we see one of the very greatest quantum mechanicians admitting that brain dynamics are not just an easy application of quantum mechanics. On the other hand, the brain is tuned to the quantum level. You can see with just a few photons. The sensitivity of hearing is adjusted just above the level of thermal noise. So the brain is a quantum-sensitive measuring device. Moreover, the brain is a universal measuring device. It takes data from all the senses—vision, sound, pressure, temperature, biochemical sensors—and builds them into unified moments of resonant consciousness. The black body radiation problem, which Planck used to introduce quantum theory, also had a universality property. But then why isn't the brain just another application of garden-variety quantum mechanics? What's different?

My claim is that what's different is the brain's self-organizing capabilities. The critical thing is that we develop and learn on a very fast time scale relative to the evolution of matter. The revolution is in understanding universal quantum-sensitive rapidly self-organizing measurement devices.

Let's look at the history of science from this perspective. In the Newtonian revolution, the universe was described in terms of fixed, absolute coordinates. Then Einstein taught us that the way in which we make physical measurements, including how fast light travels, can influence what we know about the world. Then quantum mechanics went a step further and taught us that the act of measurement can actively change the states that are being measured, as in the Heisenberg uncertainty principle. But still, in all of these theories, the theory of the measurement device itself was really outside of physics. Physics taught us how measurement could be changed by the measuring device, but it did not provide a theory of the measurement device, in this case, the brain.

Theories of mind and brain, in contrast, are really theories of measurement devices which happen to be self-organizing in order to adapt to an evolving world. Understanding such measurement devices would be a very big step in science. So why has it taken so long for such theories to get born?

My answer is in the form of a story that has comforted me greatly when I was trying to figure out why our field is so crazy. I've written about it in several papers and books, so you may already know my view. I believe that we are living through part of a century-long process that has gradually led to the recent flowering of neural networks.

If you look at the greatest physicists of the middle to late nineteenth century, you'll see that they were often great psychologists or neuroscientists too. For example, [Hermann von] Helmholtz started early in life to test whether philosophical Idealists like his father were correct. Was it really true that you can act on an idea at the instant that you have it? Helmholtz tested this by measuring how long it took a nerve signal to travel along the arm. To do this accurately, he had to compensate for factors like muscle activity and heat generation. By making very careful measurements, he discovered the law of Conservation of Energy, which is one of the foundations of nineteenth-century physics. And he did this to settle a philosophical question by using methods of neuroscience. Helmholtz was as interested in the physics of vision and audition as he was in the psychophysics of how we perceive visual and auditory events.

The same was true for [Ernst] Mach, who studied the Mach bands in vision as well as the Mach numbers that are important in aeronautics. Mach's interest in space and time helped to inspire Einstein's general relativity theory.

[James Clerk] Maxwell developed the kinetic theory of gases and his theory of the electromagnetic field, but he also developed an important theory of color vision.

All of these physicists were interested in both external physical space and time, and internal psychological space and time. Remarkably, this was no longer true in the very next generation of physicists. You might say that this was just due to career specialization, but that is not convincing, because it happened too fast. I believe that there were deep intellectual reasons for this schism between physics and psychology. In particular, these interdisciplinary physicists were discovering facts about mind and brain that contemporary physics couldn't explain.

Consider Helmholtz's experiences, for example. White light in Newtonian color theory is light that has approximately equal energy in all the visible wavelengths. Helmholtz's experiments showed him, however, that our percepts tend to desaturate toward white the mean color of the scene. This property is related to our brain's ability to compensate for variable illumination —that is, to "discount the illuminant"—when perceiving a scene. Helmholtz realized that this was a highly nonlinear, context-sensitive process. Let me call this property of context-sensitivity "nonlocal" in the good sense that it involves long-range interactions (not in the bad sense, as in the back-propagation model, that it cannot be plausibly realized by a local physical propagation of signals).

Helmholtz also thought deeply about what we perceive. He claimed that we perceive what we expect to perceive based upon past learning. This was, greatly simplified, his idea of "unconscious inference." Such a view implies that bottom-up inputs from our experiences are matched against top-down expectations through some sort of cooperative-competitive process, and that these top-down expectations had to be learned. Such learning is a non-stationary process. So one needed nonlinear, nonstationary, and nonlocal models and mathematics in order to understand vision. Helmholtz realized that the necessary concepts and mathematics were not available at that time.

Fortunately, in the early twentieth century, you didn't need a lot of new math in order to do great physics. All of the revolutions in twentieth century physics started using known nineteenth century mathematics. For example, special relativity just used algebra; general relativity used Riemannian geometry; and quantum mechanics used matrix theory and linear operator theory. The physicists' main job was to discover new intuitions with which to understand the world. Once the intuitions were translated into models, the mathematics for understanding these models was ready and waiting. In contrast, to do psychology or neuroscience, you needed to discover new intuitions as well as new types of mathematics with which to analyse these intuitions. As a result, physicists, by and large, stopped studying psychology and neuroscience because their mathematical concepts were not adequate to understand the new data from these fields. Psychologists returned the favor by not wanting to learn much mathematics anymore, because the mathematics used by physics to explain the world was often irrelevant for explaining their data. It was the wrong math. This led, I think, to a major split between physical theorists and experimental psychologists and neuroscientists around the turn of the century. There followed almost a century of great physicists who knew nothing about psychology, but enjoyed nonetheless analogizing the brain to whatever was hot in technology, whether telephones, telegraphs, hydraulic systems, holograms, digital computers, or spin glasses. On the other side, psychologists often had profound intuitions about their data, but they didn't have appropriate formalisms with which to turn these intuitions into precise theoretical science.

This led to a century of controversy during which psychologists (and neuroscientists, too) often became divided into opposing cliques or camps that mapped out the extreme positions of some dimension of the data. For example, some psychologists collected data showing that learning seemed to be gradual, whereas others collected data showing that it seemed to be all-or-none. They were, in a sense, both correct, because the learning rate is context-sensitive, but they didn't have the quantitative tools that were needed to map out in which circumstances one or the other outcome could be predicted. Likewise, one had the Gestaltists, who believed in the action of unseen electrical brain fields, on the one hand, and the Behaviorists, who believed that everything has to be observable, on the other. Etc.

The net effect was that each group collected more and more data to bolster its position, thereby leading to one of the largest collective data bases in the history of science, but none of the controversies was ever fully settled, because the conceptual and mathematical tools that were needed to describe the underlying nonlinear, nonstationary, and nonlocal processes were nowhere to be found. My own life's work has been passionately devoted to discovering new intuitive and mathematical concepts and methods with which to overcome these apparent antagonisms and to thereby achieve a new synthesis of ideas.

Why is this hard to do? Why has it been such a controversial path? I claim that, in order to self-organize intelligent adaptive processes in real time, the brain needs nonlinear feedback processes that describe dynamical interactions among huge numbers of units acting on multiple spatial and temporal scales. Such processes are not easy to think about or to understand. One of the controversies that I experienced early on was whether we needed differential equations at all. Many people wanted discrete or symbolic models, but self-organizing systems need to be described dynamically in real time. Their symbols emerge from their dynamics. Another controversy involved the use of nonlinearity. Jim Anderson and I clashed about this matter. I felt that Jim wanted to keep things linear as long as he could. So did Kohonen for a number of years. My own derivations used linear interactions wherever possible, if only to point clearly to those interactions which really had to be nonlinear.

Feedback in nonlinear systems is particularly hard to understand. It's essential to achieve the real-time self-stabilization of memory and other properties. But mathematically, it's a large step. Many people have held off as long as they could to avoid closing the feedback loop. Backpropagation illustrates this tendency, since in that model, the feedback loop is never really closed. That is why I think of backpropagation as a neo-classical model that is holding on to the old paradigm as long as it can. In backpropagation, bottom-up activation is used to compute an error, which then slowly adapts the model's weights. What you really need, however, is to close the feedback loop to reorganize the fast dynamics of the activations themselves, which in turn will alter the adaptive weights. Adaptive Resonance Theory boldly took this step, and in so doing helped me to turn Helmholtz's intuitive concept of unconscious inference into rigorous science; in particular, rigorous science that is relevant to why we are conscious.

In summary, I see us ankle-deep in a major revolution that will play itself out during the next few generations. This revolution is about how biological measurement and control systems are designed to adapt quickly and stably in real time to a rapidly fluctuating world. It is about discovering new heuristics and mathematics with which to explain how nonlinear feedback

Stephen Grossberg

systems can accomplish this goal. Along the way, we will continue to discover a lush landscape of models for explaining how intelligent and adaptive minds emerge from brain dynamics through their interactions with the world. Even now, such models are linking the detailed architectures of brain systems to the emergent behaviors that they control. Neural models are already being used to solve difficult technological problems, and have suggested explanations of debilitating mental diseases. Ours is a great field that can be of use to many people and also for better understanding ourselves.

Stephen Grossberg

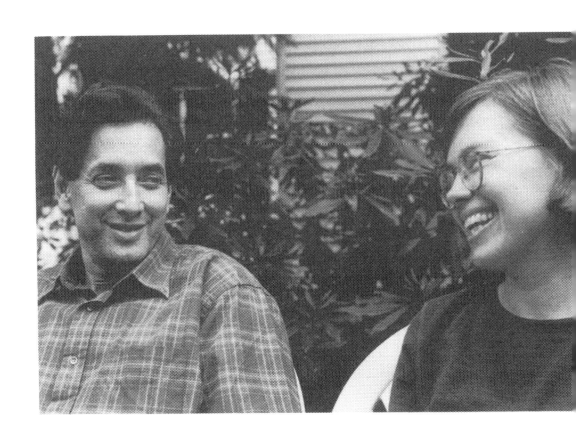

9   Gail Carpenter and Stephen Grossberg

Gail Carpenter is Professor in the Department of Cognitive and Neural Systems and in the Department of Mathematics, Boston University, Boston, Massachusetts. An article about her most recent work can be found in "Distributed learning, recognition, and prediction by ART and ARTMAP neural networks," Neural Networks 10: 1473–1494, 1997.

   Besides her own well-known research, Professor Carpenter has collaborated on a number of important papers with her husband, Professor Stephen Grossberg [see interview 8]. This interview was conducted with both Professor Carpenter and Professor Grossberg, partly to find out how such a close and productive scientific collaboration functions in practice.

July 1993, Portland, Oregon

ER: Tell us about how you know each other. How did it all begin?

GC: We met in 1974 at MIT in the applied math department. At that time Steve had been a professor there for six or seven years, and that was to be his last year there before he went to Boston University. I had just completed my Ph.D. in mathematics at the University of Wisconsin. I was starting as an instructor in applied math at MIT as my first job. At that time there were relatively few people studying neural networks. I had done a thesis on a neural model, and there was a small but very exciting group of people at MIT, including Steve, who were developing neural models. More generally, mathematical biology was an exciting area within mathematics at that time. There were also several graduate students. One of them was Dan Levine. We actually met at Dan's thesis defense.

ER: Very romantic.

GC: Right. And another student who was there at the time was Stu Geman, who is now at Brown. We had small seminars, and many people were visiting. There was a real focus of energy in the field, even though people now think of that as a time when very little was going on.

   So we first met very much in the professional context. While I was doing my dissertation, I had heard about Steve and seen some of his papers. At Wisconsin, when people would ask me, "Is there somebody at MIT that you're hoping to work with?" I remember saying, "Steve Grossberg's there now, but he's about to leave, and I'm not sure if he'll be there next year."

It turns out his appointment at BU [Boston University] had been delayed by a year, and that was the year when we met. Do you want to add something?

SG: That is how we met, so we owe something to Dan Levine.

GC: Who was at that time also a friend of Paul Werbos. I didn't know Paul then, but he was also finishing his dissertation that same year at Harvard, in applied math, and he and Dan had been friends for a number of years. I think Steve knew Paul, too.

SG: Paul was having trouble on his thesis, and I tried to advise him on how to try to work out examples to get people to appreciate what backprop could do.

ER: So what did you think of Steve when you met him, since he was someone you had known about but hadn't ever met?

GC: I liked his work very much. It wasn't too long before our romantic link started, within a couple of months. I had started out reading his articles, and I guess the rest is history. He was teaching a course at the time on learning models that he taught every year at MIT and had students from math, psychology, and other disciplines. I sat in on the course.

ER: That was the early '70s?

GC: 1974. In 1976 I went to Northeastern, where I became an assistant professor.

SG: ... and then Gail came to BU.

GC: By 1975, I wanted to stay in the Boston area so that we would be in the same city.

SG: Gail had a job offer from Carnegie Mellon, but that just seemed too difficult because I had a job at BU, and she would have been in Pittsburgh. That was just a little too rough for us, if we had a choice.

ER: I want to back up a little bit and get a couple of personal details, perhaps, about how your relationship with each other developed. Did you ask her out?

SG: It was clear to both of us that this was a very important relationship, right off, and then it was just a question of how not to spoil it.

GC: It wasn't quite that straightforward. We had talked a lot, and our birthdays are almost on the same day, so we went to dinner to celebrate.

SG: Gail had had a romance before, and I was ending a relationship ...

GC: This was one of the first things Steve told me.

SG: I told her, "I have just decided to be a lifelong bachelor. I'm not going to get into any more of these romances, because there's a little time when it's wonderful, and then you spend a lot of time separating without hard feelings. How could I break my resolution? I had just made it!" I was working out the last stages of a relationship so that we could remain friendly after it ended.

Gail and I both realized that this was very important; we wanted to go on in a nice, stately, not too hurried way because we both wanted it to work. And so our romance really started on my birthday, my thirty-fifth birthday, on New Year's Eve at a party. We didn't rush into this, but we knew …

GC: We're talking about a span of two or three months, rather than two or three years.

SG: Which for us was forever! Gail had an apartment downtown within walking distance of MIT, and I had bought a house a year or two before. I was going through a major nesting stage. I needed something solid in my life because everything else was so uncertain, especially since I kept taking intellectual risks by attacking such difficult and, then, unfashionable problems.

Over the years we've gotten closer than I thought you could get to somebody. She'll often start to say a sentence that I've already started in my head, or conversely, I don't need to bother saying it anymore.

GC: Now [our daughter] Deborah is starting to do the same thing.

SG: We went through phases where we both worked a lot, but I was so used to being alone that I never could work with anybody in the room. Gradually we got so close that we didn't want to be far apart. So Gail would work in the next room while I'd write on the dining room table. That didn't work out too well because she needed her computer terminal, which she had at home upstairs. But then I felt that she was too far away….

GC: There was a big step when the dining room table got split in half. We shared it.

SG: We worked at opposite ends of the table, in the same room, for several years.

ER: Had you moved in at some point?

GC: Yes, in 1975.

SG: We lived together for four years before we got married. We didn't really start working together scientifically right away although we were very interested in each other's work. Gail had done a lot of work on nerve impulse equations and the Hodgkin-Huxley model, and I was working more on the network level. But we realized there were strong links mathematically between networks and the Hodgkin-Huxley single cell, which is a type of network also. Then we gradually converged on projects that we wanted to work on. I'd been very interested in photoreceptor transduction; we worked on that together and then on circadian rhythms. We gradually started collaborating more and more. After we'd known each other several years, our first paper together came out in 1981, so that's quite a span. We'd already become very close as friends and lovers and colleagues before we were actually collaborating.

GC: I already had tenure before we had started working together.

ER: In what year were you married?

GC: 1979.

ER: And you were saying you took all this time when you were colleagues and friends and lovers, but not yet collaborators. And was that a conscious decision for both of you.

SG: No, it wasn't really a conscious choice. Gail had a lot of work that she was doing by herself and with others, and I had been doing a lot of work also.

GC: Our work really started out as quite distinct. When I met him, Steve was already developing the foundations of ART [Adaptive Resonance Theory], for example, and working on what became the 1978 human memory paper. And I did a dissertation on the Hodgkin-Huxley equation, which is for the single nerve cell. I was very mathematical. The focus of my published work in the early years was primarily single nerve cell models and mathematical analysis. Our work wasn't so close to begin with that there was an obvious way to think about collaborating, but we talked about each other's work all the time.

ER: Were you showing each other drafts of things that you were working on and soliciting feedback from each other?

SG: I think so.

GC: Yes.

SG: I remember Gail gave me a lot of feedback on the human memory paper.

GC: I remember the one where ART was introduced. The *Biological Cybernetics* paper is in two parts, which has turned out to be a problem because it's usually split up in anthologies. It was submitted as one, but it was too long, so just for practical reasons having to do with *Biological Cybernetics*'s page length, they said, "We want the paper split into two." I remember discussing how to do that.

SG: So we were very close in that regard. I don't remember exactly why we collaborated on photoreceptors. I had given a talk at U. of Penn., and Ed Pugh had told me some data about photoreceptor transduction. I think that's where I heard about the experimental work on the turtle cone, and it seemed to me that it was very similar to gated dipole dynamics, except that it was intracellular. That interested me a lot. Thinking that we should be able to model this, we started talking, and then we started working together to try to understand how the different channels in a single cell could generate these effects, including intracellular adaptation.

GC: You could think of it partly in terms of the size of the networks, especially in the evolution of my work, as starting out with one cell; the vertebrate photoreceptor model represented a single cell plus transmitter ...

SG: That's why it was a good interface for us ...

GC: Then the circadian models that we worked on for about three years were quite small networks. The primary work after that was the development of the ART networks. That started in 1985.

SG: It was an interface where circuits that I'd been working on in vision might have an analog or a variant in a single-cell context, and then we attacked bigger and bigger networks ...

GC: I remember very early on we would talk about fragments, and one of the things that struck us is that part of the Hodgkin-Huxley model can be viewed as a network sigmoid signal function. We were struck by the formal similarity between the single-cell formalism, where you have a shunting term, a product of conductances, and the competitive learning STM formalism. That's something I remember discussing very early.

SG: We got excited about that because if you take the axon, you can break it up into a lot of little pieces and view it as a one-dimensional network. If you take some of Gail's theorems about propagating waves, what was exciting was that, in a sense, the Hodgkin-Huxley dynamics were selecting for parameters to give you a wave, whereas in a cortical network the wave would be like a seizure, and you'd select against it. Then we began realizing that it was in this context of competitive interactions, with the potential link to ion conductances—excitatory and inhibitory, fast and slow—that we could think of the single cell as a network, you could also think of the individual network nodes as having laws that were very much like the single cell.

One of the interesting things about this for me was that it took us a long time to clearly see this. We talked to each other all the time freely, but it took us years to see this. That was a great comfort to me because I realized that even when people live together and love each other, it takes so long to understand some things, so how could I expect colleagues to understand each other easily? It helped take the edge off my frustration with how hard it was to communicate. That made me more comfortable with lots of things.

GC: Well, more patient, maybe.

SG: We've always had the great benefit that both of us are very deeply committed to science and love science, and we've had the wonderful experience of being able to talk freely about the widest range of areas.

GC: And we both had the same mathematical background.

SG: And to have that communion, it's really been great. It's not the main focus of our relationship—emotionally and in many other ways we're very well suited. However, it's been really wonderful, and it's been a comfort to us both. Meeting Gail changed my life completely; from feeling isolated and not having someone to talk to, I suddenly had the best person in the world to talk to. I couldn't believe how lucky I was, starting in 1974–75, even in the context of other stressful events like being denied tenure at BU as well as at MIT. When I was initially turned down for tenure at BU, there was such stress at the house that we would play games like *Scrabble* for hours and we would watch ... what is the show with the donkey?

GC: There was a series of *Francis the Talking Mule* movies on daytime TV. We watched these not just for a week but for the entire month of January.

SG: We were not big TV watchers, but everything stopped. We just pulled in ...

GC: We didn't want to see anybody, we didn't want to have anybody say, "Hey, how are you?" We still remember Francis fondly for helping us to get through that month.

SG: We watched Francis movies and played games and cuddled and tried to not think about the future because we didn't know what was going to happen. But at least we had each other. One of the things we computed was whether, if I lost my job, we could still keep our house on Gail's salary, which was about $14,000. I thought I might write books, and we computed that we could get by. We were bracing for that to happen.

GC: We made decisions like taking our retirement from MIT as of then. Even though I was only twenty-seven when I left MIT, I started out as a retiree because we were calculating every bit—our retirement checks would have paid our mortgage ... I was expecting to be the sole breadwinner.

SG: So that was what we were facing. If I lost tenure twice, I might, given the market at that time, not really be hireable again. And I might have to find a way to be productive outside of any academic context. Certainly many people do this profitably, but I have always thought of myself as an academic. But we had each other, and that really changed everything. It's been an immense source of energy for both of us.

ER: You have done important work together that's under both of your names. I wondered if you could characterize your collaborative style.

SG: Do you want me to start?

GC: Sure ...

SG: We talk together. The main difficulty is we're so close that it's like talking to yourself inside in a way. And I know when I'm talking to myself, I'm ruthless. I would never talk to another person the way I talk to myself. I'm not being mean; I'm just trying to get at the answer. So sometimes we would talk to each other that way, but we were talking to someone else— the person we loved—so we've had to learn how to remind ourselves that we're separate people.

GC: It's evolved. We've always talked about our separate work that isn't collaborative. Most of our collaborative work hasn't taken place where we're sitting in the same room, officially working on a problem together, in part because we have a constant opportunity to have small conversations. Although sometimes we do have to schedule appointments, or everything else washes in and takes over.

SG: We had to work out how to get together in the context of a very close, intimate relationship and do science.

GC: Part of it is you just put yourself into different compartments to some extent. We interact in our department at a much greater distance than at home. It's like being a different person, just as everybody is in different contexts. Also, in recent years, one of the things that all of us have faced is the graduate program. It has been a huge stress on everyone in our program. With lots of students and very rapid growth, having two professors work either together and or with one student became a luxury.

ER: Well, I wonder if you could choose one thing that you collaborated on, perhaps from the early '80s, and maybe trace the genesis of the idea and how you moved it back and forth between you, and what the phenomenological nature of the collaboration was?

SG: I would say in some of the earlier work, for example, when Gail was still doing more single cell modeling, I might come in with a rough idea of what I thought should be going on. My strongest skills are intuitive and mathematical. Gail has strong mathematical and computer skills. In all our collaborative work she did all the simulation studies. We would have a phase together when we'd discuss design principles and what the model should be. Then Gail would try to develop specific model simulations, to see what worked and what didn't. She also did a lot of analytic work. Then we would talk together again, and so on.

GC: I think one project that was certainly important was the ART collaboration. I could give my view of that. Steve had developed the adaptive resonance theory during the 1970s, and the theory was explicitly formulated in the 1976 *Biological Cybernetics* article. And at that time there was a computational analysis for stability, along with a series of examples of data from cognition, olfaction, and vision, and several examples of resonances. Then over the course of the next decade, he had a series of other papers that focused on the cognitive aspects. He had a paper in *Psychological Review* in 1980, for example. In the mid-seventies, I remember even his first lecture on adaptive resonance, where he had talked about a lot of data, and then in the last five minutes had given a very quick outline of the basic thought experiment of the ART system. I remember discussing it and saying, "That last part was so wonderful, why don't you make it into a whole lecture?" He did, and it evolved into the 1980 paper, "How Does the Brain Build a Cognitive Code?"

However, through all of these papers, including analyses of different kinds of data, evoked potentials, and so on, there wasn't an actual full working ART model that could stand alone, that somebody could take and simulate. There were pieces of it, and many of the concepts were there. Around 1984, our circadian rhythm work was winding down—we felt that we had modeled that literature to the extent that the data warranted. I was looking for something new to start and had always liked the ART work. I sat down saying, "Let's try to write something out that's an actual system."

In the 1987 ART 1 paper, which was written in 1985, some of the problems that the architecture solves seem simple in retrospect. However, it took months to see how to design the stand-alone model. One issue was: how do you encode a pattern that's a subset? I remember talking about written character E and F or E and L, where one pattern is embedded in another as a subset. In the course of designing the model, new theoretical ideas, such as vigilance matching and gain control, were also introduced.

SG: Even the decision to design ART 1 only for binary input patterns took a lot of discussion. The goal of the theory was to encode more general analog patterns. However, ART 1 was intended to be the simplest possible model that nevertheless realized key theoretical properties. With winner-take-all coding and binary input patterns, a real analysis of the system became possible.

GC: In ART 1, and I think in most of the models since, the role of simulation has basically been supportive. Much of the work was done with pencil and paper, and the simulations illustrate properties rather than prove them. A lot of the work, the core, not only of our joint work, but an approach that's characteristic of Steve's work and other work in the group, is to focus on a series of design principles or critical problems. In the case of ART, one of the critical problems was one pattern being embedded in the other where they had to be coded distinctly. That was one of the driving computational problems. ART 2, for analog inputs, was published the same year, although it had taken another year to develop.

Although ART 2 was based on the Euclidean distance, the model development later came full circle to fuzzy ART, which is a direct extension of ART 1. Fuzzy ART is more natural computationally than ART 2 and is what most people now use, I think. The contemporary ARTMAP systems use ART 1 or fuzzy ART in the supervised learning context.

ER: Is ferreting out the architecture a very collaborative effort that you both work on in a variety of different ways? I'm wondering about the writing.

GC: Typically, in all our group efforts, I think somebody does a very early first draft after some discussion, then it goes to somebody else, who makes changes, and then it goes back. I know in some groups, one person writes and that's it. But I don't know of any of our papers where that's been so ...

SG: We have the rule that if you don't like something, you've got to re-write an alternative. You can't just say, I don't like it and send it back. You have to ...

ER: Make a suggestion ...

SG: ... make a definite improvement ... We eventually reach a consensus. Now it's a little more remote because we're both so active with students. Now, we might write and rewrite before giving a draft to the other.

GC: The ART 1 paper was the first scoping out of many themes, plus theorems and simulations. Going through the thought processes of how to organize these things became very complex ...

SG: What I'm trying to remember is how we organized the front end of the paper. I think that we had to prepare for talks, and that always helps. That paper was a big struggle because it was much more mathematical than some readers really wanted, so we made sure the main ideas would be up front. Not everyone could get to the end of the paper, but they could at least get the main ideas.

GC: That was before the neural network field had crystallized. The paper was also written for more than one audience, psychologists, for example. I've had engineers say to me, "Why did you write all this stuff? Why didn't you just cut right to the equations?" And other people would say, "Why did you have the equations?" We would always try to give a road map at the beginning. It would say, "If equations are your language, skip to section 30." They were irritated that there were all the other sections that they had to leaf through. This situation is better now; there's more of a body of knowledge that's common to the field, although there are still communications problems.

SG: We realize that some of our papers create special difficulties. Our goal is to try, however imperfectly, to get as many potential readers as possible to know what the story is about, even if they don't want to follow the details. But then, who is the reader? As Gail said, there are some people who want the equations and not the psychological and neural interpretation, which for us is very important for guiding one's intuitions and design choices.

ER: You've succeeded with me. I can usually read the front ends of your papers.

SG: That was really a main goal. Over the years, I took very seriously criticisms such as "I have to read all your papers to understand any one of them." In fact, you might not know everything that led to a certain paper, but if you read it on its own terms, the model does what it does, in a self-contained way. But it is better up front to give the reader heuristics that will try to repeat and refer to other things. Some people say, "Why do you refer to all these papers?" But that's for people who want to know where to find background material. You can't win.

GC: One thing we've been putting in more and more, especially the last two or three years, is terse algorithmic specifications so that somebody—in almost a cookbook fashion if they want to replicate—can simulate each system. Back with ART 1, we still weren't doing that. Although you could pick the algorithm out of the paper, it took some effort. You'd have to read most of the paper to be able to do that. Implementing the algorithm is another way for somebody to read it, get a feel for the model, really learn it. That has helped a lot. Now, I also find huge demand from people who also want a packaged program, even if it's simple; they want to be able to start without even going through the step of programming.

ER: You had talked about how difficult it had been recently in the last few months, that you hadn't been able to do as much collaborating . . .

SG: We're really overloaded. What happened was that the Department of Cognitive and Neural Systems has grown very quickly. We're added nine professors since 1988, which in these times is a big investment for the University. Many smart kids applied and often we didn't have funding for them, but they were too good to reject. We said, "If you want to come, come." They came! We take very seriously our responsibility to train them. We meet with them in regular research meetings, and we help them to learn how to prepare lectures and papers and give them a lot of advice. We've really been working very hard to give them the level of support that we feel is necessary. Some of the collaborations have been running for some time.

GC: The graduate program has been a kind of collaboration between us that has been extremely important. In the sense of research, its results are just barely beginning to show. This has been very much a long-term capitalization of effort. Before the department was formed, Steve and I were co-directors of the graduate program. Then it became a graduate department, where Steve is Chairman, and I'm the Director of Graduate Studies. We split up responsibilities in much the way people split them up at home. It's been nice because among other things it's the first time I have ever taught in anything remotely like my research field. Before coming to BU, I had always taught mathematics.

SG: Gail helped me found the Center and the graduate program, and now she really is a co-chair with me, and I'm also director of the Center. It's been very much a team operation. However, one of the things we've been sensitive to is that, although we're married, we don't want people to resent that fact. I think it's worked pretty well. We really have a very friendly group of colleagues. We try to support one another personally and intellectually in a lot of different ways.

ER: Is there scientific work in the future that you're looking forward to collaborating on?

SG: We've already started talking about a variety of problems, like scene understanding and other higher-order cognitive processes for which basic understanding is lacking. We worked together on a problem related to how you generate multiplexed spatial maps. One reason we did that was because in dealing with problems of visual search and attentively organizing information to recognize objects, you need both spatial representations and categorical representations. We've already started talking about how you do complex scene understanding. That requires spatial analysis, categorization, temporal organization, plans. But, there were so many things going on already that we had to stop that for the moment to clean things up.

GC: I think some of the pieces that we're now working on individually with students are informed by these ideas as a longer-term goal. We used to have regular appointments and research meetings, but neither one of us had any time between the appointments to do anything. I think the very fact that we laid out these goals helps us to think more clearly about some of the individual components we're working on.

SG: I would say that a lot of the projects are heading toward higher-level system integration, even as we're developing, as a Department, new pieces of the brain puzzle. And one of the nicest things, one of the keys to the productivity of the Department, is its way of organizing cooperative, collaborative work.

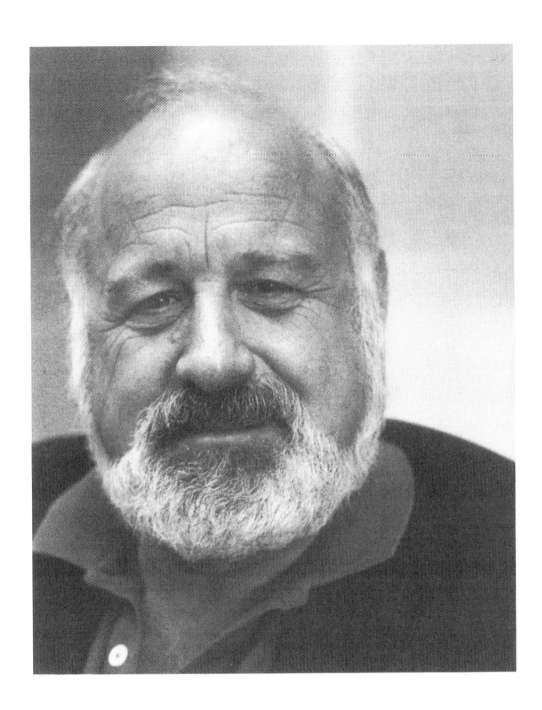

10   Michael A. Arbib

Michael Arbib is Professor of Computer Science, Neurobiology, Biomedical Engineering, Electrical Engineering, and Psychology and also Director of the USC Brain Project, both at the University of Southern California, Los Angeles, California. A good introduction to his work is in his 1989 book The Metaphorical Brain 2: Neural Networks and Beyond, *Wiley-Interscience. He was also Editor-in-Chief of the 1995 collection* The Handbook of Brain Theory and Neural Networks, *MIT Press, which contains brief articles describing the work of many of those interviewed for* Talking Nets.

September 1993, Providence, Rhode Island

ER: Why don't you tell me a little bit about your parents and your childhood?

MA: I was born in England in 1940 on May 28, which was the day of the evacuation of Dunkirk. My father had recently joined the army and had been in training camp and had managed to travel the length of England to come and join my mother. He then went off to war and served in the tank corps in North Africa. He had a South African general who capitulated rather too easily to the Germans and was shipped off to Italy, to a prisoner of war camp where, he told me, the only meat he got to eat was the maggots that rose to the top when they boiled the rice. Then the Italians capitulated and told their prisoners to wait and the Americans would come in the morning to liberate them, but the Germans came in at midnight and shipped them off to Germany, so my father had two years in a German prisoner of war camp. Rather a difficult time. One time the Germans asked for the names of all the people who were Jewish, including my father, but it turned out that being a British officer was sufficient protection, so he made it through the war. My mother must have done a wonderful job because I don't remember any problems when my father returned. He'd always been somehow a part of our life.

England was rather depressed in '45, so my father decided that we had to emigrate to get a better economic future and after considering just about every part of the world chose New Zealand. We got there in '47, but my parents found it very provincial, and my mother cried every night for her home and friends and family back in England. After a couple of business trips to Sydney, Dad decided that was a better place for us, so in '49 we moved to Australia, which is where I grew up. I was in high school there and then an undergraduate at Sydney University. When we get to it, that's where the story of neural networks starts for me. And then I went to MIT.

ER: What did your parents do? Your mother was at home?

MA: When we moved to Australia my father started by selling army surplus buildings and then eventually became a master builder, making or designing prefabricated buildings, mainly for factories, also shearing sheds. I remember working at a sheep show in Sydney, helping on the display stand for the shearing sheds. They also made copra dryers for New Guinea, so at one time Dad used to commute up to New Guinea from time to time on the flying boats. That was his career until he retired. My mother was always a very active person in the community. Then, at about the age of fifty-five she started a whole new career and became the Julia Child of Australia, publishing cookbooks. I think her cookbooks sold something like three hundred thousand copies. Given that that's just the Australian market, which is 5 percent of the American, that's a pretty incredible performance. She got to be quite a fixture on TV and the radio and the papers. I think that career lasted about eight years, and then she retired. She died three years ago. My father's since remarried. I had three sisters. One died at the age of eleven. She'd been born with a small hole in the heart and finally died of complications during surgery. The other two sisters are alive and well in Australia.

ER: And where are you in birth order?

MA: I was the oldest. Still am.

ER: And what were you like as a child growing up. How did you end up at MIT? Were you interested in things technical?

MA: Well, from the earliest age I was interested in mathematics. As a six-year-old, I was already reading the Meccano magazine. Meccano is like Erector sets. You build little things with pieces of metal and screws and pulleys and so on. Meccano put out a magazine which had lots of science articles as well as jokes and things to do with Meccano. So, I remember at about the age of eight giving a lecture on V-2 rockets, which I don't think was a great success with my schoolmates. When I went to Sydney, I went to a private school on scholarship because one of my dad's fellow prisoners of war had been a student there and had recommended it. And when I was eleven, I went to the high school. I had the good fortune of having a mathematics teacher named Fred Pollock, who normally just took the last two years but decided he would take one class all the way through the five years. In my first year of five years of high school he lent me *Mathematics and the Imagination* by Kasner and Newman, which is an introduction to everything up to topology. I would borrow it from him once a year and read it.

I had a very strong interest in mathematics. At the end of my five years at high school I came top of the state of New South Wales in the statewide examination on mathematics and then went to university. I started my freshman year in engineering because the father of a friend of mine had said that this was a good thing to do, but both of us quickly discovered we did not like engineering. I think for me the high point of my year as an engineer was that we had a course on stress and strain in beams. We went through the most incredible algebra and computations to come up with how thick the beams should be to carry the load. After all this, the lecturer then said, "But engineering practice says we make it twice as big." I realized this was not for me.

I founded an organization in the first year of university called the Useless Mathematics Mob, with the idea that, to be fun, mathematics should be totally inapplicable. It rather horrifies me that I did not remain true to the credo of my own organization. Anyway, computers were very primitive at that time but very alluring. There were lots of articles on computers as giant brains. We're now talking about 1957 through '60 when I was an undergraduate at Sydney University. This was long before the transistor had had an impact on computers. People like Edmund Berkeley wrote extrapolations that the computer of the future would need all the power of Niagara Falls to operate and cool it. We had a close family friend, a physicist named John Blatt, who was one of the most serious early users of computers in Australia. He would, every summer in Australia, fly off to New York for the winter where he would work at the Courant Institute at NYU, with their incredibly powerful 7090s, or whatever they were at the time. Incredibly powerful then, but some abysmal fraction of what your personal computer has these days.

Through him I learned something about computing. He arranged during my first summer vacation in Australia for me to work at Sydney University, where they had something called the Silliac, which stood for the Sydney version of the Illiac 2, the Illinois Automatic Computer. I must confess I don't remember very much about it except that all the programming was done on punched paper tape and that they had one program which would play "Waltzing Matilda" through the loudspeaker of the computer, doubling the speed on each repetition.

Anyway, that got me into computers, and then the other two summers that I was an undergraduate I worked at IBM, which was then newly established in Sydney. The IBM 650 was my computer, with all of two thousand words of memory on a rotating drum. Perhaps more important, I never really learned how to program well. In fact, one friend of mine said he was hired the following summer to debug all the programs I'd written the previous summer.

At that time I devoured not only Norbert Wiener's book, *Cybernetics*, but the original McCulloch-Pitts articles from '43 and '47 in the *Bulletin of Mathematical Biophysics*, and a lot of other things of that kind. It was about that period, during my third year to fourth year as an undergraduate (1959 and 1960) that I became very serious about neural networks and cybernetics. Networks at that time were a subset of cybernetics. I got very interested in automata theory. A paper by Rabin and Scott had just come out on the semi-group approach to finite automata in the *IBM Journal of Research and Development*. There were other papers. Copi, Elgot, and Wright had a paper in the *Journal of the ACM*, linking finite automata to formalized neural networks. A book called *Automata Studies* that was fairly new at that time, published in 1956 and edited by Shannon and McCarthy, was another influential book for me. Also at that time I found Martin Davis's book *Computability and Unsolvability*, [1958] which was a formal account of Turing machines and the theory that went with them and which had one joke in it—namely, the only figure was labeled "A Square of Turing Machine Tape." Everything else was immense formalism.

At that time we did not have Xerox machines, so either you wrote things out or you had photographs made of the pages. I read and wrote out Turing's original paper and found about thirty errors in it. I translated Gödel's original '31 paper with the help of a friend who was a student of German. At the same time I started reading a lot of heavy mathematics. I taught myself Lebesgue integration so I could read the proofs of the ergodic theorem because Khinchin, a Russian mathematician, had put out two little books, one on information theory and one on statistical mechanics, which made heavy use of ergodic theory. In Australia, the system at that time was that an undergraduate degree was three years, and then you took a fourth year if you wanted to do honors. It was not at all like the American system in which you got a general education. Basically, you enrolled in four subjects the first year, three subjects the second year, two the third, and then one the fourth, where each subject of a course expanded the number of lectures to more than fill the week. I think we were doing well over twenty hours of lectures a week.

So my first year was engineering, mathematics, physics, chemistry; my second year was pure mathematics, applied mathematics; and statistics; my third year was pure and applied mathematics; and my fourth year was pure mathematics. In my fourth year, I started looking for where to go for graduate school. By that time, through my reading, I knew of Wiener and Shannon and Minsky and McCarthy, who were at that time all at MIT, so MIT was very high on my list of places to go.

ER: McCulloch was there too.

MA: But, you see, I didn't know that at first when I applied. I had read all the classic McCulloch papers, which were from the University of Illinois Medical School. In Wiener's book he talks about McCulloch as a colleague back at Illinois. I had become friends with a lecturer, which is sort of like an assistant professor, in the medical school, a neurophysiologist named Bill Levick. Levick was working with Professor Peter Bishop on the visual system of the cat. Bill had decided he needed to know more mathematics, so we did a deal where I would help him with his mathematics and he would let me watch him and Professor Bishop do terrible things to cats. It was he who showed me, for the first time, the 1959 paper, pretty much hot off the press, on "What the Frog's Eye Tells The Frog's Brain," by Lettvin, Maturana, McCulloch, and Pitts [reprinted in *Neurocomputing 2*], which is a very significant paper in my life. That was when I learned that McCulloch, and Pitts were at MIT; they'd moved there apparently in 1952.

In terms of applying to graduate school, at that time the tradition was for essentially all mathematicians from Sydney University to go to Cambridge, England, for their Ph.D.s. I had applied there and never got a reply. Then twelve years later a professor, the same professor with the son who had recommended that I go to engineering in my freshman year, Professor V. A. Bailey—I don't think that anybody knew what his first name was; he was just V. A. Bailey—died, and they emptied out his mailbox, and there at the back was the reply from Cambridge to my application for Ph.D. studies, which had somehow gotten lodged in the back of his box and never been found. I wrote them a letter declining their offer on the grounds that I'd already received my Ph.D. ten years earlier. They never replied.

So that was why I didn't go to Cambridge. I did get admitted to NYU on a full scholarship, but MIT admitted me too, and it was clear by that time that everyone, so to speak, was at MIT. It was the end of the golden age of cybernetics. So I went.

Australians live at home, usually, when they go to University, so this was the first time I had been away from home except for an occasional journey. I remember traveling halfway around the world, leaving the summer of Australia and arriving in one of the bitterest winters in living memory in Cambridge. I visited relatives in New York, took the bus up to Boston, and then took a cab to MIT. We went along Storrow Drive, and there was the totally frozen Charles River, with this wonderful view of MIT on the other side. I remember just looking out of the cab thinking, "My God, you'd better be worth it." But it was, it was.

A friend who'd preceded me by a year or two to study chemistry at Harvard helped me find an apartment on Massachusetts Avenue. The first thing I did when I arrived was to visit the mathematics department and met Gian-Carlo Rota and Ken Hoffman, the first two mathematicians I encountered. Somewhere along the line I went into the main lobby just off Mass. Avenue and phoned McCulloch, with whom I'd had no previous contact. He was very welcoming and told me to come right over. I was sure I had made a mistake because his voice sounded so young, but when I got there, there he was with his famous white beard. Some time later he explained how he had once been in a southern town and a little boy had come up to him and looked up and said, "Are you de Lord?" I can't remember whether he said yes or no.

As an undergraduate, for my fourth year paper, my senior thesis as you'd call it here, I had written what later became a paper published in the *Journal of the ACM* in 1961, called "Finite Automata, Turing Machines, and Neural Networks." That was my first publication in neural networks.

In my first term at MIT I was a TA and was disappointed that a TA didn't teach; all I got to do was grade homework in linear algebra. I remember being amazed at how bad students at MIT were. I had had the fantasy— well, the fear, really—that I would go from being one of the top students in Australia to being at the bottom of the pack because here was MIT with the crème de la crème. Once I started grading undergraduate linear algebra, all my fears were destroyed!

McCulloch adopted me, and I became an RA in his group. Those were the good old days when there was lots of money around so that being an RA was not particularly onerous. Basically, the Navy and other agencies gave lots of money to MIT and MIT funneled it to various people, and Warren was one of the good guys, so he had quite a lot of money to support bright young students.

The big thing that Warren McCulloch was worried about at that time was reliability: how is it that neural networks can still function although we know there are lots of perturbations? His favorite story on this line was a midnight call from John von Neumann from Princeton saying, "Warren, I've drunk a whole bottle of absinthe, and I know the thresholds of all my neurons are shot to hell. How is it I can still think?" That was the motivating problem.

That's what Jack Cowan was working on at that time with Shmuel (Sam) Winograd, who later became a very high level person at IBM. What McCulloch had done was to handcraft small networks, making little Venn diagrams and then showing how, as the threshold shifted, if you designed the network right, you could have reasonable insensitivity to the change in threshold and still get the network to perform pretty much as advertised. Jack and Sam took a different approach, where they took Shannon's theory of reliable communication in the presence of noise and said, "What if we think of the neurons as doing a process of computing, rather than coding, and we try to make the redundancy in the network fit in with Shannon's ideas?" Their book came out a year or so later, *Reliable Computation in the Presence of Noise* [1963].

I think that the most influential thing in McCulloch's group for me at that time was his partnership with a guy named Bill Kilmer, who I think had come in from Michigan, later went to Montana, and eventually joined me at the University of Massachusetts. Bill was working with Warren on the idea of the reticular formation as a mode selector. Warren had been influenced by the idea that the reticular formation is involved in switching the overall organism between sleep and wakefulness. These were ideas from Magoun on the waking brain, and Warren had extended that to the idea that there were various modes of behavior.

There's a joke in neuroscience, which is due to Karl Pribram, about the limbic system being responsible for the four Fs: Feeding, Fighting, Fleeing, and Reproduction. It was Warren's idea to extend the sleep-wakefulness idea so that perhaps the reticular formation was responsible for switching the overall state of the organism. There would be one part of the brain that would say, well, is this a feeding situation or a fleeing or whatever situation, and then the rest of the brain, when set into this mode, could do the more detailed computations. Mode switching.

The other part of the equation came from Arnie and Madge Scheibel, who were a husband and wife anatomy team at UCLA. Arnie is still alive and well, but his wife died many years ago. They had done some lovely studies of the reticular formation and had observed that the anatomy was such that the dendritic trees ran roughly parallel to each other and orthogonal to the fibers running up and down the axis of the reticular formation. They had suggested a poker chip analogy—that you could replace all the detail by a stack of poker chips, where there'd be a lot of cells in each chip, but because of the way the dendrites were placed, they would have roughly homogeneous input and output. This suggested to Warren and Bill Kilmer the idea of modeling the reticular formation as a stack of modules corresponding to the anatomical poker chips. Each one would have a slightly different selection of input, but each would be trying to make up its mind as to which mode to go into. They would communicate back and forth, competing and cooperating until finally they reached a consensus on the basis of their divergent input and that would switch the mode of organization.

In looking back, I think that the ideas in that paper were a tremendous influence on me because they said two things. One was that if you're going to study very complicated neural networks, you shouldn't do it all at one level, that you need an intermediate level, in this case their modules. This later became the basis for my theory of schemas, where I replace the anatomical modules by functional schemas, but the idea was that you need a high-level language in which to explain the functional interactions rather than mapping everything immediately down onto the neural net. And the second thing was the notion of competition and cooperation.

At that time there were two ways of thinking about neural networks that I was aware of. One was the stuff that I'd done my first paper on—namely, the fact that you could build any finite automaton using a neural network. You could express the state of the system as the firing of the neurons in it, and then the input together with the state would determine the next state. You could set up the wiring in such a way as to represent any finite-state transition you cared to look at. Then of course if you added it to a control box to run a tape, you had a Turing machine and universal computation. That was the result that really went back to the '43 McCulloch-Pitts paper but written there in an unintelligible way.

In fact, one of the first things I did when I got to MIT was go to see Walter Pitts, to go over with him the '43 paper because there were some obscurities in the logic. Pitts had adopted the logical notation of Rudolf Carnap and had written an almost impenetrable paper, so in many cases I had to rederive the results rather than follow their proofs. I wanted to check with Pitts that I had got it right. It was a terrible meeting. We got about two sentences into the conversation, and Pitts started shaking and wouldn't stop, so I had to leave. It turned out he was already far gone into the DTs.

McCulloch's story was that Walter Pitts, as a fourteen-year-old, had been about to be forced by his family—which was very poor at the time, early in World War II—to leave school and go and work to raise money for the family. By chance, he was sitting on a park bench when he got into conversation with an elderly man, and fortunately for him the elderly man was Bertrand Russell, who introduced him to Carnap. Carnap knew that Warren McCulloch, who was then in Chicago, was interested in making a logical theory of the brain and brought the two together, and that's what led to the classic McCulloch and Pitts partnership. That led to a long period in which Pitts, who was an ugly but very bright person, became sort of an adopted son of the McCullochs. Unfortunately, he was terribly insecure and wasn't prepared to be loved for his brilliance; he wanted to be loved for his looks, and he had no looks. It was a very strange relationship, I think, where Pitts was the child and yet, in some ways, intellectually the more powerful of the pair, though McCulloch knew an incredible amount about the brain and had been a very successful anatomist and still was at that time. Apparently, because of all these different psychological pressures, Pitts eventually went the way of drink. I think for many years Lettvin became essentially his guardian and managed to have him maintain a research position at MIT even though he was long past being a brilliant achiever.

As I was saying, there were two views about neural nets at the start of the '60s. One was that you could build any finite automaton and the other was the beginning of learning theory. That time was pretty early. Basically, we had the perceptron from Rosenblatt, there was some work from Taylor in England, and a few other beginnings. We were just making the transition into thinking about what has become the sine qua non for most people of neural nets today—learning theory. What was missing in the two conceptions—(a) you could do anything, and (b) you could learn how to do it—was the notion that you should think of a more complicated system in which there were subsystems interacting. Those could be not necessarily doing the same thing, with each having well-assigned jobs; each could be competing. It might have part of the truth, and then some process of interaction was required, so then there's competition and cooperation. The notion of the multilevel view was I think the biggest lesson I got from my time with McCulloch.

I also met Norbert Wiener very early in the piece and ended up as his Ph.D. student, but it turned out to my disappointment that Wiener was not very interested in cybernetics anymore and was devoting himself to statistical mechanics. But, since he was the great founder of cybernetics and I really wanted to understand how his mind worked, I signed up to do a thesis in his area. Then Norbert Wiener went on sabbatical, and during about six months I only got one letter from him. It was a charming letter, which I've kept, saying that he'd visited Cordoba in Spain where he had paid homage to Moses Maimonides, the great medieval Jewish philosopher, whom he claimed as an ancestor, but this really wasn't advancing me very much in the field of statistical mechanics. I turned to Henry P. McKean Jr., who was a superb probability theorist with some interest in statistical mechanics and transferred to him. After a while we decided this was not the right subject, and I ended up putting in a thesis proposal for fractional integration, which ties in very much with the current mathematics of fractals. The idea was that in a lot of applied mathematics there was a great interest in white noise–driven processes. McKean and Kyoshi Ito had written a lot on an approach to stochastic integration, so I proposed to generalize it to a much broader class of stochastic processes. But, unfortunately, I succeeded too well and found a very simple way of doing it. The day before my Ph.D. defense McKean asked me to take a walk. I knew what he was going to say, but cruelly enough I let him go ahead and suffer through saying it—namely, please write another Ph.D. thesis. So I said OK.

This may have had a very big impact on my orientation as a scientist because I had already been accepted for a full summer course at the Rand Corporation, run by Allen Newell and his colleagues, on his approach to artificial intelligence [AI]. Had I spent the summer at RAND I might well have ended up with a much more conventional AI career than I have had. Instead, I went off from Boston to rural New England because McKean lived in a small village north of Hanover, New Hampshire. Hanover was where Dartmouth College sat, and since that was the nearest mathematics library, that's where I spent the summer, driving up to McKean's house once a week past the little red school house and through the covered bridge, and turning left at Waldo Peterson's place—and so grew to love New England. I managed over that summer to write another thesis and finish. The one sad story about that was that when I went to pick up my diploma in September of '63, I discovered that MIT had written the title of the thesis on the diploma itself, but they had the title of the rejected thesis not the actual thesis. What I regret is that at that time I made them change the title. I wish now, of course, that I had the amusing diploma rather than the correct diploma, but never mind.

Actually, a lot happened in the two and a half years that I was at MIT, besides the Ph.D., which was just a small part of it. There was a lot of involvement with McCulloch's group. One of the interesting things about the involvement was that McCulloch had told me not to tell Wiener about it.

Wiener had been a child prodigy and had to the end of his days retained many of the marks of his childhood as a prodigy. He was in many ways insecure, would need a lot of praise, and was in no way a judge of human character. He had published two books called *Ex-Prodigy* and *I Am a Mathematician*. Cruel people said they should be called *Ex-Mathematician* and *I Am a Prodigy*, but, in fact, he was a very great mathematician until the end of his days. In this century the American Mathematical Society has only twice published memorial issues of its "Bulletin," one to honor John von Neumann and the other for Norbert Wiener. I think it's very interesting that they did that because these are both men who helped found the study of cybernetics and neural networks. They're also men whose work spanned from applications to very deep pure mathematics. Wiener was a great man, but perhaps a defective human being.

McCulloch had been a very strong neuroanatomist and the work he did with Pitts and the later work on the reliability problem showed his lifelong devotion to trying to see how to bring the methods of logic to bear in the appropriate way to probe the nervous system. On the other hand, he was a romantic, and he would rather tell a good story than be totally shackled by all the facts.

I remember once a plane ride with Jack Eccles, the Australian Nobel Laureate in neurophysiology. We both had been at a meeting in Boston. At that time I was living in Stanford, he was living in Chicago, and so we flew as far as Chicago together. He was really anti-McCulloch because of McCulloch's somewhat romantic way of handling the facts. What I pointed out to him was that most of us who worked with McCulloch had enough sense to accept the inspiration of his ideas but knew that we then had to do the hard work of finding out which of his ideas were supported by the literature and which weren't. In this way, a lot of young people had really gained a great deal of insight into the nervous system and a great deal of inspiration for their careers from Warren. The other thing about Warren was at that time he was drinking a lot. But where it caused the DTs in poor Pitts, for Warren a bottle or so of Scotch was just the key to loquaciousness. For people like myself who saw a lot of him, it was a bit of a pain because the same stories would come out again and again, but for people who were seeing him for the first time, it was always extremely stimulating and motivating.

I finished my Ph.D. and was going around MIT paying my farewell respects and found myself in Norbert's office for the last time. So we're chatting, and he says, "What else have you been doing while you're here?" and I think to myself, "Oh, it won't hurt to tell him," and I said, "Well, I've been working with McCulloch," and immediately Wiener went into an apoplectic fit and said, "Why, that man, that wretched man, why, if I had the money I'd buy him a case of whiskey so he could drink himself to death." Wouff!! So I spent the next fifteen minutes trying to be loyal to McCulloch while soothing Wiener.

I discussed this reaction with a number of colleagues. The best explanation I have—I have no independent confirmation of it, but it rings so true with the characters of the protagonists that I refuse not to believe it—came from Pat Wall, an expert on the neurophysiology of the pain system. Many years before, in the '50s, buoyed by the success of his book on cybernetics, Norbert had decided to develop "the" theory of the brain. So he had gone to Warren and said, "Warren, tell me all about the brain, and what the open problems are," and Warren had told him. But, of course, Warren had told a somewhat romantic story, and Norbert, being no judge of human character, had not understood this and took it all as a totally objective presentation of the state of play. He had then spent two years developing a theory to explain all these "facts," and when he presented the theory at a physiological congress, he was howled down. Instead of realizing what the situation was, he thought McCulloch had deliberately set him up, thus robbing him of two years of his life and his chance to establish a great theory. This is Pat Wall's explanation. I must say it jibes so well with the character of both men that I'm prepared to believe it.

A year and a half into my graduate studies (in mid-1962) I went back to Australia for a summer. I left the summer in the northern hemisphere for the winter in the southern hemisphere. I gave a course called "Brains, Machines, and Mathematics" at the University of New South Wales. At that time they had a radio station that broadcast courses, so they asked me to write up notes for this, which could then be sent out to subscribers. I would speak over the air with the notes in front of me to refer to figures and so on. When I came back to MIT, I showed these notes to McCulloch, and he encouraged me to go ahead and publish them. I had the interesting experience of sitting in McKean's office discussing my Ph.D. thesis with him when the McGraw-Hill representative came in to talk to the student, not the professor.

We could talk the whole day just about MIT. We haven't talked about the ineffable Jack Cowan yet. Amongst the other people I immediately went to see were Minsky and McCarthy, who I knew from the automata studies book which came out in 1956, the year that McCarthy, at a conference held in Dartmouth, gave the name "artificial intelligence" to a new offshoot of cybernetics. In that book Minsky was still writing on neural nets, material from his Ph.D. thesis, while McCarthy was talking about logical issues that continued throughout his career to the present day. Anyway, I arrived at Minsky's office the day in 1961 he got his reprints for "Steps towards Artificial Intelligence," which is one of the two or three founding papers in the subject of artificial intelligence. It's actually an interesting paper to go back to now because although it is one of the opening salvos in the battle for artificial intelligence, it has a lot of very good neural net theory in it, reflecting some of his work with Oliver Selfridge.

Jack Cowan did not have a Ph.D. at the time, although his knowledge and experience made him essentially a postdoctoral researcher in McCulloch's group. I've already mentioned that he had taken a novel approach to the work of McCulloch on reliability and with Winograd had pushed it a long way further through bringing in ideas of information theory. When I went back to Australia and gave my lectures on "Brains, Machines and Mathematics," one chapter was an exposition of Shannon's information theory and of the new work with Winograd. Jack seemed more upset that I had got some mileage out of his work in my book than he recognized his luck that his work was being publicized in a way that went beyond the circulation of his MIT Press monograph.

I remember a conference held in Dayton, Ohio, at about that time, on bionics. This field comes up with different names. It was cybernetics for a while, then it was bionics, now it's neural networks. Who knows what it will be next year? What I remember vividly about this meeting in Dayton, Ohio, was a man named Jack Steele, who was one of the monitors of the bionics program for the Air Force. He had a delicious definition of bionics: "The life sciences in the service of the death sciences."

The Minsky and Papert book *Perceptrons* came out of that period. Minsky and Papert basically said that if you limit your networks to one layer in depth, then, unless you have very complicated individual neurons, you can't do very much. This is not too surprising. It's hard to see why this was taken as a serious critique of neural networks. It's like saying to computer hackers that if you can't have any loops in your code, and you only have ten instructions, then serial computers are really very limited!

Many people see the book as what killed neural nets, but I really don't think that's true. I think that the funding priorities, the fashions in computer science departments, had shifted the emphasis away from neural nets to the more symbolic methods of AI by the time the book came out. I think it was more that a younger generation of computer scientists who didn't know the earlier work may have used the book as justification for sticking with "straight AI" and ignoring neural nets. I don't think it played a role in the actual power struggle that was only reversed in the early '80s.

After getting my Ph.D. I did a lot of traveling. I hired a car and drove all around the States and got to meet a lot of people. Then, in the first half of '65, I did a sort of postdoc with Jack Cowan, who had returned to Imperial College, where he had done his diploma before going to Warren. He was now in the department of Dennis Gabor, the inventor of the hologram. When I arrived at Imperial College, Professor John Westcott, head of control theory there, announced that in a couple of months they were having a conference on control theory, and would I like to give a paper? With complete flippancy, knowing almost nothing about control theory, I said, "Oh, sure, why not?"

And he said, "Well, what will you talk about there?"

And I said, "Well, the rapprochement between automata theory and control theory."

And then some weeks later, not having known my twisted sense of humor, he said, "Where's your paper?"

I said, "What paper?"

He said, "The one on the rapprochement between automata theory and control theory." So I got cracking on a book by Zadeh and Desoer and on Kalman's papers and came up with a paper on the rapprochement between automata theory and control theory! (I had met Lotfi Zadeh in Berkeley and Rudolf Kalman in Baltimore during my post-Ph.D. tour of the United States.) That became very important for my non–neural net life. Jack Cowan and I were not totally compatible, and he was working on his Ph.D. thesis at the time, which was on statistical mechanics. We never clicked in terms of doing any joint work together.

I did get to know Dennis Gabor, which was a pleasure. *Brains, Machines, and Mathematics* [1964] came out while I was there, and to my pleasure and amazement Jacob Bronowski, a very well-known writer on the history of ideas and the implications of science, wrote the lead review in *Scientific American* on the subject of my book. I think this was not so much because of the merit of the book, but the fact that Wiener had just died, and so cybernetics was a hot topic at that time. Similarly, Stephen Toulmin, a very well-known philosopher, wrote an article on "The Importance of Being Wiener" in the *New York Review of Books*, which referred to my book, and it included the phrase "even Michael Arbib says," which made my twenty-four-year-old day. The review then went to disagree with what I was saying, but the idea that I was referred to as if I were a known authority was very gratifying indeed. It's sort of sad when you peak at twenty-four! None of my books has ever sold as many copies or been so prominently reviewed since.

Until about June of '64 it had been my intention to go back to Australia to teach. But around May or June I got offers from both Zadeh and Kalman to postdoc with them. Kalman had just moved to Stanford. In the end I decided to accept Kalman's offer. In June of '65 I went to Stanford.

Kalman, Peter Falb, who was in the applied mathematics department at Brown for many many years, and I gave a series of lectures that summer. Peter's ambition was always to get on the faculty at Harvard. He was very rich but was a big gambler and one of those people who hate to fly. One weekend we flew to Las Vegas, and he was terrified the whole way. He gave me a system for playing craps. I happened to get lucky. I had taken, I think, a hundred dollars, feeling that was an immense stake at that time in my fiscal career. I was doling it out in five dollar increments, and there was a guy at the table with a roll of hundreds, peeling them off. I made five hundred dollars, which at that time was probably about half a month's salary. On that basis, I increased the frequency of transpacific phone calls to a young woman, Prue Hassell, I had met a month before leaving Australia for Stanford. That proved fateful. When I went home for Christmas, I proposed to Prue on the seventeenth of December '65, we married on the twenty-ninth, and then she went back to her parents in Western Australia. I flew off to Stanford, and we haven't seen each other since. No, no, she came three weeks later, and we're still together.

Anyway, those lectures at Stanford became another book, called *Topics in Mathematical System Theory*, which is a fairly classic book in mathematical system theory. That started five years at Stanford. I don't know how it happened, but after six months as research associate for Kalman in the Department of Engineering Mechanics, I suddenly became an assistant professor of Electrical Engineering at Stanford, despite my dismal experience in first year engineering at Sydney University.

Back to neural nets. About this time, automata and neural nets were really sort of the same thing. Neural nets didn't have an independent life. They were part of automata theory. But the paper on "What the Frog's Eye Tells the Frog's Brain" had been gnawing at me. I got in contact with David Ingle at McLean Hospital in Boston, who had been doing more recent experiments on frog vision. The one that really got me going showed a frog two flies, and the frog snapped at one of them. This may not seem surprising, but it struck me that this was the real transition from Lettvin's theme of "What the Frog's Eye Tells the Frog's Brain" to "What the Frog's Eye Tells the Frog"—that is, how the frog uses this visual information to guide its behavior. This was a real turning point for me.

I had a student named Rich Didday in electrical engineering at Stanford who did a Ph.D. thesis with me on modeling this stuff. He spent some time in Ingle's lab, and the thesis came out in '70. I haven't checked the history, but the thesis certainly provided one of the first Winner-Take-All [WTA] networks, if not the first. We wanted to know how the frog's brain could take a map of where the flies were and, without serial computing, decide which one to snap at. I think some people in Reichardt's lab came up with another Winner-Take-All circuit at about the same time.

The other thing this work really established was the notion of action-oriented perception. At that time, work on vision was dominated by Hubel and Wiesel, by Horace Barlow, and so on. Even at that time, vision was an area in which modelers and physiologists talked to each other. I think the dominant view of vision then was to look at it as an autonomous module, extracting information to reconstruct the structure of the environment. By contrast, I was concerned with how vision was used to control action. It is only in the last few years that the theme of action-oriented perception has reemerged to become a very powerful paradigm in the vision community at large. Finally, people in vision and people in robotics are really talking together about the notion that you don't want to do general purpose visual computing, but, rather, want to have different modules extracting different types of visual information. Jumping ahead a long way: in the late '80s people like van Essen showed the visual system in the brain is not a hierarchy, as Hubel and Wiesel thought, where you start with visual area V1 and then just extract a series of more and more abstract descriptions. Instead, vision involves many areas linked in different pathways. One area knows a lot about color, another knows a lot about motion, another knows a lot about depth, and so on. The idea is that the brain is extracting many different aspects of the world, related to different types of processes, in some cases fairly directly related to motion and to action, in other cases much more abstract. This is a paradigm that has now reemerged and fits well with my frog-inspired view of action-oriented perception around 1970.

By the time I left Stanford in 1970, there was a balance between trying to understand the real brain, as shown in the work on the frog, and abstract neural network theory. I took two Ph.D. students with me to my next place —Parvati Dev, working on depth perception, and Curtis Boylls, working on cerebellum.

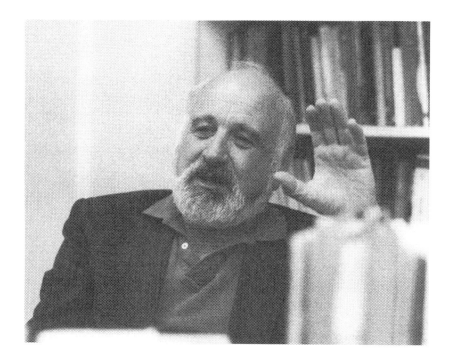

I moved to the University of Massachusetts to become chairman of computer science. This happened because I'd had to spend the summer in New England to finish the Ph.D. thesis. A man named Bill Marsh had been a graduate student at Dartmouth at the time I was there finishing my Ph.D., and we had become friends. He had moved to Amherst to help found a new college, Hampshire College. In 1969–70, the year before Hampshire College opened to students, the faculty had set up a public lecture series core as a way of getting the other colleges to begin to integrate Hampshire College into their intellectual life. I'd accepted an invitation on the basis of our friendship of six years earlier. A little while before my trip east I received a phone call from Conrad Wogrin who had become the director of computing services at the University of Massachusetts at Amherst. We had met about a year or two before, when he was still at Yale. He'd come to ask the faculty at Stanford if they had any hot young Ph.D.s to nominate for recruiting for Yale, and the half hour we'd spent together had stuck in his memory so that, when he had the charge of looking for a new head of computer science at U. Mass., he thought of me. I was twenty-nine at the time and should have said no, and would have said no, but I was going to be in Amherst anyway, so why not go for an interview? Then I think ego got the better of me, and the idea of being appointed chairman and full professor before I turned thirty was too much for me. I think what really gratified me, apart from the crude ego trip, was that they did not have a Ph.D. program, and the charter for the new chairman was not only to be chair but to put together the proposal for a new Ph.D. program. What I proposed to them was that they were already reasonably strong in computer systems, but didn't have much in theory, and nothing in what I was still calling cybernetics. So I proposed a three-part view of the department: systems, theory, and cybernetics. The dean agreed to it.

So I left Stanford and moved to U. Mass., where I established this department, a sort of bittersweet story in a way. I was able to hire Bill Kilmer, who had been a colleague at MIT in the McCulloch days. The first year or two after Bill arrived things worked very well, but then he went through a period where there was just no money available for the sort of brain modeling he wanted to do. He became incredibly depressed and basically left the field of brain modeling and started doing ecological modeling. So, unfortunately, there I was with a full professor I had hired to work with me on neural modeling, and his research had stopped. Another coup, it seemed at the time, was to hire Nico Spinelli, who had been a colleague of Karl Pribram's at Stanford University, a very inventive visual neurophysiologist with a real interest in modeling. I don't know what happened. We had a few productive years from him, and then he just stopped doing any science. However, one good thing that came out of this was that Spinelli and I were able to attract some money from Harry Klopf at the Air Force. At that time, Klopf had a theory of the hedonistic neuron, which was really a metaphor rather than a theory. We were able to show him that with Nico's work on the plasticity of the visual system and the modeling skills that Kilmer and I had, U. Mass. would be a good place for him to deposit some money and try to turn his metaphors into solid science. Unfortunately, I can't take any credit for this, but Kilmer and Spinelli hired a young man who had finished his Ph.D. at Michigan and moved to SUNY Binghampton—namely, Andrew Barto. With the help of a graduate student named Rich Sutton that Harry Klopf had recommended we support after he graduated from Stanford, Andy really figured out how to take these relatively wild ideas of Harry's and turn them into an interesting theory of learning in neural networks that has now established itself as the immensely influential approach called reinforcement learning.

For three years, Kilmer, Spinelli, and I had funding for what we called the Center for Systems Neuroscience from the Sloan Foundation. For me, the first year of the Center (1975–76) was the most fruitful, since I had the pleasure of working with two superb visiting Fellows—with Shun-Ichi Amari of Tokyo on "Competition and Cooperation in Neural Nets," and with Israel Lieblich of Jerusalem on the World Graph model of motivated learning in spatial behavior.

The money ran out for the center after three years because the Sloan Foundation decided to switch its support from neuroscience to cognitive science. So I decided that, what the hell, what I was doing could be called cognitive science. Meanwhile, Barbara Partee, who had been a fellow graduate student at MIT—she in linguistics, I in mathematics—was then on the faculty of linguistics at U. Mass., with her husband Eamon Bach. She had been on one of the panels that Sloan had brought in to discuss cognitive science, and I think I had been on another one. We each talked to Ken Klivington, who was then our contact at Sloan. He told us we should talk to each other! And so we put in a series of proposals for three rounds of cognitive science funding. We were successful on the first two, but not on the third. This led to a very good period in which, first, it was linguistics and computer science, then we brought in psychology and philosophy, and then we brought in people from the other colleges in the area. I believe the cognitive science program is still doing well, although unfortunately since my departure computer science has become much more straight computer science rather than interdisciplinary.

Perhaps the most surprising outcome of that period was from a conversation in Edinburgh (where I spent a sabbatical year in 1976–77) with Donald Michie, who was both the grand old man and enfant terrible of artificial intelligence, or machine intelligence as he called it, in Edinburgh. There's something called the Gifford lectures in natural theology, which have been running for about the last hundred years. They've generated some wonderful books like *Man on His Nature* by Sherrington and *Process and Reality* by Whitehead. I said to Donald Michie—in one of those joking tones of voice one uses for something which one sort of means, but when one doesn't want to be offended if the person laughs if they don't take it seriously—saying, well, it would be fun to give the Gifford lectures.

Instead of laughing, he said, "Yes, that would be great. We haven't had anybody in artificial intelligence except Longuet-Higgins," and so he started lobbying for it. He lobbied, but he also suggested that a theologian share the lectures with me.

After about three years I got the invitation to give the Gifford lectures in natural theology at the University of Edinburgh in 1983 and the news that they would be shared with Mary Hesse, who was not a theologian, but a philosopher of science who had a big interest in philosophy of religion. We had never met each other, we didn't know each other's work, but it turned out to be a good choice. We had three years to get ready to give the lectures together.

I put to Mary the notion that we would write a book together, and then each of us would base our lectures on certain chapters that would have already been our joint effort. We met twice in Cambridge in her college and once at U. Mass., and slowly built this book.

The theme was "The Construction of Reality," which is a Piagetian theme, looking at the way in which the schemas we already have shape the way we make sense of the world to create new schemas. I approached that as a person who has done brain modeling and artificial intelligence and robotics in terms of the schemas in the head, whereas Mary, from her work in history and philosophy of science, was more concerned with the social construction of reality: how do a group of scientists come to agree on a theory given its underdetermination by the facts? We finally forged, I think, a coherent epistemology where we brought together the schemas as social structures and the schemas as things in the head, with, for example, language learning being a nice case: it's not that there's a canonical grammar somewhere that you're instructed in; rather, you interact with the whole community using language. You build up in your own head a representation of that language, and then you become part of the environment for somebody else acquiring the language.

We took seriously the natural theology charge for the lectures, and we agreed to disagree about two small issues. One was the freedom of the will, and the other was the existence of God! On the freedom of the will, I took the view that freedom is basically a social construct, whereas Mary wanted there to be some quantum indeterminacy of the type Jack Eccles uses. As for God, she believed, and I did not.

JA: I still don't know what natural theology is.

MA: Natural theology is the attempt to infer the nature of the Creator from the nature of His creation. You look at nature and say, "What would God have to be like to have created the world or the universe or humans this way?" It was the attempt of nineteenth-century theologians and scientists to reconcile their knowledge.

There was a precursor of the Gifford lectures in the early 1800s called the Bridgewater Treatises. One of those is a wonderful book that I've used in my work, by Sir Charles Bell. He wrote it before Darwin. He looked at how the fin of the whale, the hand of different animals, and the hand of the human share a basic ground plan. In a few years Darwin could see this as evidence for natural selection, but Bell saw it in terms of the parsimony of God's design. There were ten Bridgewater Treatises, and Babbage—he of the universal computing machine of the early 1800s—wrote the eleventh Bridgewater Treatise, which was not an official one, where he expressed his views on natural theology in light of his discoveries on the computing engine.

In 1983, these ideas became the series of lectures that Mary and I gave together in Edinburgh and a few years later became a book, *The Construction of Reality*, [1986] which never took off, but seems to crop up from time to time.

I was in Amherst for sixteen years. Unfortunately, Kilmer and Spinelli had dropped out of neuroscience. Andy Barto was very good, and eventually transferred from research associate to assistant professor and so on, but there were no new slots opening up for neural nets. However, our reputation grew, so we attracted lots of very good students.

In the early to mid-1980s, some of the people in biology and psychology decided to put together an interdisciplinary neuroscience program. The first proposal they put out had the word "empirical" in front of the noun "neuroscience" at each occurrence, and neither Andy Barto nor I were on the list of faculty. The dean hit the roof when he saw this and got me in to help rewrite the proposal. For once, I was diplomatic and restrained, but in a sense it put the writing on the wall. We had a computer science department that was very good. I had very good relations with my colleagues. There were lots of interesting ideas in computer vision, distributed artificial intelligence, robotics, cognitive science, but it wasn't going anywhere in terms of the number of faculty available for neural networks in the department. Meanwhile, the experimentalists in neuroscience, instead of being excited at having a distinguished program of brain modeling on campus, saw it as either irrelevant or threatening.

Prue and I, with our son Benjamin (our daughter Pippa was away at school) spent a year's leave at UCSD in La Jolla in '85–'86. The chancellor there, Richard Atkinson, had been a colleague at Stanford, where I'd run a faculty seminar on memory and perception which he had attended. Shortly after we arrived in La Jolla, I went and had a short conversation to pay my respects to Atkinson. About five minutes into the conversation he said, "Would you like a job here?"

So I said, "Well, I'll have to discuss it with my wife." Prue comes from Perth in Western Australia, which has a southern California climate, and she expressed the opinion that sixteen New England winters were quite enough. So I went back to Atkinson and said, "OK, great, Prue and I would really like that, what do we do?"

He said, "Well, you have to realize that this is a very democratic university, so I can't do anything about it myself, but I'll set up an appointment for you with the dean of engineering." So about a month later I got my appointment with the dean of engineering. I go in and I know things are not going to work well when the first thing he says is, "Somebody sent me your CV," not, "The chancellor sent me your CV." Anyway, I have an hour in which I tell him how great it would be for UCSD and me if they hired me, at the end of which I say, "Well, what do we do next?"

I heard, "Oh, well, I can't do anything. You must understand, this is a very democratic university. The invitation has to come from the computer science department."

Eventually, the one contact I had in the computer science department set up a dinner at which he invited the chairman, and I had this incredible feeling of sort of crawling across the floor and saying, "Excuse me, but, er, the chancellor says maybe I'd like a job here, and the dean says he can't do anything about it, so could you possibly interview me for a job here please?" So I had an interview and the faculty, with the exception of my friend, voted unanimously against me. I suppose the generous theory would be that they decided that the study of the brain and neural networks was not a proper part of the charge of the computer science department. My wife's theory was that they felt threatened by my energy. So that was the end of UCSD.

By this time, Prue had gotten it into her head that we really were going to leave Massachusetts and live in sunny California. At that stage, another Stanford contact, an Australian who was by then head of electrical engineering at Santa Barbara, invited us up, and I interviewed there. Everything went wonderfully. Then some faculty blew the whistle on the chancellor, who had, it turned out, spent $135,000 dollars of university funds renovating his kitchen on the grounds that he had to do a lot of official entertaining. As a result of this, the upper administration was turned off, and only routine assistant professor appointments could be made. That was the end of Santa Barbara.

The next UC campus was UCLA, where another friend from Stanford, with whom I'd set up the bioengineering program there, was now head of the Crump Institute of Biomedical Engineering. They had advertised in *Science* for a full professor. I phoned him and said, "Well, could I apply for this?"

He said, "Oh, well, actually we weren't thinking of somebody in your area, but if you're available, that's it."

He talked to his colleagues and then phoned me and said, "Yes, everybody wants you to do it." But when I went to UCLA, instead of being set up as a proper interview, my visit was set up as a sort of love fest, where they would show me how wonderful they were so I would want to come. Unfortunately, the rules were that some department had to give me a position, even though the institute was paying my salary. The department was computer science, the chairman was out of town, and there were no appointments with the appropriate dean. Although the visit went very well in other ways, it was clear I had to go back for a proper interview. However, the department canceled the interview before it occurred. The official theory is that the department had never hired somebody with tenure before and so voted unanimously that they would not create a bad precedent by hiring me as a full professor. So that was the end of UCLA.

At this time, we were pretty clear we were going back to U. Mass., but Ed Blum, whom I had known through work in automata theory going right back to '66, had been on sabbatical down at La Jolla, visiting from USC, the University of Southern California. We had some conversations, and he said, "Oh, well, we must have you up to interview because we're setting up a new interdisciplinary program in neuroscience." Nothing had come of it; it was already May 1, and so we thought that was it. But then, suddenly, I was summoned to USC. I gave a couple of talks and everything went well, so I became a professor of computer science and neurobiology and a few other things at USC. I was one of the first two people appointed as part of the new program in NIBS: Neural, Informational, and Behavioral Sciences. At the time, I saw this as a consolation prize compared to the UC system. In fact, although it would have probably been nicer to live in La Jolla full time, subsequent history has shown that, intellectually, USC has turned out best in terms of the level of interaction. The Brain Research Institute at UCLA has been in trouble for years, and at UCSD there are lots of good people but no real community.

At USC I feel that I'm both a real professor of computer science and a real professor of neurobiology; USC has worked out very well as a place in which to do really good brain modeling. With George Bekey, chairman of the computer science department when I was hired, I've built up a robotics lab in which we go back and forth between neural strategies as studied in the monkey and neural strategies as implemented in the computer to control the robot.

A research strand that started up at U. Mass. was work with Parvati Dev, an Indian woman who later became chief scientist for a biomedical imaging firm in Palo Alto. She made a model of stereopsis, in the course of which she spent a summer with Richard Gregory in England. Richard Gregory and I tend to have punning matches. The last time I visited him, he was very excited because he just had a new book coming out called *Odd Perceptions*. So I said, "Ah, Richard, now you're committed to a sequel called 'Even Perceptions.'" But he trumped me. He said, "No, no, it's going to be called 'Even Odder Perceptions.'"

Back to Parvati Dev. She came up with a model of stereo vision. A little later, David Marr and Tommy Poggio published a paper in *Science* [reprinted in *Neurocomputing*] which was a minor variation on Dev's model. They compounded the injury by actually knowing about her paper. In the twenty-third—I remember the number to this day—in the twenty-third footnote they said, "Oh yeah, there's been some unimportant work in the past" and then cited Parvati's work along with a couple of other papers. David was an extremely bright, extremely charming, extremely persuasive person, but he had the idea that the reason neuroscientists hadn't appreciated modeling enough was because a lot of it had been bad. Rather than show them that there was in fact a lot of good neural modeling, which was my strategy, he agreed with them that everything else was poor and then showed them his stuff as the first round of really good modeling.

David Marr and I had an interesting relationship. We were very good friends, and yet it was one of these love-hate things because there was always this thing of, "David, why don't you just admit there's other good work?" Around 1980, I think, we had reached a sort of pact. I was then editing a thing called the *Brain Theory Newsletter*. I was ahead of my time. It was very hard to get more than a few hundred subscribers. If I'd kept that thing running till now, it would be selling in the tens of thousands, but I gave up before connectionism really took off again. I persuaded David that he should write an article for the *Brain Theory Newsletter* that would put his work in a perspective that showed that, yes, his work was wonderful, but also that other people had been doing good work and that his work did have antecedents. A month or so later, he came up to Amherst and had Thanksgiving dinner with us, and I vividly remember going out after dinner with him for a walk along a country road under very bright stars. After the dinner, we didn't hear from him for a while, which was surprising. When we finally got in touch with him, we learned he'd been diagnosed with leukemia. One thing about David was that he had a group of acolytes at MIT who worshipped everything he did. The good side of that was that, while he was incapacitated from chemotherapy, they were immensely supportive. He had decided he would write a book on vision, and the preface of the book has this incredible bit of English understatement. It says, "Certain events have occurred that forced me to write this book a few years earlier than I had planned" [David Marr. *Vision.* San Francisco: W. H. Freeman, 1982 p. xvii]. That's the only mention in the book of his disease.

The wonderful thing was that Tommy Poggio and Shimon Ullman and other people in the group would work on the book while he was sick. When he came out of hospital, instead of having to catch up on three or four weeks of lost work, the book would have progressed and he could jump in again. In fact, the last time Prue and I saw him at the Copley Plaza in Boston, he was very happy because the book had finally gone to press. I don't think he lived to see it published, but he did at least live to see it in press and feel that he had this legacy to pass on.

For me, it's sort of bittersweet in the sense that it's very powerful work and very influential, and yet has given many readers the impression of being de novo, which destroys what I think is the integrity of scientific work. There is a network of people working in science, and even if you are Einstein, you have to acknowledge your predecessors. No matter who you are, I think you make your progress by acknowledging what has been done, and then you show what you have added, whereas in machine vision, there are a lot of people who really believe, in the words of the writers of an *Economist* cover story many years ago, that machine vision is the creation of two men, David Marr and Tomaso Poggio of MIT. In fact, most of what they did built on things that people in the community already knew about in essence. They added some nice things. The story of zero crossings was, I think, definitely theirs. Their later "non-Devian" work on stereo was in fact interestingly original. There was no doubt that Marr and Poggio were very important contributors to computer vision, but they were by no means the creators of the field.

At U. Mass., building on my early work with Rich Didday, and continuing at USC we've built up what we call *Rana computatrix*, "the frog that computes." We have gone on to develop many different ideas. How does it habituate? How does it recognize barriers and detour around them? How does it recognize enemies and jump away from them? Many of these aspects of action-oriented perception are really trying to grow a whole animal, as it were. We try to think about the way in which more and more parts of the brain interact to give wider and wider behavioral repertoires—work that continues to this day.

It's interesting reflecting back on my career to see the sort of serendipity that occurred. Certain things were really planned out. I would say the frog work for a long time had been planned out. But, on the other hand, there were other topics which occurred for the most bizarre reasons. For example, my interest in hands was really an accumulation of coincidences. It started around '79 when I went to a meeting at Brandeis that David Ingle, whom I knew through the frog work, arranged on neural mechanisms of visually guided behavior. One of the speakers there was Marc Jeannerod from France, whom I had not met before, who gave a wonderful talk on his work with an Algerian named Biguer on the control of hand movements. The big point he was making was that when we reach for an object, the brain has to simultaneously figure out the control of the arm and the shaping of the hand. It's not that you get there and then figure out what to do with the hand. The brain is preshaping the hand at the same time that it's coming up with the trajectory. Then he went into some of the things that could go wrong with different types of brain lesion. I was fascinated by this.

A little later, Vernon Brooks, who was then editing the volumes on motor control of the *Handbook of Physiology: Section on Neurophysiology*, decided to ask me to write the one theoretical chapter that would appear in these two fat volumes. It's one of the most painful papers I have ever written in my life. Brooks kept coming up with this wretched view held by many neurophysiologists that the purpose of theory is to design new experiments, whereas I always thought the purpose of experiments was to verify new theories.

It was a real battle, but in the end the editorial attentions of Brooks helped me produce quite a good article. While trying to extend the coverage of the article, I decided to think through the things I learned about the hand from Jeannerod. I wanted to develop my idea of schemas to include a fairly simple diagram of the interaction between perceptual schemas—figuring out where the object is, what size it is, and what orientation it is in—and the schemas for control of the arm, control of the hand, and so on, and how they all interacted. This diagram in the handbook is probably the most successful thing I've done, in terms of the number of reproductions that have occurred in textbooks and papers, although it was basically a paper and pencil exercise, rather than a detailed model.

Subsequently, when Ian Darian-Smith was arranging a symposium in '83 in Melbourne, Australia, on the subject of the control of hand movements, he invited me to be a speaker on the strength of that picture of mine that had come out two years earlier in the *Handbook*. But that was basically all I had, this one figure. Then I mobilized two of my students at the time, Thea Iberall and Damian Lyons, to work with me on developing these ideas. That led to a very interesting series of papers on thinking about how the brain would represent an object, not in terms of recognizing what the object is, but in terms of figuring out how to grasp it. For Thea, that led in to a lot of thoughts about human behavior, and for Damian, it led into the development of a new language for schemas called RS, for "robot schemas," which tied in with my work with Ernie Manes on the categorical approach to programming language semantics. (From 1959 to about 1987, I maintained an active research program in automata theory, mathematical systems theory, and theory of computation. But that is another story!) Thus, hands became an important theme of my work, but only because I'd heard this talk, then had to write this *Handbook* article, and then somebody thought I was an expert and invited me to a meeting, and I determined to make myself an expert by the time the meeting occurred.

A recent series of models with Nicolas Schweighofer was triggered by the data that shows that if you wear prisms on your eyes, you can eventually learn to adapt. Your eyes will eventually swing to the appropriate place, as seen through the prisms, but you can only learn this if you have a cerebellum. We modeled this using Albus-type adjustments of the synaptic weights, but with much more of a systems view in terms of how you apply corrections to a downstream motor generator, rather than how you use the cerebellar cortex to pick out movements.

The way your saccadic system works is that normally when you make a rapid eye movement, you're very often wrong, and then you make a quick corrective movement, without your noticing it. It feels as if you've turned your gaze to one place. But if you were to measure with coils or take a movie or whatever, you'd see that in general there are going to be corrective saccades. Mickey Goldberg at NIH [the National Institutes of Health] would show a target to a monkey, and while the monkey was saccading towards it—it seems there's no effective visual input during this fast eye movement —Goldberg would move the target to a new place. So the monkey's brain would say, "Oh, not on target yet," and make the corrective saccade. Eventually, the monkey learns to make the saccade in one step if you're consistent in the displacement; the monkey will saccade not to where the target is seen, but to where the target ends up. It's like a virtual prism, if you will.

Normally in our theories we talk of learning as if it were a trial-by-trial thing. I make the trial. If I'm wrong, I make a correction using a classic learning rule of some kind. But if you look at the timing in the brain, the brain issues a command, the command follows, then the erroneous results follow; errors have to be sensed and then get back into the brain, where the neurons that were firing have finished their related activity maybe a hundred milliseconds before. In their model of classical conditioning, Barto, Sutton, and Klopf invented the notion of eligibility: the synapse has some sort of internal memory, so it remembers that it was active. So now if you send a reinforcement signal to this part of the brain, if you assume that it hasn't done anything else since, then the only eligible synapses are the ones that were involved in making the mistake, and the correction goes to them. This is a very nice idea. However, notice the problem for us. In Goldberg's preparation, you have a saccade and then a corrective saccade. If you have the "usual" form of eligibility, you will apply the correction not to the synapses involved in the saccade that was wrong but to those for the saccade that applied the correction. So Nicolas Schweighofer and I had to invent a new kind of eligibility, a window of eligibility. The eligibility starts at zero, then goes up, and then decays again. Instead of just having a simple decay so the most recent thing wins, in our case the most recent thing won't yet be eligible. In this way the synapses for the first saccade will be eligible for correction, and those for the second saccade will not be eligible for correction. The system works.

This very powerful idea is exciting in two ways. One is that the notion of eligibility that Klopf, Sutton, and Barto came up with was very powerful for bridging the conditioning literature and the neural network literature. The fact that we've shown the idea has to be made somewhat more subtle for different applications is interesting for the neural nets community. The second point for me is that, until recently, there's been a burgeoning world of neurochemistry which I've tried to stay away from, quite distinct from the world of relatively large-scale neural networks. Now, suddenly, we're seeing that we need to tailor the learning rules. Now, if you tailor the learning rules, you have to get into the biochemistry and understand how the playing off of the different mechanisms can change the time parameters of the second messenger system, which presumably underlies eligibility. I now for the first time really have an integrated view in my work which shows the need to unify the neurochemistry with the systems modeling.

We're beginning to do PET [positron emission tomography] and functional MRI [magnetic resonance imaging], which in the long run will be a very powerful method for looking at overall human brain function. We are also pushing the other way, with all this neurochemistry. Neurochemistry forms the bulk of papers presented at the society for Neuroscience meeting, but I've been ignoring it. Shame on me, but there wasn't a way to really use it at the systems level. It was just so much detail. But now we begin to see how second-order details of these synaptic and other mechanisms become crucial to understanding real functional questions. I think the next few years will be tremendously exciting in that way.

ER: Do you have other comments about the future of the field?

MA: I think that there was a worry around the early to mid-1980s when people who had been doing neural networks all along suddenly found thousands of new people pouring in with immense enthusiasm. We thought that this might be a flash in the pan. But I think what has happened since is irreversible. For whatever reason, a lot of physicists have come in and now the level of mathematical ability in the field has gone up.

One of the other main changes has been hardware. There is so much fast-computing hardware around that a lot of ideas which were purely theoretical in the '70s are now eminently practical in the '90s. If one had to lock up the machine for a week to run a learning algorithm, that might be fine for an academic putting out a paper, but it had no practical relevance. Now people are getting good results for many different applications. A lot of work now has to be either very focused, on a very specific application, or you have to develop a hybrid system where you apply some standard signal processing and some standard AI expert systems stuff, using a neural net for a module or two. I think the day of the magic single neural network has gone. From the practical side, you build a hybrid system, and you find that making some of those modules neural networks is really a very smart thing to do.

In terms of neuroscience, there were always a few people enthusiastic about theory, but they were a real minority. After I got my Ph.D. in 1963, I drove around the U.S. for a few months. That was when the first lab computer, the LINC, which later became joined with the PDP 8, had just hit the neurophysiology labs. It was very interesting to talk to the neurophysiologists at that time because some were very enthusiastic and others swore they would never let computers into the lab because it would destroy the touch they had as they were putting in the microelectrode. Of course, in the ten years or so after that, computers became absolutely indispensable. People just realized there was no way they could control their experiments or keep track of the data without computers.

I think the workstations of the last five years have made a similar change for simulations. Until five years ago, you were an experimentalist who had learned to love his or her lab computer, but it was a primitive little thing, and it didn't have the power to do anything except run the data. Now you can buy a massive workstation for a few thousand dollars that can let you have time left over to run lots of simulations. I think more experimentalists are beginning to have either themselves or someone in their lab who can play with the models and think about them in relation to the data.

That's leading to some double-threat people, but it's also leading to consortia, where experimentalists and modelers are really talking to each other seriously so that the analysis of the experiments involves the modeler, and what the modeler comes up with suggests new experiments.

There was an initial period, in the second coming of neural networks in the '80s, when people would just do neural networks uncritically. Now people will compare them with signal-processing approaches or conventional control theory. We just had a competition where there was an attempt to predict the power consumption of a building. The winner was a neural network designed around Bayes theorem. This is interesting in two ways. It was a neural network that won it, but it was a neural network based on a rather sophisticated probability theory analysis.

I don't believe that neural nets are a magic panacea. I think there's still a place for knowing how to add numbers exactly, rather than using a neural net. I think in the future we'll see hybrid systems where we have something like schema theory or modular design to understand how to take a complex problem, break it into pieces, and then for some of those pieces find that neural nets will do the best job. As we learn more about neural nets, we'll be able to do better and better.

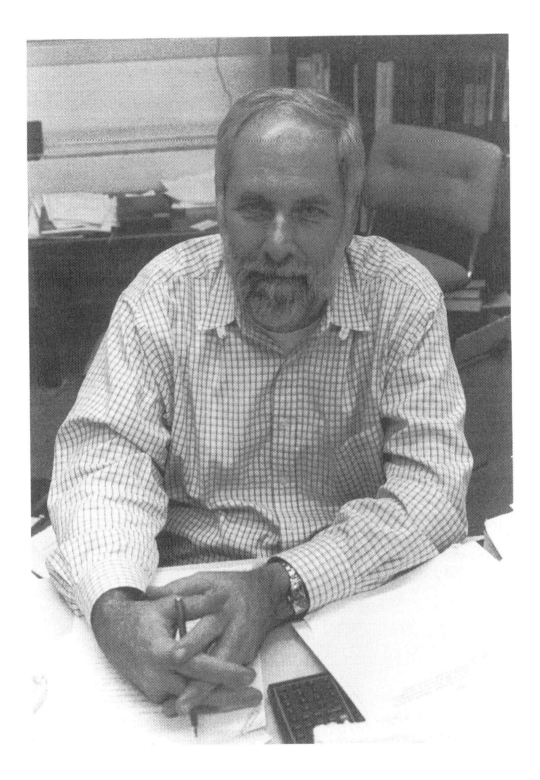

11 James A. Anderson

James Anderson is Professor of Cognitive and Linguistic Sciences at Brown University, Providence, Rhode Island. The best source of further details about his work is his book, An Introduction to Neural Networks, *MIT Press, 1995.*

Written Interview

I was born July 31, 1940, in Detroit, Michigan. My father's family was from Sweden. My grandfather was born in 1876 and arrived in New York in 1892, at the age of sixteen. My grandfather and some of his brothers founded a furniture factory in Jamestown, New York, and went on to become wealthy businessmen, although, unfortunately, most of this money was lost in the depression. My father learned Swedish before he finally learned English. The family were devout Swedish Lutherans. My father said that most of the sermons he remembers were devoted to proving that the Pope was the Antichrist.

The furniture factory produced enough money to send my father to Dartmouth, where he was an English major and graduated in 1931, in time for the worst part of the depression. He married my mother just after graduation from Dartmouth.

My mother was from a family that had lived in New England since the pilgrims. They had never been particularly rich, nor particularly poor either, and lived in a small town north of Boston on Cape Ann, Manchester, Massachusetts.

My father managed to get a college teaching job at a small college in Cleveland, Ohio—Fenn College. He eventually received a master's in English from what is now Case-Western Reserve. My parents' extremely low combined salaries forced them to live in slum housing in a dangerous neighborhood. For many years afterwards they had trouble eating spaghetti because that was what they mostly lived on during the depression years. My father was a very good writer, and after a few years was offered a good job with a group making motion pictures in Detroit.

Six months after I was born, we moved to White Plains, Hastings-on-Hudson, New York, because my father was offered a better job in Manhattan. When I was a bit over a year old, the Japanese attacked Pearl Harbor.

My father tried to enlist soon after war was declared but was rejected because he was an extremely nearsighted thirty-five year old in poor physical condition. Because of his persistance, he was finally accepted by the United States Army Air Force. After reflection, the Air Force decided that his writing and advertising talents could be put to good use; in any case, with eyesight as bad as his, he should be kept far away from anything to do with physical airplanes.

He was first sent to Wright Field, in Dayton, Ohio. In 1943, my father was assigned to the First Motion Picture Unit, based at the Hal Roach Studios in Culver City, California. One of the other members of this unit was a moderately successful actor, Ronald Reagan. My father became one of the script writers in the unit, and one of his proudest accomplishments was writing a film called *Air Power and Armies*, which was shown to Stalin at the Yalta Conference.

We arrived in Beverly Hills along with many others who went west because of World War II and stayed on after the war. During that period, real people lived in Beverly Hills. When Beverly Hills was originally formed, the idea was that the rich folks would live north of Wilshire Boulevard, and their maids and servants would live south of Wilshire, so there were modestly priced houses and apartments available for the help. The area I grew up in was therefore a reasonably average middle-class neighborhood. The loose living of the motion picture industry impacted my consciousness only when I noticed that my classmates tended to have frequent changes in their last names.

My mother got a job as a nursery school teacher at the Beverly Vista Community Church on South Elm Drive, a beautiful 1920s church building that I liked because it was quiet, empty, spooky, and smelled good. The church suffered the sad fate of many older Southern California buildings. Its beams were found to be infested with dry rot, and the place where the church building, nursery school, tiled courtyard, and community hall once stood is now a parking lot. In 1950 we moved to a new house in the Santa Monica mountains in the area now called Brentwood, close to the sites made famous by O. J. Simpson.

For forty years my mother was a nursery school teacher at the Beverly Vista Nursery School and later at the Crestwood Hills Nursery School near our new house, and was almost worshipped by her students. Every Halloween for many years a constant stream of present and former students would come to "Kit's house" for candy. One year, I remember, we had nearly a hundred visitors. She taught three-year-olds. When asked for the secret of her success, she replied, "Just keep an eye on them and make sure they don't kill each other."

My first grade teacher, Mrs. Wilson—in those days school teachers did not have first names—was indirectly responsible for the beginnings of my interest in brain function. In first grade we spent a good deal of time drawing pictures with crayons. Mrs. Wilson insisted that in a proper drawing every image should be surrounded by a black crayon line which she called an "accent line." The classroom stock of black crayons was soon worn down to tiny stubs and eventually could only draw very thick accent lines.

I had a problem. I could clearly see that objects in the world—people, for example—were not surrounded by thick black lines. But, upon closer introspection, they did not seem to be surrounded by thin black lines either. So I concluded, regretfully, that Mrs. Wilson, a pleasant lady and a good first grade teacher, was simply wrong about accent lines. They weren't there. However, she was a little bit right as well because I could clearly see that there was something special about the edges of things. They seemed to be much more distinct than they should be, as if accent lines existed but were vanishingly thin. They were there but not there. I found this a great puzzle and spent considerable time looking at objects, trying to see if I could figure out what made their edges special. It wasn't until many years later that I learned about lateral inhibition and orientation selective units in visual cortex. I believe this experience left me, first, with the deep suspicion that things out there in the world were not always what they seemed in here, in our heads, and, second, that adults, even nice ones, were not always correct.

In those days, the Beverly Hills and later the Los Angeles public school systems were far better than they have become since. In retrospect, I can see that many of my teachers all through public school were outstanding. They knew their subject and often displayed great enthusiasm for it. They were willing to spend a lot of extra time with promising students, particularly in the sciences and in mathematics. I was fortunate enough to have high school mathematics teachers who would have been an asset to many college faculties. One of my favorite high school math teachers, Miss McDonald (no first names!), had a master's in physics from Berkeley. In those days, there were special math classes for the better students, where we moved fast and learned a lot of advanced topics.

I have always been interested in why people end up doing the things they do. As far as I am concerned, there were two major reasons why I got interested in science at an early age.

The first influence involved what I read. I read voraciously all during elementary school: comic books, encyclopedias, books about dinosaurs, books about castles, Hardy Boys novels, war stories, catalogs, books about virtually anything. I was completely uncritical until I was about eleven and ran across a copy of *Astounding Science Fiction*. From that first issue I knew this kind of writing was for me. I wanted to understand even the stories I didn't understand. I read every science fiction book in our local library on San Vicente Boulevard, even the dreadful ones. I have had a continuous subscription to *Astounding Science Fiction* (now *Analog*) since about 1952 as well as to *The Magazine of Fantasy and Science Fiction* and to *Galaxy* when it was around. There was a period in college when I believe I could honestly say that I had read a significant fraction of the entire genre.

Science fiction, particularly during the 1950s was vibrant. Exciting people were doing exciting things. Even when the science the stories described made no particular contact with reality, it was still sufficiently plausible to make you think that it might really have been that way if God had been a little more venturesome.

And science fiction was, and still is, full of ideas. Some were crazy, but some were so good they might be correct. Some actually were correct. The ideas were about everything, not just science: politics, history, physics, biology, sociology. The powerful libertarian bias that is now so prominent on the Internet and among computer professionals was present then in the stories of Heinlein and many others. Governments were invariably stupid, bureaucrats were beneath contempt, liberal arts majors were hopelessly ineffectual, and the only repository of common sense in the known universe was among scientists and engineers. Yeah! Since the daily newspapers provided data supporting most of those conclusions, it was hard for a twelve year old not to be impressed.

What really came across in science fiction was that ideas mattered. The bolder the ideas, the better. Received wisdom was probably wrong, and if authority figures said it, it was certain to be wrong. Problems had solutions, usually technical, if the problem was looked at in the right way. Even though I know now that things are not quite this simple, my subconscious still believes it.

The second major influence on me was amateur radio. Somehow, probably due to the accidental purchase of a copy of the radio magazine *QST* when I was about twelve, I got the idea that radio was something that looked challenging and something I might be able to do. I had developed some skill making model airplanes out of paper and balsa wood, and making electronic gadgets seemed similar, except that instead of winding up a rubber band and flying the product, you talked to someone else with it.

No one around where I lived knew much about electronics. I built a single tube radio from a kit. I read some more, accumulated some parts, and in one of the feats that still gave me the most satisfaction, built a primitive but working one-tube radio of my own design, with a coil wound on a two-by-four, a variable tuning capacitor taken from a discarded radio, and a vacuum tube, a 117L7GT. The vacuum tube was one of the few made that had a filament that worked directly off household voltage, so I didn't need a transformer. It didn't work very well, but it did work. I remember using it and listening with great pride and pleasure to the local radio stations.

I got my novice amateur license when I was thirteen and bought a simple crystal-controlled transmitter kit. I put the transmitter kit together, and it worked, or at least it lit up the light bulb I tested it with. One day after school, I managed to communicate via Morse code with a station in Van Nuys, located about five miles away in the San Fernando Valley. Maybe it wasn't very far, but my first contact was both exciting and traumatic. I was afraid that I would disgrace myself completely in this new culture with some kind of grievous faux pas, but I managed to get through it.

For the next few years, radio opened a new world that had a lot in common with science fiction. By the end of 1954, with the help of a couple of equipment upgrades, a general-class license, and a barely adequate antenna, I was talking to people all over the world. I managed to make friends among the local amateurs, including several roughly my own age who lived within walking distance. I developed a taste for DXing—that is, contacts with far away stations—the more obscure the location, the better. Even if it is good for nothing else, DXing is wonderful for knowledge of geography, and I knew exactly where British Somaliland, the South Sandwich Islands, and the Bonin and Volcano Islands were because I had talked to someone there. Maybe the conversations we had were not very profound, but, by God, they were genuine exchanges of information. And technology did it. The potential was obvious. The Internet has produced no real surprises for radio amateurs, just obvious extensions of what we were already doing decades ago.

At this point I have an attractive plaque on my wall in honor of having managed to "work them all"—that is, talk to another amateur in every country on the official amateur DX countries list. This difficult accomplishment means absolutely nothing to anyone outside of a small number of enthusiasts. But then most of science follows an identical pattern of reward.

One lesson I learned from this history was that nerds are eternal, probably corresponding to a particular combination of alleles on the human genome, but the expression that nerdiness takes depends on the technology of the time. In my day we were radio nerds, though we did not use that term: pasty, unhealthy, either thin or fat, and antisocial. I remember an acquaintance during high school who used to carry several vacuum tubes along with him as conversation starters. ("Look at this one! It's a beam power tetrode!") Girls were not impressed, and he could not understand why. Nowadays, the computer provides the means for the fulfillment of inherent nerd potential. In my day it was electronics or sometimes cars. Same genome, different expression. I wonder what we did in the Middle Ages?

My father was an alcoholic and a screen writer. The combination led to severe financial problems. Though we lived in Brentwood, a comfortable upper middle-class suburb, our family financial condition was perilous and significantly worsened during the time I was at University High School in West Los Angeles. When it came time to apply for college, I remember the school's college advisor was dismayed at how low our family income was. In January of 1958 my father joined Alcoholics Anonymous. This stopped his drinking, and my family's financial position started improving rapidly, although it was still difficult for quite a while. Currently, my father has been in AA for thirty-eight years. I have been to many open AA meetings as a family member. AA meetings usually involve one or more talks by members describing their lives when they were drinking. Back in the 1950s and early 1960s people were much more reticent about describing their personal problems than they are now. Many of the AA talks were hilarious, and some were eye opening. Not much about human behavioral pathology has surprised me since.

When it came time to apply for college, I had a problem. I was interested only in science or engineering. Money was tight, so I would need considerable financial support. I knew there were two famous science and engineering schools in the country, MIT and Caltech. As someone who grew up in Los Angeles, I believed nothing important existed east of San Bernardino. I applied to both MIT and Caltech and was accepted at both. MIT gave me a generous financial package, including an Alfred P. Sloan scholarship that guaranteed a high level of support for four years. Caltech did not make an offer in that league, so, somewhat against my desires, I ended up going to MIT. I had no idea where MIT actually was, except that it was located near Boston. Everything on the East Coast seemed remote and confusing, with bad weather and juvenile delinquents.

The first year at MIT at that time resembled Marine Corps boot camp—with physics, calculus, and inorganic chemistry taken by all freshmen. The entire MIT freshman class had an hour quiz every Friday morning at 9:00. We all trooped to our assigned rooms, in my case a large engineering drafting room furnished with large drafting tables and uncomfortable, high stools. We lived or died based on how we did. The process was competitive, stressful, and dehumanizing, but it did communicate a lot of information. There was also a required course in the humanities, but no one took it seriously, though I found it entertaining. I discovered a thorough background in science fiction prepares you for reading other stuff, including lit-ra-choor, though serious mainstream novels seemed unimaginative in comparison. They still do.

I was now faced with the problem of finding a major. Good science fiction asks big questions: What is the nature of reality? What is the nature of the mind? What is the place of man in the universe? Those were the questions I wanted to answer.

In 1958 there was only one choice: physics. I knew what engineers did because I had been part of a high school summer program at Hughes Aircraft Corporation plant in Culver City. Electrical engineers built clever gadgets but didn't tackle the big questions. I was an OK but not great mathematician, and, besides, mathematics was too abstract. So physics was it.

I already knew what I wanted to be when I grew up. I wanted to be Hari Seldon, the central thinker in Isaac Asimov's *Foundation* series. Hari Seldon was the first psychohistorian, living at the start of the decline of the twelve-thousand-year-old Galactic Empire. Seldon was able to predict the future of the empire through the equations for human behavior he had developed. MIT did not offer courses in psychohistory. Physics seemed like a good, temporary substitute.

Along with a staggering amount of information, MIT also provided a way of thinking about problems. Sometimes this way was good, but in retrospect, it now seems misleading and dangerous. Around 1960, computers were just starting to have an obvious impact on the way science was done. As undergraduates, we did not even have pocket calculators, only slide rules. More, our instructors were products of an earlier generation of science education. What this meant in practice was great emphasis on cleverness and ingenuity in analyzing problems. The MIT hour exams were perfect examples of how this worked. A hopelessly complex test problem would be given. If the right bit of insight was applied, the problem yielded, and the answer was obvious. Finding the key to the problem could be very hard, but there was always the assumption that it was there and could be found by being clever.

There were two major problems with this approach to life.

First, cleverness is not always combined with depth of insight. Students who did extremely well on tests could be quite superficial in their understanding. Of course, this is an acknowledged problem in all higher education. Later experience with graduate admissions at Brown has led me to be very wary of straight-A students.

The second problem was more serious. This approach to college exams could easily become a way of life. Before mechanical ways of handling complexity—like computers—were available, a simple equation that arose from a clever approximation or a deep insight was often the only way to handle real systems. However, this requirement could undesirably restrict the class of systems that could be analyzed. It also tended to grossly undervalue the work involved in coping with details. Both the MIT hour exams and theoretical physics—with, for example, the Schrodinger equation as a model—taught us to search for the "big theory," the master equation that would break the problem wide open. It is far too easy to use a computer as a substitute for thought. Why think when you can simulate?

I did quite well my first two years at MIT but then became more and more disenchanted. My grades were marginal my junior and senior years, especially in physics, my major. This was because I found school in general and physics in particular more and more boring and less and less relevant to anything I was genuinely interested in. I took a number of the limited MIT offerings in the humanities, brooded, and was unhappy with the prospects for my future.

By this time, I had considerable experience with private industry. I had worked in the Los Angeles aerospace industry for several summers. Sophomore year I worked for North American Aviation, at their plant just south of the Los Angeles Airport. This old building was where the P-51 Mustang had been designed. They still had dramatic pictures of it on the walls. My project involved study of reentry heating on the X-15 rocket plane. My job was to write computer programs to calculate heating of bits of the plane during various reentry conditions to see if the wings would overheat and fall off. I had to learn an early version of Fortran, Fortran II, in order to write the programs. We would submit our jobs on coding sheets, anonymous key punch operators would transfer our code to punch cards, the jobs would run overnight, and the next day we would get our results back, or, if the jobs did not run, get actual core dumps, which in those days were printouts on wide fanfold paper of the entire memory of the IBM 7094 that we used. We could often tell where we went wrong by checking the core dumps. The second floor of the building was an enormous "bull pen" with hundreds of desks and drafting tables lined up in rows.

My two last summers involved working for the Aerospace Corporation in El Segundo, which was fun but was also a lot like physics. I had to wear a suit and tie like the other technical personnel. I suspect somebody had sold management on the idea that it would be good to hire college students for the summer, but there were no particular projects that needed their help. No one was quite sure what to do with me, so mostly I played around with the lab equipment.

I had to make a decision during my senior year in college. I had to decide to do something with my life, but my experience with the aerospace industry led me to conclude that I definitely did not want to spend my career refining the electronics on missiles as a small part of a giant team in a bull pen.

In addition, all young men of that era were faced with a major problem: the draft. Some of my earliest memories were of World War II. The Korean War had influenced my junior high school career. I had read *All Quiet on the Western Front* a half dozen times. The Cold War was in full swing. It did not require much geopolitical savvy to see that the U.S. Army was not going to be a safe place. In addition, my extensive reading had convinced me beyond all doubt that my personality type was completely unsuited to the military. Teamwork had never been my strong point.

If I was not going to work for the military industrial complex with its many deferments, the only way to be reasonably sure of staying out of the army was to go to graduate school. However, I had no particular desire to go to graduate school in physics, though I applied to several of them through inertia and was rejected by them all. This was clearly the right decision from the point of view of the graduate programs involved.

I had always been interested in the big questions that science fiction physics addressed but real physics ignored. The biggest of these big questions, I felt, was how the mind worked. I knew the MIT physics department pretty well by that time, and I knew that with my grades there was no chance I would be admitted to their graduate school in physics. So I switched my application for graduate school at MIT from the physics department to the biology department. I felt I probably would not get in, but if I did, it would give me a chance to work with something that might be interesting while I stayed out of the army. For some reason I have never understood, the MIT biology department admitted me to their graduate program and even provided financial aid.

In retrospect, I think that my shift to biology was one of the two or three most important and most correct decisions I have made in my life, but at the time I felt like I was taking a large step down in status. My friends did too. Physics was considered the model for all the other, lesser sciences. The only people smarter than physicists were mathematicians, and they were weird. If you had some reality contact and were smart, you became a physicist. If you were really smart, you became a particle physicist. If you were really really smart, you became a theoretical physicist and confronted the universe head on, armed with just your naked intellect. We knew, based on movies and novels, how this kind of prototypical physics was done: brilliant, disheveled, mildly eccentric academic, alone in a room with a blackboard covered with equations. It was the apex of our fantasies.

Biology was somewhere down there with home economics and theory of sewers in the MIT pecking order. I received condolences about my demotion from my friends who were going on to do real science.

I started graduate school at MIT in biology in September 1962. Since I had no background whatsoever in biology, I was required to take a number of undergraduate courses. Somewhat to my surprise, when I was doing something I liked, my grades picked up substantially. This period was before grade inflation, and one of my proudest academic achievements is the A I received in the major introductory computer-programming course, competing with a horde of MIT undergraduates. The other great event of that first year in graduate school was being required to take Hans-Leukas Teuber's "Introduction to Psychology." Teuber had just arrived at MIT, and this was the first year he taught the course. I still can remember Teuber's large, expressive eyebrows moving up and down when he made an important point. This course made such a strong impression on me that I still use a number of his ideas in my own teaching. Teuber first introduced me to the work of my hero William James, who, I soon discovered, thought of almost everything first and usually expressed it better and more clearly than anyone since.

Teuber's course material covered what we would now probably call cognitive science. It was concerned with neurophysiology, animal behavior, clinical neurology, and big ideas—in equal measure. The course was a revelation. It described exactly what I wanted to do, except it seemed to be called psychology and not physics.

Now graduate school became an exercise in learning all the stuff I was interested in and convincing the biology department to give me a Ph.D. as soon after July 1966 as possible. The date was important because I had learned that nobody got drafted after they reached the age of twenty-six. Apparently, experience from World War II had convinced the military that raw recruits beyond that age had too much common sense and and too little physical capacity to make good soldiers.

In my second year in graduate school I met George Moore, who was spending a year visiting from UCLA. George introduced me to the "sea hare," *Aplysia california*, an animal only a neurophysiologist could love. *Aplysia* are large gastropod molluscs that live in the kelp beds off the coast of California. Ecologically, they are a molluscan cow, grazing serenely on seaweed. Like most herbivores they are severely lacking in cleverness, initiative, and motivation, a point for vegetarians to ponder. The *Aplysia* nervous system has a small number of very large neurons that are easy to record from with microelectrodes. These so-called "identifiable neurons" recur with the same location, function, and connections from animal to animal—an ideal arrangement for experiments.

Much neurophysiology involves the search for the perfect preparation—that is, the particular "simple" animal or system that gives clear, illuminating results about an important function. *Aplysia* is such a valuable preparation. It is easy to work with, easily available, and emits behavior occasionally. One of its behaviors is a whole series of withdrawal reflexes. When an *Aplysia* is touched unexpectedly, it pulls the touched part out of the way. Many animals, including us, behave similarly. I thought it would be worthwhile to study the tentacle withdrawal in a whole animal preparation. I made an incision in the animal to expose the cerebral ganglion that controlled the tentacle response, recorded from neurons in the ganglion, and provoked the *Aplysia* to withdraw by touching it with a probe.

George Moore's original plan was to leave UCLA and come to MIT permanently, but he ultimately decided not to, so I did a Ph.D. thesis on *Aplysia* with very limited advising. It was educational to do everything myself, but inefficient, and I missed a lot of obvious points. Eventually, however, all this resulted in a Ph.D. thesis that I referred to myself as the "Unified *Aplysia* Theory" but that carried a more pedestrian title. No one else seemed very interested in a unified *Aplysia* theory.

My feeling was that *Aplysia* was a good example of one possible and highly successful form of nervous system organization using a small number of very complex neurons, largely hardwired. I felt that mammals were likely to show a different organization: one that was also successful, using a very large number of neurons organized and connected with some number of statistical rules, but without the degree of individual soldering of connections by God (or his agents) present in *Aplysia*. These statistical rules were likely to be simpler than the ad hoc connections that would probably be found in small numbers of complex *Aplysia* neurons performing complex functions. So this was the direction I started to explore since I thought that mammals were far more interesting than *Aplysia*. Interestingly, more recent work strongly suggests that the core, hardwired reflex is only a small part of the actual strength of the reflex, even in *Aplysia*. Although there is a core, there also seem to be a large number of interneurons contributing to the reflex, showing a much more diffuse and much more mammal-like, distributed organization.

So even while I was working on *Aplysia* for my Ph.D. thesis, I was quite sure that my future did not contain more of it. It was an interesting detour.

I had always been fascinated by memory. Thanks to the computer courses I had taken, I had a pretty good idea how computer memories are organized. I could see that human memories and computer memories are organized completely differently. That was intriguing to me because I knew that they both store information but in very different ways. Ours works faster and a lot better in some ways, but worse in others.

Sometimes when I get stuck or want to think great thoughts about big problems, I will go for a long walk. My first year in graduate school I took several walks like this. I knew about the paper on the frog eye by Jerry Lettvin, who I also knew as a charistmatic and controversial figure in the biology department. He was the faculty member who had dared to say in an orientation talk to a crop of serious first-year graduate students, "The main thing is to have fun doing science." I was starting to learn about the work of Hubel and Wiesel on the cat primary visual cortex. I returned from one long walk convinced that all mental functions in mammals were spatial to a large degree—that is, many neurons distributed over a sizeable region of space were involved in doing any mental function of interest. A single neuron did not count for much. We had selective neurons all right; Hubel and Wiesel and Lettvin had found some of them. But a perception of any complexity at all involved a widespread spatial pattern of the activities of many neurons.

This may not sound like a very profound insight now, but it led me to focus on the properties of patterns shown by many units operating together and not on single units, an emphasis I still believe to be correct. This was somewhat counter to the received, though rarely articulated, neural theory of the times, which said roughly, "Well, if the frog has bug detectors, and the cat cortex has orientation selective cells, then we will find more and more selective cells as we march through the brain." This approach led to a search for "grandmother" cells, which did not seem to exist. This experience also emphasized to me the fact that every neuroscientist, even the most empirical, is a theoretician, except that they are rarely aware of it. The worst kinds of theories are the ones that do not rise to consciousness, but which through dark subterranean influences determine what data are to be considered important and what kinds of experiments get done. Keynes once commented that "practical men, who believe themselves to be quite exempt from any intellectual influences, are usually the slaves of some defunct economist." Most neuroscientists, believing themselves to be servants of the data above all else, are not even the slaves of the ideas of a real, but dead human, but rather of a vague unarticulated cultural consensus.

So we were dealing with activity patterns of many neurons. Patterns involving many neurons are hard to deal with conceptually. For example, a single unit may participate in many different patterns. Selectivity is lost. More speculatively, if the same is true for memory, then the strength of a single synapse may be a function of many past events, rather than one—a break with the notion that memory is a vast file cabinet with everything in its place. When I started exploring the literature, I found that Karl Lashley, Sir John Eccles, and even William James had come to similar conclusions, confirming my belief that however clever and original your ideas, someone else thought of them first.

The first time I tried to do anything with the idea that memory is a distributed, pattern-based operation was in a graduate seminar on memory in the psychology department. I had a very clear visual image in my mind of the kind of system I wanted. I saw a bunch of input lines, something like guitar strings connected to a hazy, somewhat three-dimensional set of lines and connections. In operation, a chord was struck on the input strings, and after a brief period a different chord, based on past learning, appeared on the strings. This device was basically an associative memory device, where an input pattern combined with a bit of network magic gave rise to an associated output. I knew from my psychology courses that association was something people were very good at. It should be possible to reproduce it with an artificial system.

I had run across perceptrons in a class taught by Murray Eden, but perceptrons were presented as a pattern recognition device that, for example, would tell you what letter corresponded to a particular spatial pattern. The basic perceptron architecture seemed pretty reasonable based on what I knew of neuroanatomy, but pattern recognition seemed far too rigid. Pattern association, however, was something else. I could see right away that associations were essentially arbitrary and formed what might be called an "alogical" computing style. I wrote these qualitative insights up for a term paper and got a B on it, probably more than I deserved considering the haziness and confusion underlying my model. I went back to work on *Aplysia*, the animal that would both keep me out of the army and maybe get me a job.

I received my Ph.D. in January of 1967, right on schedule. George Moore had managed to obtain support for me as a postdoc at the Brain Research Institute at UCLA. I wanted to return to L.A. where I grew up. Unfortunately, just as I arrived at the BRI, George Moore left to go across town to USC as part of their new bioengineering program, so I was again left on my own, with no advisor, no lab, no equipment, but with financial support for a couple of years.

I was delighted. This was the 1960s. I wanted to do my own thing, and I had two years of support. I figured if I couldn't make it in science, I would do something else for a living. I managed to find a few linear feet of lab bench space on the seventh floor of the BRI, courtesy of Jose Segundo and Alan Grinnell, that I could use as a desk. Dr. Segundo was extremely helpful to me and seemed to understand what I was doing, a wonderful person to whom I owe a great debt. He was interested in models of neuronal interactions, and he, George Moore, and Don Perkel, then at the RAND Corporation, had written several papers on spike train analysis, with examples taken from *Aplysia*, that have become classics.

Once I was settled in my little space on the seventh floor of the BRI, I needed to decide strategy. Even then, there was a torrent of experimental papers in neuroscience. There was so much data that no one could absorb it. The situation is ten times worse now. I decided that someone had to become the audience for which those papers were written and that someone was going to be me. I would try to figure out what was going on and make sense of it. If I couldn't make sense of at least a little of it, I would find a new job. It was the '60s. Anything was possible.

I chose memory as my topic. I had told people I was going to work on *Aplysia,* but I never believed that, and since I had no lab, I couldn't even if I wanted to.

I thought that memory was really peculiar. We knew something about the neural hardware and something about the way memory worked functionally. It certainly wasn't a file cabinet, though there were a few papers around that suggested it might be. It was time for another long walk, this time around the beautiful UCLA campus.

I have always liked to buy used equipment. First, it is cheap. Second, it is interesting because it has a history of previous owners who left their traces on it. And third, it is challenging to make things work that others have discarded. Similarly, I like ideas that others have rejected as unreasonable. Conversely, I am suspicious of ideas that have been accepted just because they seem so reasonable. My reading of history and my own experience has convinced me that the place where theory goes most seriously and undetectably wrong is in the most basic assumptions: What are you actually trying to do? Is that the right thing to do? Are you assuming a function for a system because it is the right thing to do or because it is convenient and makes analysis more manageable?

If I was to take my pattern associator seriously as a model for memory, then it suggested that the responses of individual units and even the individual storage elements, probably synapses, reflected their entire past history —that is, distinct memories mixed together by the very act of storage. This seemed very odd. I was aware of several memory models that drew similar conclusions but that then went to some pains to develop mechanisms to keep things separate. So in my long walk I said to myself, "Suppose we just accept instead of reject the fact that things mix together in the act of storage and see what happens."

Lots happened. For one thing, if we simply added patterns directly to each other, the sum could indeed act as a memory and quite a good one if there were enough storage elements involved. The analysis tools required to see this were in books I was just then reading: Lee's *Statistical Theory of Communication* and Davenport and Root's *Random Signals and Noise.* All we had to do was apply correlation functions or matched filters to the sum, and the memory could answer a number of interesting questions—for example, recognition questions, or "Have I seen this pattern before?" I could even compute how accurately it could answer this question. More, this idea predicted the existence of a whole host of interference effects and related enhancement effects in the operation of memory. For example, if we saw a lot of noisy examples of a pattern, the memory would effectively take the sum in the storage process, thereby applying automatically one of the most effective noise-reducing signal-processing techniques. Somewhat to my surprise, most of the predictions of this model were made at the level of the patterns themselves—that is, at the level of gross behavior or, dare I even think it, of cognition. Worse, if this model was even vaguely true, it would be very hard to see in operation at the level of single neurons or synapses because each individual part formed only a small bit of a larger pattern.

Another nice thing about the approach was that the strength of a lot of effects like interference and enhancement depended on the details of the data representation—that is, the way information was represented in the distributed activity patterns. As a neuroscientist, I knew that the brain essentially *was* data representation—that is, finely tuned, genetically determined preprocessing.

Anyway, this simple, unpromising assumption—that information specificity is lost by the act of storage—turned out to open up a series of interesting speculations.

I was inspired to write a brief paper pointing out some of these implications, which I submitted to the journal then called *Kybernetik*, now called *Biological Cybernetics*. It was accepted almost immediately and became my first real scientific publication. This encouraged me to think that I might manage to make a living at science, on my own terms.

Once you start thinking along these lines, it is hard to stop. From a single memory where everything mixes together, it is an obvious step to a memory with lots of units—a little like neurons—where every unit contains a memory of this summed type in its connections, forming a connectivity matrix that couples one group of units to another. The weights, or connection strengths, of the units are the summed recognition memories. This became the associative memory that I had visualized for my term paper in graduate school, except here it was and it worked. It also had both the desirable and undesirable qualitative properties of the simpler memory. This associative memory got described poorly in a 1970 paper and more clearly in a 1972 paper.

Thanks to several different sources of funds—the BRI's Mental Health Training Program, a Public Health Service Fellowship, and a postdoc at the Space Biology Laboratory courtesy of Ross Adey, who liked my modeling work—I was able to stay at UCLA for four years, from 1967 to 1971. This period was the height of "the '60s" and was a time of intense political and cultural activity, particularly in California, fascinating but strenuous.

From a personal point of view I now needed a steady job. I was newly married, and after November 1970 I had a new son. (Hi, Diana and Eric! You are the most important people in my life.) So I had responsibilities. The election of my father's wartime coworker, Ronald Reagan, as governor of California had an immediate impact on the University of California, a hotbed of radicals and malcontents. Academic job prospects in California were dim.

Again thanks to Segundo I found out about a postdoc at Rockefeller University, and in June 1971 my wife, son, and I left for New York in our Volkswagon Microbus. After driving through the Rockies at 25 m.p.h uphill, max, we arrived at Rockefeller University, where I was to work on pigeon cerebellum at a laboratory in Theobald Smith Hall, a short way from the copper-lined lab constructed by Lorente de Nó.

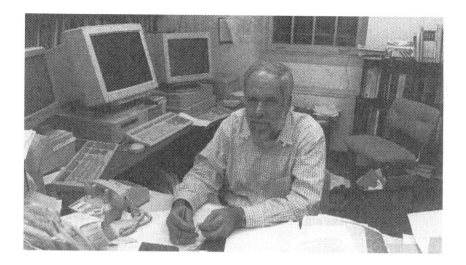

Rockefeller was a mix of good and bad. The physiological experiments I participated in were tedious and, I felt, without significance for understanding how the brain might work. The lab director made it a point to crush any faint sign of speculation as being unscientific.

At that time, however, Rockefeller was a true university. It had physicists, psychologists, and mathematicians on its faculty, along with the biologists and medical doctors that it was originally designed to house. Among the psychologists was William K. Estes, inventor of statistical learning theory and a leader in the field of mathematical psychology. He had a large group of coworkers, at first located on the floor above mine in Theobald Smith Hall, moving a little later to the third floor of a new building on the other end of the Rockefeller campus. Since that golden era, Rockefeller has regressed to its original role as a biomedical research institute.

Just before I left UCLA, Bob Barrett, who shared my laboratory-office and who worked on the physiology of pit vipers, pointed out to me an article by Saul Sternberg in the *American Scientist*. The article reviewed what became known as the Sternberg list-scanning experiments. The main effect is strong and reproducible. If a subject learns a short list of items of almost any type, and then is asked as to whether or not a test item was on the list, the response time is a linear function of the number of items on the list. This seemed perfectly resonable if one assumed that there was a list of items in memory, and the list was scanned to look for a match between test item and learned items. If an additional item was added to the list, it should take longer to scan the list, about 35 milliseconds an item, in fact. However, what made the Sternberg results interesting was that for many cases the time required to respond—"Yes, the item was on the list" or "No, the item was not on the list"—had the same slope as the number of items was changed. An efficient computer program to do this task would presumably do learned item—test item matches and then exit the program when a match was

James A. Anderson

found. But this would imply that the slopes of "No" and "Yes" would be in a two for one ratio because on the average only half the list had to be scanned for a "Yes" but the entire list had to be scanned for a "No." But what was seen experimentally was a one-to-one ratio.

It seemed clear to me that this pattern of results was consistent with my model for memory. If everything mixed together at the storage elements, a nice clean list was not present anywhere. And the most reasonable ways I could think of to extract the information from the memory would have a time course consistent with Sternberg's experimental results.

I had several discussions with members of Estes's laboratory and with Estes himself about this. I was very unhappy with my neuroscientific work brutalizing pigeons. I asked Estes if I could join his laboratory to develop these ideas for the second year of my stay at Rockefeller. He was kind enough to say yes. This decision also involved a pay cut of some magnitude, but I felt it was more than worth it. Just after my decision to join the Estes laboratory, I remember reading in the *New York Times* that the starting salary of a New York City garbage collector was exactly twice what I would be getting the next year.

I spent a happy year in Estes's laboratory learning a whole lot about psychology and writing a paper on my model for the Sternberg effect. I was struck by a number of things in that laboratory. Psychologists were far more open and responsive to new ideas than were neuroscientists. This was during the period sometimes called the neural network dark ages, after the Minsky and Papert book on perceptrons had dried up most of the funding for neural networks in engineering and computer science. Neural networks continued to be developed by psychologists, however, because they turned out to be effective models in psychology. It is no accident that much of the early work on neural networks—most notably the PDP group at UCSD—was done by cognitive psychologists. What happened during the dark ages was that the ideas had moved away from the highly visible areas of big science and technology into areas of science that did not appear in the newspapers.

Another nice aspect of experimental psychology was the fact that a number of striking, robust, and lawful experimental phenomena were known. No one outside of psychology seemed to know this. It was clear that many of the strongest predictions of neural networks were observable at the behavioral level but not at the neural level. As only one example, the Minsky and Papert book had as its primary theoretical result that a simple perceptron could not tell whether a visual pattern was connected or not. Yet, for a figure of any complexity, in our immediate perceptions humans cannot either. The cover of the Minsky and Papert book made this point by having two spirals, one connected and one not. However, almost no one realizes this until it is pointed out to them, and even then it is difficult to see. The conclusion was that perceptrons indeed have some severe processing power limitations, but those limitations seem to correspond to the strengths and weaknesses shown by humans. Perhaps neural nets are not very good engineering devices, but they are great models for mental function.

During my stay at Rockefeller, I made contact with a small group at Brown that had started to become interested in brain models: Leon Cooper, Ulf Grenander, and Jim McIlwain. I was introduced to them by Cooper's graduate student, Menasche Nass, who burst into my office in Smith Hall one day and asked me to tell him everything known about memory. Cooper liked my matrix-based associative memory model. All this discussion led to a number of visits to Providence and eventually an offer of a job in the Brown Division of Applied Mathematics. After my appointment at Rockefeller was up, I compressed my family and all our possessions into our VW Microbus and moved to Providence in the summer of 1973.

I was clearly not an applied mathematician or any kind of mathematician for that matter, and after three years my contract was not renewed by applied math. I moved my office to Hunter Laboratory, which contains the psychology department. My organizational affiliation shifted to the Center for Neural Science, an interdepartmental center, largely the creation of Leon Cooper. The center was formed just about the time that Cooper won the Nobel Prize for his work on superconductivity. He was the "C" in the BCS theory of superconductivity, a theory that correctly explained virtually all the properties of classical low temperature superconductivity. Cooper was able to use his considerable prestige and influence to obtain support for his new intellectual interests, which after about 1970 lay primarily in models of the nervous system.

Since 1973 I have remained at Brown, though my stay at a single institution has been enlivened by several shifts of department. Since 1973 I have not gone anywhere in particular other than to meetings, except for a summer in 1979 spent in La Jolla at UCSD. The major event of that summer was a conference that Geoff Hinton and I organized with sponsorship from the Sloan Foundation as part of their attempt to get cognitive science to be as big a success as their earlier support of neuroscience. [This small workshop/conference is mentioned by several of the participants in this book as an important influence in reigniting interest in neural networks.] It accomplished a lot just by bringing an eclectic group together who discovered at the conference that they were all doing similar things. It also led to the publication of a conference proceedings book, *Parallel Models of Associative Memory*, which turned out to be quite influential.

When I arrived at Brown, I was still intrigued by the large number of solid experimental effects seen in cognitive psychology. Many of them seemed to me to be exactly what you might see arising from operation of the kind of parallel, distributed computing machine that I felt the brain to be. Particularly interesting were a number of effects seen in the formation of what psychologists call concepts.

One of the most important and useful features of human cognition arises from deliberate distortion of the information presented to us by our senses.

We see the world not in its true amorphous unanalyzed glory but as composed of discrete objects. A firehose of information comes in through the senses, and we can handle not more than a fraction of a drop of it. If you look at any sensory modality at virtually any time, there are enough correlations, dependencies, structures, and relations to overwhelm any computer, including ours.

One effective way to handle this flood of information seems to be radical simplification. Throw everything inessential away. It is a fact about the physical world that it responds well to this treatment, at least for our purposes as humans. Language is the mechanism where this operation can be seen in its strongest form.

The marvel of language is that it seems to give a flexible and adaptive set of approximators that can be used to communicate "enough" information to be useful. Of course, in many cases the approximations are wrong or misleading, and this is what keeps lawyers and philosophers in business. Language is data compression with a vengeance. We don't just throw away a little information; we throw away almost all of it and manipulate the pathetic remnant we have left. That is often enough for practical purposes.

Consider a common noun like "table." Then consider a particular table—say the one sitting in our dining room. The real table might be rectangular, with rounded corners, 62 inches by 42 inches, mahogany veneer, split in two sections so additional leaves can be inserted, each section supported by a central pillar with three curved legs ending in small, decorative brass caps, making a total of two pillars and six legs. The table is reddish brown containing many hues. This table has several surface defects, including places where a child years ago did his homework on it in pencil and indented into the wood surface words and word fragments, mostly unreadable. And so on, and so on.

Although such a description can be extended to virtually any length at will, the "essentials" are picked up in a few seconds by our visual system. Further details are almost completely irrelevant to the question of where to put the cranberry sauce on Thanksgiving.

I first ran across this problem when I was a child. Because I read a lot and my father was a writer, I thought I would give writing a try. I discovered that it was virtually impossible to describe anything accurately. The skill of a writer is to get the level of detail just right, so it includes enough to allow an "adequate" mental reconstruction by the reader, but not enough to get in the way of the plot.

An analogy from the world of mathematics is a technique, like the Taylor series or the Fourier series, that approximates complex functions as sums of simple ones. Since the eighteenth century, people have known that complex functions can sometimes be very well approximated by a small number of terms in a series expansion, with a consequent great simplification. Much of applied mathematics, theoretical physics, and practical engineering is devoted to the problem of just what is the best way to approximate complex systems so that they can be analzyed "accurately enough" for the purpose at hand. (We might define God as the great nonapproximator who sees the series in its full expansion, the program at its full length, the information stream unconstricted.)

So the issue becomes, How is this process accomplished? Obviously, experiments will let us see only the barest beginnings of it. How is it lots of different physical things can become described by the same name? The classic name for this process in psychology is concept formation.

There are numerous models for concept formation. One of the most difficult problem in making any concept model work lies in discovering where the boundaries are. The assumption that there are objects and they can be treated to some degree in isolation is a remarkably powerful and constraining assumption. It is such a strong assumption that I wonder sometime at how easily it is accepted. It seems "natural," but, of course, isolated objects do not exist in the world. As a practical approximation, however, it is useful to assume that the world contains discrete objects that can be handled independently of other objects. Computing this powerful abstraction is hard and involves perceptual mechanisms like "figure-ground" separation that are not well understood. However, there are provocative aspects of lawfulness to the whole process.

I became intrigued by the "artificial concept" experiments done by Michael Posner and Steven Keele in the late 1960s. They constructed patterns of nine dots, randomly placed first on a piece of paper, later on a computer screen. They constructed a few different random patterns they called prototypes. The prototypes were then distorted by moving the dots around in random directions and distances. Experimental subjects were presented with pattern examples and were led to categorize them so that all the examples of prototype one were associated with the number "1" on the computer keyboard, and so on. Humans are good at this task, even for sets of highly distorted examples.

After the learning phase, subjects were tested with the patterns they had just seen, with new examples generated from the prototype, and with the prototypes themselves, which they never saw during the learning phase. Subjects were fastest and most accurate categorizing the prototype and were also more sure they had been shown the prototype during the learning phase than the patterns they actually had been shown. These striking distortions of memory are quite easy to produce and are sometimes called "prototype effects."

This experiment seems to demonstrate the presence of an adaptive process in which a noisy category is represented by an average of the category, the prototype. This process seems to arise automatically from the memory storage process. It is clearly a distortion of memory since what was actually seen was supplanted by something that was never seen. So much for accuracy in memory.

There is a huge body of psychological data suggesting the ubiquity of such benign, even useful, corruption mechanisms, so I found it a matter of some amusement, and also exasperation, when the classical mathematical analysis of neural networks emphasized minimizing errors of reconstruction and retrieval—for example, the least mean squares algorithms or back propagation. This is fine for some kinds of learning machines, but for real people it is more like "Distortions 'R' Us."

I had a perfectly nice memory model in the linear associator. It was almost trivial to show that when the associator learned correlated ("similar") patterns, it generated memory prototypes in the act of storage. As Andy Knapp, a talented Brown undergraduate, and I showed, the resulting model did quite a nice job of fitting much of the experimental data in the Posner and Keele experiments, though the underlying idea was far more general and interesting than learning random dot patterns.

The major problem with the linear associator was that it was linear. The definition of linearity means that a linear system like this forms sums of possible output patterns. Humans tend to be much more categorical in their responses: it is a letter "E" and not an "F" even though the patterns are physically very similar. The linear associator cannot do this discretizing. There are other reasons not to like linearity that involve difficulties in computing certain classes of functions—for example, Exclusive OR—but I always thought those were specious arguments because people also compute those functions poorly.

However, there is considerable evidence for what looks like small signal linearity—that is, when the process of, say, word recognition first starts, all meanings of an ambiguous word are represented and only later is the contextually appropriate word meaning chosen.

We needed a response selector that allows only a single response at the end of the computation. Real neurons were obviously nonlinear for large signals since they can't fire too fast and also can't fire slower than a zero firing rate. Therefore, the state vector representing an activity pattern is constrained by limits on the activities of individual elements. It was partly this observation that also gave rise to the sigmoidal activation functions that are so popular with modelers.

When it was time to nonlinearize the associative model, this was the approximatation I used: a purely linear model for small signals, but one where the responses of individual neural elements was limited. It was called the BSB model, meaning "Brain State in a Box"—that is, the state of the resulting system was contained within a box of limits.

Because the BSB model was partly linear with a simple nonlinearity, it was easy to analyze. The architecture chosen was "autoassociative," and the dynamics of the system involved positive feedback. The system state would start somewhere inside the box, and the operation of feedback through the connectivity matrix would push the system state into the corner of the box, which became stable states, or "attractor states" in the jargon of nonlinear dynamical system theory.

For those who like these things, the dominant physical analogy involved in using a linear region with limits was only secondarily neurons, but primarily the behavior of operational amplifiers, which tended to "latch up" if not handled carefully in circuits—that is, go to either the positive or negative supply voltage.

At that time I knew virtually nothing about nonlinear dynamical systems except that it was a nice name, but I could see what the qualitative behavior was going to be. A great many starting points would end up in the same final state, the attractor. What a great concept model! It started off with a sum of possible output states, and then the dynamics of the network chose the most appropriate one.

To my regret, I completely lacked the ability to analyze these networks in terms of energy minimization or Lyapunov functions, which became so important in the later history of neural networks. Many thanks to lots of very smart people like Geoff Hinton and John Hopfield, who showed how useful that mode of network analysis was. What was important to me was the result of the operation of the network. The discrete network final states distorted an underlying and much richer continuous representation. The nonlinear network reduced input information but gained great power. It was also possible to show that the operation of the network did the discarding in a way that in some cases seemed to be statistically valid. The resulting discretizations could then be used for cognitive operations.

I always thought neural networks were pretty boring devices. Using them to do things in functional systems was interesting. Seeing the footprints of these mechanisms appear in data was very exciting. We looked for the traces. For example, the first BSB paper used the network to give a potential explanation for what was called "categorical perception" in the speech literature, an effect seen for very short phonemes. Experimental data strongly suggested that fast initial processing operated so as to keep only the categories, the phoneme names, and discarded the memory of the detailed physical stimulus. The BSB model, in common with most nonlinear attractor models, could be made to act like this.

Another more speculative application of this notion of discrete stable states appeared in multistable perception—for example, the several possible stable interpretations seen for the Necker Cube or in many other optical illusions. Disambiguation of multiple word meanings was another good compuational example, as Alan Kawamoto showed in his Ph.D. thesis. Kawamoto showed quite nicely that the system started off showing a superposition of states and then settled on one for the final state, with the other meanings going away. The experimental data on disambiguation suggested this process took at most a couple of hundred milliseconds, which seemed to me to be consistent with the time parameters expected for a settling neural network.

We have learned a lot about the brain over the past thirty years, but most of this information has been about the details. It is only recently that we have started to have more than the vaguest idea of the larger-scale computational organization of the brain—that is, what the brain might be doing when it is working. And our major discovery seems to be an awareness that we really don't know what is going on.

This is curious. To use an analogy, it is as if we know great amounts about the parts that comprise an automobile. We know many of the finest details and even have some ideas about the functions of a few component parts, like an oil filter or a fuel pump, not to mention the ubiquity of the nuts and bolts that tie the pieces together. We know something about the chemistry of combustion. What we lack is understanding that the major function of the parts, when working, is to transport the vehicle and its contents from one physical location to another.

In many respects, a car is a better analogy to the brain than a computer. A car is composed of a number of specialized modules working together to perform a useful overall function. No one asks it to be a general purpose machine. Why do we ask the brain to be one? I suspect because we don't like limits on the abilities of our personal biological computer.

I have now participated in several practical projects involving neural networks, both as a consultant and as a subcontractor. Applications are wonderful discipline for academics because difficult issues cannot be avoided. Academics like to look at problems that might have solutions that are elegant or informative. In engineering, a device has to work and do something. Some parts may be more elegant than others, but the whole system has to work. There are lots of considerations like cost, reliability, and robustness that affect the way things are done.

My first real experience with a project of this type was a joint study with a group at the Texas Instruments Central Research Laboratories in Dallas—originally Andy Penz, Dean Collins, and Mike Gately. The original problem was to analyze a segment of the microwave spectrum to see how many radar transmitters were present. Many neural net problems involve pattern recognition: say, if given a microwave receiver output, suggest the best classification of the signal. This one was different. There was a flood of data, and the object was to make sense of it. In a complex radar environment there could be hundreds of thousands of radar pulses a second. Signal-to-noise ratio of individual pulses was not the issue. There were a small number of transmitters out there, and since this was a military application, the problem was to determine the number of transmitters, whether or not the transmitters were threats, and if they were threats, which was the most dangerous.

My first thought was that this was very much like the biological concept-forming problem that I had looked at before for the Posner-Keele experiments, where the adaptive system saw a number of noisy examples. I also had a useful attractor network in BSB. The two could be combined so as to form an unsupervised learning system, where all the examples of a single transmitter ended up in the same attractor. The key to getting it to work was finding a good data representation for the data coming from the microwave receiver. The data representation used was based on the ubiquitous topographic maps of sensory properties seen in the cerebral cortex. The value of a signal parameter—say, frequency, intensity, direction of arrival, and so on—was mapped into a blurry location on a map of the parameter. This kind of representation is sometimes called a "bar code" because a moving bar of activity, like a meter pointer on an analog speedometer or a voltmeter, indicates the value. I was delighted to find that this technique essentially worked the first time it was tried. The neural network—based model itself is being developed further for use with a wideband acousto-optical spectrum analyzer built by Photonic Systems.

I thought this project was a good example of how some common ideas from cognitive science could be applied directly to engineering. We assumed microwave signals acted like objects, and we applied ideas like concept formation and object recognition to do the analysis. It was also a system that was specifically not interested in accurate classification, but in extracting commonalities and deliberately distorting the details of individual examples to produce a constant representation, the attractor.

The radar project suggested some interesting scientific questions. One attractor network did useful clustering and data simplification. Suppose we had a whole array of attractor networks, what could they do? How would they do it? This project turned into an example where an applied project led back into less-applied science.

Perhaps the single most significant observation about the mammalian nervous system is that it is very large, and the larger it gets the better it seems to work. We know a great deal about the properties of individual neurons. We know less, although we do know something, about the average behavior of large ensembles of millions of neurons by use of technques like evoked responses, PET scans, and functional magnetic resonance imaging. We know virtually nothing about the properties of intermediate-size groupings of neurons. This gap results from the best example I know of in science of the "lamppost phenomenon." This name refers to the old joke about the drunk looking under the lamppost for his car keys because that is where the light is best, even though he lost them somewhere else.

We focus on single neurons because we *can* focus on single neurons. Experimental and analytical techniques are available to do amazing things with single neurons. However, once we start to record from more than one neuron, especially in the dense forests of the mammalian cerebral cortex where the cells all look more or less the same, our techniques fail us. Even if we record from a handful of neurons, say ten or twenty, we have little idea about how to handle the resulting flood of data.

It would be inconceivable to analyze a large corporation like IBM or organizations like the U.S. Army or the U.S. government if we restricted ourselves to the behavior of single employees. The real structure of large organizations appears at the level of work groups, departments, and divisions, or in the case of the U.S. Army, at the level of squads, companies, regiments, battalions, divisions, armies, and so on. Single members come and go in the organization and over time may move from group to group or even retire, but the organization itself remains stable.

Almost everyone believes, based on vague hints and suggestive neuro-anatomy, that there are important groupings of cells that can act as functional units. Most people who think about it at all feel that these functional groupings of many cells are where the real computational business of the nervous system takes place. Single-unit responses report only the dimmest shadows of the real mechanisms of neural computation. Hebb believed this, and based his notion of cell assemblies on it. I believed it too.

Based on the power of small attractor networks to usefully distort by dis-cretizing, I became intrigued with networks composed of many attractor networks. Attractor networks are characterized by their relatively small number of attractors more than by the large numbers of interacting single units whose dynamics give rise to the attractors. Therefore, it might be pos-sible to assume that attractor networks interact by passing information about their attractor states back and forth. The connections between individual networks become matrices of weights that couple states together, rather than the single scalar values assumed for the couplings between single units in traditional neural networks.

Surprisingly, such models are quite easy to analyze. Since individual net-works are coupled locally, the "network of networks" gives rise to traveling waves of activation across the surface of a model cortex. And where two traveling waves excited by elementary features of an input collide, a learning system can easily learn a new attractor state, based on a nonlinear combina-tion of old states. Networks at the location of the "interference pattern" thereby develop an expanded repertoire of states, forming new attractor states that correspond to combinations of features. Such combination states are spatially localized and exceptionally useful for pattern recognition. Models for brain function that made use of traveling waves, interference patterns, and so on were common in the 1950s and 1960s—for example, in the work of Harry Blum and Karl Lashley, among others, and more recently Jack Cowan.

The resulting models are easy to simulate and work very well. It is much more difficult to connect them directly to experimental data from either physiology or psychology. But the models seem to have great computa-tional power in limited domains based on the underlying data representation, exactly the kind of strictly limited generalization power that seems to char-acterize the cortex. We had done an earlier study on the learning of arith-metic facts that suggested that generalization ability was much more a function of details of the data representation than the network architecture. One conclusion, which has a great deal of support, is that most human "abstract" thought seems to be firmly based on perceptual representations.

The great question for the future, the most important question and the most difficult to solve, is consciousness. In spite of my grounding in mysticism in the 1960s, I am convinced that consciousness is a scientific question that has an answer, though I have no idea what that answer might be or what form it might take. My hunch is that this is where the laws of physics as derived for very simple and very small systems will have to be extended. Maybe there is just something special about systems of great complexity—many informational states lying very close together in energy, lots of noise, and a physical size somewhere between a BB and a basketball. There is no way to find out with current technology.

It is remarkable how thoroughly the question of consciousness is avoided. In the early 1980s, there was a wonderful and similar controversy in cognitive science on visual imagery. If you experience pictures in the head in some form, and almost everyone does, then you know what visual imagery is. But can you actually prove to someone else who doesn't have it that you have it? It may seem like a picture, but it is easy to show that for most people the imagery is highly malleable and of low spatial resolution, so many questions that could be easily answered if we had a real image (is San Diego west or east of Reno?) are very hard to answer from our remembered maps. Our imagery is contaminated with other processes. Perhaps our intuitive feeling that our imagery is visual in the same sense that an external picture is visual is erroneous. There are a number of smart and articulate people who claim to have little or no visual imagery, and how can the rest of us convince them? How do they even think? Maybe *they* are lying.

I suspect that consciousness is a little like this. Everyone has an opinion and an experience, and since we have little in the way of data, there is no way to tell whose opinion is better. Most arguments about consciousness consist of discussing whether it actually is anything or not. Would we know it if we saw it acting in the physical world? If it was an intermediate-level phenomenon like the network of network models, how could we detect its operation by looking at single units? Right now we could not, even if it was there.

There is a very strong tendency to confuse consciousness with particular mental functions just because our kind of consciousness seems to require and use them. A good example would be short-term memory, which has been suggested as a hallmark of consciousness. Another use of consciousness would be as a deus ex machina to solve the binding problem. This approach notes properties of consciousness typical of our kind of cognition, but doesn't actually say anything about consciousness, just what is required to recognize our kind of consciousness. If a conscious being had no short-term memory, it might be unable to talk about much of interest to us, but would be no less conscious.

Another good question is whether consciousness is binary—that is, there or not there—or analog—i.e., that is, graded. I think few would deny that a dog or a chimpanzee is conscious if we are. But how about a mosquito? or a virus? Maybe they are conscious too, just a little bit. Does consciousness appear with a hearty "splat!" sometime during evolution or gradually increase in strength? If you have a bad day and lose a few neurons, does your consciousness decrease, like turning down the voltage on a light bulb? This would allow for quantitative estimates of consciousness based perhaps on nervous system connectivity or the energy landscape of the state space, and so on. Maybe computers are just as conscious as we are; they just don't talk about it.

The generation of consciousness through a nonlinear neural net that tries to solve the binding problem to provide more effective computation strikes me as unconvincing and almost insulting. Is that all consciousness is there for? What does it do? If it doesn't do anything physical, why is it there? But does it have to do practical things to be there? Is there any special computational function that a conscious system can do that an unconscious one cannot? I suspect any particular well-defined function could always be produced by a mechanical system.

It is worth noting that the most desirable mystical state in most traditions is characterized by loss of cognition, loss of categories, loss of memory. As Huang Po says, "The mind, which is without beginning is unborn and indestructable. It is not green or yellow.... It does not belong to the category of things which exist or do not exist.... It is neither long nor short, big or small.... It is that which you see before you. Begin to reason about it and you at once fall into error."

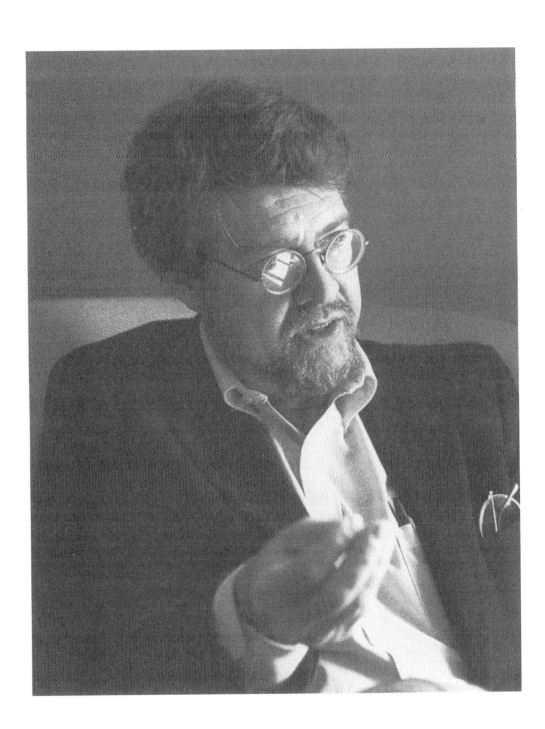

12   David E. Rumelhart

David Rumelhart is Professor of Psychology at Stanford University, Stanford, California. He is co-editor of and helped write many of the chapters in the classic "PDP" books, the two volume 1986 set of books that helped create the resurgence of interest in neural networks. (D. E. Rumelhart and J. L. McClelland and the PDP Research Group, Parallel Distributed Processing, *vol. 1. Foundations , J. L. McClelland and D. E. Rumelhart and the PDP Research Group,* Parallel Distributed Processing, *vol. 2. Psychological and Biological Models, both from MIT Press.)*

March 30, 1993, San Francisco, California

ER: Maybe we could start with the circumstances of your growing up, things like that.

DR: I was born in South Dakota, in a small town called Wessington Springs. Its size was about 1200 people. I was born June 12, 1942. I went to the University of South Dakota for my undergraduate work. I started out there in philosophy.

ER: Can we back up a little bit? I'd really like to know more about what the atmosphere was like at home, how you got interested in ideas ...

DR: How do I start? I have two siblings, both younger, two brothers. My parents were born and were raised in the same small town and lived there their whole lives. My father was a printer who worked in a print shop from the time he was fourteen until he retired. My mother has been a librarian for the last forty years, something like that, and the only librarian in the town library. The town is a small town, and the area around it is all rural. The main point of the town is to serve the farmers in the area.

I lived in town. The high school I went to was a high school of about two hundred people, about half from the town and about half from the surrounding area. I suppose in terms of academic interests, my parents had both been good students, but neither of them went to college. In fact, I was about the first in my family to go to college. My mother had been a schoolteacher for about a year, but in those days that meant going to six weeks of training, and then you could go and be a schoolteacher until you got married, and then you had to quit. Once you were married, you were somehow not fit to be a teacher anymore. In any case, she was a schoolteacher for a year or two after she got out of high school. School was an important thing in our family. My father was always proud of the fact that he was good at mathematics. Basically, he went through high school and that was about all, although he was in the Navy. In the Navy he did work that involved studying some more mathematics.

ER: When you were growing up, when you were in elementary school and high school, were you interested in things that became part of your career?

DR: I always did well in grade school and high school. I wasn't particularly a book reader in the way that some people are. I liked sports. This was one of the things that my father thought was very important, so I played football and basketball and baseball and ran in track. Of course, in a high school of two hundred people, that was not so difficult.

I did well in school in spite of the fact that I wasn't very oriented toward studying. Of course, this was the '50s, when I was in grade school and high school and people's views of things were different. The idea of doing homework was something that nobody ever thought about. I remember I used to read the encyclopedia. We had the *World Book Encyclopedia*, and I read the entire thing over a period of time.

ER: Alphabetically or at random?

DR: Not at random, exactly. I had topics of interest, and I would read about those, and then I would just pick up a volume and read it. A bit odd, I suppose. I was always interested in things. My father was a person who believed in a kind of apprenticeship, and I always thought, well, if something was in a book somewhere, I could read about it and figure out how to do it. I didn't really need to bother with learning at my father's knee about how to hammer nails or all the different things that he did.

My father was a great debater. I learned to be a debater as a child. We would debate politics; we would debate religion: we would debate, you name it, everything. He had a kind of anti-intellectual bent to him. He thought that intellectuals didn't really know about the real world. This was a common thread of debate because I always felt that we could figure things out by thinking about them.

ER: Where do you think that notion came from?

DR: Probably my mother. My mother is a person who is relatively quiet. She was a librarian. She was much more oriented toward books and intellectual pursuits. I suppose it was my mother who had this idea. It was a valid idea, just trying to figure out how to do things. It wasn't anything she ever said, any discussion we ever had. It was, I think, just her attitude. In school, for whatever reason, I found teachers easier to interact with on the whole than my peers. I always had good relationships with my teachers. I remember spending hours after school talking with teachers when I was in elementary school, about all kinds of things. In particular, I remember discussing the Korean War with my teachers, the death of Stalin, all these things that were occurring in the early '50s.

I had some teachers who were important in my life. They were always very encouraging. I did well in school, even though it was sort of not the right way to be—to be particularly bookish or particularly oriented toward succeeding in school or doing well in school. It was just that I did it. That was not a problem for me one way or the other. I was able, nevertheless, to be as undisciplined as anyone else.

I might say a little bit about high school. It was interesting because one of my teachers in high school, a math teacher, had never had calculus. There was only one person in the high school who had ever taken calculus and that was the typing teacher. I remember that my math teacher, who had never taken this advanced subject, felt that this other person was somebody like a god because he had taken calculus.

The other thing that I remember about this teacher was his teaching me to use the slide rule, which was sort of fun. Years later, he became a car salesman or something. My father encountered him once. He had moved, lived in a different town. This happened to be at the time when I was at the Institute for Advanced Study for a year, and I still had my little slide rule. He was impressed that I still had this little slide rule I had gotten when I was a sophomore in high school.

In high school, as I say, I did well. I was the salutatorian, the second highest–ranking student in my class of about fifty. I had this image when I was going off to college, I remember well. I figured, "Well, gee, if I'm second out of fifty at Wessington Springs, what will I be when I go to college?" I figured that, you know, maybe the top ten percent would go. I estimated that that would be second out of five, if we're talking ten percent, so that puts me at about 60 percent. So I figured I'd probably be a B or a C student in college; that's what I imagined.

Of course, when I went to college, it turned out that maybe people in my high school were a little better than I thought, and I actually did very, very well. As I said, I started out in philosophy. My father wanted me to study engineering, and I just didn't want to do engineering. It sounded boring to me, something I just didn't want to do. That was the only real conflict—that is, serious conflict—I ever had with my father. They also wanted me to go to the local junior college, in the town, which had about eighty students or something. I had an athletic scholarship to this college, but instead I went to the University of South Dakota and started studying philosophy.

ER: That was the first time you were away from home?

DR: Yeah, it was. I moved away then, and I more or less never went back. I didn't spend more than a week or two at home in a stretch after I went off to college. I started out in philosophy until I got bored with that and decided that the philosophers were too much into just debating and not enough into thinking about things or doing anything. I moved into psychology. I took it as a kind of empirical approach to epistemology. My idea was that the psychologists were looking to see what was going on, whereas the philosophers were only talking about it.

David E. Rumelhart

I had several jobs, since I really didn't have any money. I worked as a cook in the cafeteria for my food. I lived in the basement of a church, and I was the church janitor, which is how I managed to pay for my room. I had scholarships that paid for my tuition. That was it. I worked the summer before I went to college; I worked in a grocery store and earned some money to pay for going to see a movie or something.

ER: Were the scholarships all athletic? Or were some of them academic?

DR: No, no. They weren't athletic scholarships. I won a scholarship in a math contest. It didn't pay very much. It was like $150 a semester or something.

ER: It was the late '50s, early '60s, then.

DR: I graduated in 1960 from high school. I took math without thinking about it because it was easy for me. I was three years an undergraduate, and I ended up getting a major in math and psychology in the end. And not knowing what to do at that point—saying, "Gee, I have a major in math and major in psychology," I ran across a book that had an article in it about a topic called mathematical psychology. I thought, "Hm, this seems like a sensible thing for me."

I looked, and the author of this article was a man named William K. Estes, and I thought, "Whoa, that's interesting." I looked and he was at University of Indiana, so I applied to Indiana University for graduate school, thinking I would go and study mathematical psychology. More or less at the last minute I discovered that Estes was not there any more, that he had moved to Stanford University. I knew nothing of Stanford University; I'd hardly even heard of it. But I had done very well in college, and I had an NSF [National Science Foundation] fellowship, and I had a Woodrow Wilson and a Danforth fellowship. I managed to get lots of fellowships, so I could pretty much go wherever I wanted. So I thought, "Hm, I'd better apply to Stanford University." I did, and fortunately I was admitted.

I went to Stanford, in their program at that time called the Institute for Mathematical Studies in the Social Sciences, which was their program in mathematical psychology. I worked there with Bill Estes, with Dick Atkinson, Pat Suppes, and Gordon Bower. Those were the people in those days who were working in this field called mathematical psychology.

It was there that I first encountered the idea of a perceptron. I've forgotten now where; it may have been described in the *Handbook of Mathematical Psychology*. I remember first reading about perceptrons as a graduate student. I went to graduate school in Stanford in the fall of '63.

In the whole field of mathematical psychology, the idea of things like perceptrons were not prominent. That wasn't the direction that people were looking in. I was doing Markov models of learning and memory, pretty much standard stuff. My thesis was on building some of these models. It was interesting, to me anyway, because what I showed was that about five different models, which everybody thought were different, turned out to be all the same. My conclusion was that the field of mathematical psychology had focused far too narrowly. The idea in those days was that, well, we were going to focus down on a very simple problem—paired associate learning. We would focus on this very simple problem and then solve that, and then we would look at what the real structure was, and then we would know what the right models were, and we would then know where to go.

It turned out that models evolve, and so maybe ultimately they all converged. With the database that people were looking at, I was able to show mathematically that all these models were in fact identical, at least in their predictions of the mean. They predicted different things about the variances of things, but they were all identical in mean, and that was all anybody ever looked at anyway. Yet people were arguing "My model is better. My model is better." But, of course, there was no way that they were even different.

This was my Ph.D. thesis. I might mention one other thing that happened during my years at Stanford. Steve Grossberg did his thesis in around '65, I think, maybe '66. In any case, what I remember well is that he sent his thesis to Stanford, to the Institute for Mathematical Studies in Social Sciences. He had vaguely been associated with them before I came. In any case, he sent them a copy of his big, fat dissertation, which had all of these differential equations and everything, and this big cover letter in which he explained how he had solved all of the problems in psychology. Of course, the people at the Institute for Mathematical Studies in Social Sciences were a little perplexed about what this could all be about. I remember we spent a great deal of time and effort trying to figure it out and failed completely, I should say, to understand what it was that Grossberg had actually done. In the end, I guess I gave up on it. The most remarkable thing really about it was the cover letter, in which he explained how all of the hard problems in psychology had been solved. That was my second brush with what's come to be called neural networks. It was very hard to figure out what it meant. There were those who thought that, well, "There is something very deep here, and it's beyond us. We just can't figure it out." And there were those who thought that this was just a story, and it meant nothing, and we shouldn't pay any attention to it.

ER: Did either of those two contacts with neural networks inspire you to read more at that time?

DR: At that time, it was pretty much just encounters. I was busy; I was working on Markov models, and I hadn't really focused on any of these other kinds of models yet. It wasn't until I went to San Diego and Jim [Anderson] came down once from UCLA, I think in '69, and gave a talk to Don Norman and me about some sort of correlational model. I remember being very intrigued by it and impressed with both the simplicity of the idea and the power that it looked like was there. I remember that Norman and I were working on memory and had done memory models and were quite intrigued by this general idea.

ER: Just to back up for a minute from there, you got your doctorate from Stanford?

DR: Right, in '67, and then I went down to San Diego. I was in the psychology department at UCSD, and I worked there fairly closely with Don Norman.

ER: How did you choose San Diego?

DR: That's a good question. At the time when I graduated, in '67, mathematical psychologists were popular for a year or two. There was a group of them the year before me, all of whom got very good jobs. Then in my year, there were a few jobs. At the end of the '60s, things were beginning to dry up in terms of jobs for psychologists, but mathematical psychologists had a place for a while because nobody knew quite what they were going to do or who they were and thought maybe they should have one.

One of the people I met during the years that I was a graduate student was Bill McGill, who spent a year there. McGill is a very, very interesting man. I was very impressed by him when he was visiting at Stanford. I discovered that he and some others had started a department, a brand new department, at UCSD. In those days, jobs were a little bit different. Your advisor would call somebody up on the phone and say, "I have this student you should hire." And apparently something like that happened in my case. I guess Bill Estes talked to the people at UCSD. They had a job opening, and he said, "Hey, you ought to look at this guy."

I interviewed at three or four places, but UCSD was a new department; they had really interesting people there, and there was just no question that if they offered me the job, I would take it. And they did, so I went to UCSD in the fall of '67. Right away, McGill became chancellor of the university, so I ended up not interacting much with him, but rather with Don Norman, who was very active in those days working on memory. Attention and memory were his fields. I have always been a collaborator. I've always enjoyed working with people. It's just the way I think.

I worked with Peter Lindsay, who was an assistant professor there. He and I did a lot of things together, also with Norman. The three of us had a research group called LNR, Lindsay-Norman-Rumelhart, which actually maintained the name LNR long after Peter Lindsay left.

But in any case, at San Diego I started this project that resulted from my work on my dissertation. Psychologists were too narrow I thought. We had to have a bigger picture. Mathematical psychology was, I thought, limited because in those days we required closed-form solutions to things. I began to get the idea that a better method would be computer simulation. So really from the time I went to San Diego, I was thinking about computer simulation. In addition to Jim's work that I mentioned, which I found very interesting, I also was inspired by the work of Ross Quillian, who in those days was doing computer models of so-called semantic networks.

I always had one course that was like a free course in which I would choose a book of the year and teach out of that. In 1969, I think it was, or maybe '70, I chose *Perceptrons* by Minsky and Papert as the book of the year. We then carefully went through it and read it in a group. There were some people from the math department, the graduate students, and me. This, by the way, was something I learned from Bill McGill. He always liked this idea of reading a particular book and going though it with a group.

This was my most in-depth experience with things related to neural networks, or what were later called neural networks. I was quite interested in Minsky in those days because he also had another book which was called, I think, *Semantic Information Processing.* That book was a collection, including an article by Ross Quillian. It was a collection of dissertations from his graduate students.

In a way, it was Minsky who led me to read about the perceptron more than anybody else. In those days, in the late '60s, Norman and I got the idea that artificial intelligence was an important direction. We went off and got into the AI community. We got to know the people and, although we were psychologists, we became associated with artifical intelligence as an approach. It was part of my philosophy that we needed broader theories. We needed to have theories which were not tiny little micromodels, but were bigger models.

ER: This also seems to fit your notion that computer simulations were the way to go.

DR: Right, exactly. Around 1970 I said, "Look, this looks like an important thing. I'll devote five years of my life to trying to see if this project will work out"—that is, the AI approach and the computer simulation approach. That's pretty much what I did for those years. I did lots of different AI-oriented things, psychology and AI, and out of that work came several things. One of them was the book that Norman and I did, *Explorations in Cognition.* That book was the model for the book that McClelland and I did, the PDP [parallel distributed processing] volumes. In any case, *Explorations in Cognition* was also in a way based on the Minsky model. It was us and our students working together and writing this book as a group. By the time we were done, I had decided that we had to go on. We still weren't broad enough. We were broadening, but there was still more we needed to do.

A couple of other things happened, interesting things with respect to my later work on neural networks. I had a student named Jim Levin. He got interested in a system that he called Proteus. Proteus was inspired by Carl Hewitt's actor system, but it turned out to be as close as anything to neural networks. Instead of having complex actors, we had simple actors. They were little linear devices that today could easily by characterized as more or less linear neural network-type systems. We had some nonlinearities too, as I recall, but I can't remember all the details. His dissertation was on Proteus, which turned out to have a lot of interesting properties.

The other thing that I did in the late '70s or mid-'70s was devise another model. I was quite interested in reading. I took as my area of work what I called linguistic information processing.

In psychology it was commonplace to say, "OK, I study memory," or "I study perception," or "I study attention," or "I study vision,"—you name it. I can view those as slices through the system. I had this idea that we were interested in information processing. What we should do is follow the information from the time that it hits the eye until the time that you do something. But I felt that was an enormous problem, so I decided to focus on linguistic information. In particular, reading was a good case because in reading we have visual information processing: we can study perception, we can study comprehension, we can study the whole process. I devised a model called the interactive model of reading, which was published in the *Attention and Performance* volume for '75, I think.

The model was intended, among other things, to challenge the work of a couple of people who had models of reading. One was David Laberge. I went to a conference, and David Laberge was there. I had a conversation with him, and he said, "You know, your model is a fine model; it's very interesting model." But he also said, "You know the brain couldn't do that."

I said, "What are you talking about?" And I thought, "Hm," and I stored that away in the back of my brain. "What do you mean, the brain couldn't do that? Of course, the brain could do that."

He said he thought his model was more plausible. It was a purely feed forward model. My model involved all kinds of interactions. That is why it was called the interactive model. Information had to move in both directions in order for it to work. I stored that comment away, and it later played a role in my thinking.

Another important thing happened in 1974, I think it was. Jay McClelland came as an assistant professor to UCSD. Jay and I got along quite well. We jointly taught a course together for a couple of years. This was valuable, both in terms of getting to know each other and also just in general in terms of building a common understanding of things. I remember, I taught a mathematical psychology course at the time. Jay decided to take this course while he was an assistant professor. He thought that he could learn to do modeling.

So he took the course from me, and he built a little model, which in the end turned out to be closely related to a kind of a neural network model by the time we got done. The model that he built was what he called the cascade model, which was a feedforward model with saturation. He used it to explain reaction times.

I think in '76 or '77, there was a conference at Minnesota which I attended and which Jay attended and which Jim [Anderson] attended. I was in and out pretty much, but gave my talk. In those days I was working on story understanding, and I gave a talk about that. What I remember is that Jay was at this meeting and apparently had a number of conversations with Jim.

JA: We had dinner together practically every night.

DR: Jay became quite interested in some of the neural networks ideas. After Jay came back, we were talking about the cascade model, and we had this thought. You know the interactive model that I had developed could be formulated in much the same way as his cascade model, if we allowed feedback. We had systems that had connections that went in both directions. We then spent the next two and a half years or so refining this model, which later became the interactive model of word perception or word recognition. It had various titles. We published it in two parts in *Psychology Review.* It was inspired by all of these different things.

In the end it turned out to be very much like these models that settle into stable states. Indeed, it was those features that we eventually worked out. But what I remember are hours and hours and hours of tinkering on the computer. We sat down and did all this in the computer and built these computer models, and we just didn't understand them. We didn't understand why they worked or why they didn't work or what was critical about them. We had no important theory yet. We struggled and struggled and began to get insights into the nature of these interacting systems and became totally obsessed by them. We wanted to make this all work.

Another important thing happened in roughly that time frame, while McClelland and I were working on this model. We had a postdoctoral program that came from the Sloan Foundation. They were then beginning to invest money in cognitive science. We looked around the world to find people to come to our postdocs. We had, I believe, five slots. One of the people we found to come was Geoffrey Hinton. In those days, Geoff had been working on vision and had developed a relational model of visual perception.

When I read his thesis, we were trying to decide whether to invite him or some other people, and we thought, "Gee, this is pretty intriguing stuff." I remember reading his thesis and seeing relationships between it and a Proteus system, and relationships between it and the kind of stuff that McClelland and I were thinking about.

So anyway, Hinton came, and Don Norman and I had this idea that we would hold meetings—I have this impression of them being daily meetings —with our postdocs. At these meetings each postdoc would have a week to tell about his vision of things because these were interdisciplinary groups, with people from linguistics and computer science and psychology and anthropology—all these areas.

So in my interactions with Geoffrey and Jay and the others I began to understand better about relaxation and better about how our networks might be working. The network that McClelland and I were building could be viewed as a relaxation mechanism. Geoffrey originally came from Edinburgh and worked with [Christopher] Longuet-Higgins. Longuet-Higgins in his early years had been interested in various kinds of distributed memory. One of his students was David Willshaw. Geoffrey had for a long time been interested in brainlike models. He went to work with Longuet-Higgins in part because of this distributed model. He spent a year there. By then Longuet-Higgins had gone on and was interested in other things and wasn't very supportive, but Geoff did work for a year or so with David Willshaw. He was finishing his dissertation and became quite knowledgeable about these network mechanisms and how they worked, but then he was discouraged from doing this work further. This was in the early '70s. And so he went off and used relaxation methods, which were essentially the same ideas, but that was the way he framed his work.

When he was at San Diego, he came to the decision that he wanted to go back and think a lot harder about perceptrons and about learning. At that time I separated the work on learning mechanisms from the relaxation ideas. I had this idea the relaxation methods were one class of problem solving, and then there were learning methods, which were basically perceptron learning.

The other thing we did as part of our program was we allowed each of our postdocs to invent a conference, any conference that they wanted. So Geoffrey wanted to have a conference on parallel associative memory. Jim [Anderson] came and was part of our program, the Sloan program, for three months. Jim and Geoffrey put together this conference, which was held in June of '79.

This conference was really quite interesting because Jim knew a lot of the people who were doing neural network things, and Geoffrey had lots of interesting ideas. We brought in really a lot of people. Although I was not a major participant, I became increasingly intrigued by the work that was going on—Geoffrey's and the work that Jay and I had been doing and then this conference. It all was percolating in my head that this neural network business was something that I'd better pay attention to; this was really interesting stuff.

I thought, "Somehow my work with Jay and these neural networks are related. I ought to be able to put all this together." So I continued discussions with McClelland and Hinton, and then Geoffrey went off back to England for a while. Jay and I kept talking. Then I went to Stanford on a kind of a sabbatical leave. My goal when I was there was to write a book. I was supposed to write a book on schema theory, but I couldn't manage it. I instead kept thinking about this work on neural networks, parallel associative memory or whatever we called it. I don't think we did call it neural networks. But anyway, whatever it was, I kept thinking about it.

I didn't write the book. I had built this computer language called SOL, semantic operating language, which was designed to do semantic networks. I modified it entirely so that it would do matrix operations and do all this modeling of essentially neural networks. I simply couldn't manage to do the work that I was supposed to do.

I decided while I was away that I just had to get this out of my system. I had to figure out what was going on. It seemed like there were all these interesting things, and they really must be related to each other in some way. I remember there was a meeting in the summer after this. APA [American Psychological Association] met in Los Angeles. This was the summer of '81.

I went up to see the books. It was an outing. My wife came with me. I said to her, "You know, there's something going on here. I really want to learn about this, this whatever, neural network, parallel associative memory stuff. I have this book I'm supposed to be writing, but, you know, I think I don't want to write it now. I'm going to put it off. I think this is important." I said, "I think it's important enough that I should spend at least five years figuring out what's going on."

I had these five-year plans—at least five years for figuring out what was going on here. So by the time we finished our train ride, I had committed myself to saying, "OK, this is it. I want to learn about this stuff."

When I came back to San Diego from this trip, I went to see McClelland, and I said to Jay, "Look, Geoffrey's coming back in December. Let's spend two quarters going over all the stuff on these neural network things." UCSD used a quarter system. "Let's spend the winter and spring, while Geoffrey's going to be here. We'll have meetings every day. I'm on sabbatical. I can do this." Jay was on a Young Investigator Award, and Geoffrey was coming as a kind of a postdoctoral continuation. We thought we would just really focus on this, and by the end we would write a book. We'd sort all this out; we'd write it down and tell people about it. "Six months, that's plenty of time for doing this," we thought.

We sat down starting in early January, and we brought together the people who were most interested. That was Geoffrey, Jay, me, Francis Crick, and a couple of graduate students. Richard Golden came to some of these meetings—I think also Mike Moser and Mike Jordan and Paul Smolensky, who by then was a metapostdoc on the Sloan program. We decided we would sort out what was going on, and we would use it as a guide, and then we would write a book when we got done. We would be working on the book during all this time.

So we went to the literature, and we read more or less all the work we could find: Jim's work, work by Steve Grossberg, work by Leon Cooper—all the people we could think of who were doing work in this general area. We would try to put it all together. My memory now could be wrong, but what I remember is that we met essentially daily, for two quarters, not quite six months. We met every day, and we met for several hours a day.

The first order of business was to say, "Well, what are we going to call these things? What are they named?" We ended by deciding that we should call them parallel distributed processing [PDP] systems. We were interested in them being parallel, and we were interested in them being distributed, so we devised this name, PDP. That was one of our first orders of business, to come up with this name. So then at least we had a name to call this whole family of things.

We read Rosenblatt; we basically informed ourselves as much as possible of all the literature that that we could find. We couldn't help but keep thinking about how we could put it all together. It was during that spring I went off to a meeting in Florida. It was an ONR [Office of Naval Research] contractors' meeting.

In San Diego we were talking about the difficult problems, like solving the X-OR [exclusive OR] problem. Geoffrey said, "OK, here's the problem. Here's a classic problem that the perceptrons don't work on." I had read a little bit in Rosenblatt about his ideas on how to build multilayer systems. Of course, I'd read *Perceptrons*. And I thought, "Well, somehow we have to figure out how to teach, how to train, a network that has more than one layer. Why can't we do this?"

McClelland and I had done a trick, we thought, and that trick was the following. We wanted to have nonlinear systems that could learn with sigmoidal units. We were worried because we didn't know exactly how to train them. So what we thought was we'd pretend they were linear, and we would compute the derivatives as if they were linear, and then we could train them. We did this on a one-layer system. That was what we called delta learning. It was like the Widrow-Hoff model except that we used sigmoids instead of linear output units. They were more like the kind of thing that Jim did, which was to use sharp thresholds.

Every time I go on an airplane trip, I set for myself a problem to solve. And on this particular trip to the ONR meeting, I set for myself the problem, "How can we train these multilayer networks?" I knew about, as I say, the work of Rosenblatt and about the way he tried to do it. He had this idea of sending error signals back across layers, but he didn't have a very principled way of doing it.

So I thought, "Well, suppose we pretend that this is a linear system. Could we solve it?" Sure. We would know how to train it if it were linear, but of course a linear system doesn't have the right properties. In the linear system, we might as well not have any hidden units. They don't do anything in a linear system. So I thought, "Well, we'll just pretend like it's linear, and figure out how to train it as if it were linear, and then we'll put in these sigmoids. In that way, we can make a system that would work."

In those days I was doing everything in LISP [a computer language]. I hacked up this idea, and as far as I know the first time I ever worked on the X-OR problem was by using my LISP code to train one of these back propagation networks to solve the problem. The very first problem I worked on.

When I did it, I was disappointed by a number of things. It worked, but it took maybe a thousand iterations to learn. I thought, "Gee, that's pretty bad." Geoffrey pointed out, "This is a big problem. There're going to be all kinds of local minima. It just isn't going to fly very well."

Shortly thereafter I became a bit distracted. McClelland and I wanted to work on past tense learning. I thought I needed multiple layers to do the problem of mapping from the phonology. I wanted to do past tense learning, and I thought, "Well, you know, we might want to have a hidden layer that would learn the past tense marker somehow." I didn't call it a hidden layer, but an intermediate layer, like a variation on the Gamba perceptron. That was what I had been focusing on.

But then McClelland and I figured out another trick for learning past tenses, the so-called "Wickelfeature" representation. We thought, "Oh well, we don't need multiple layers." So I put that aside and went off, and we realized that if we made fancier input representations, we wouldn't need this intermediate layer. I began working on that.

David Zipser came to San Diego in the summer of '82. He was interested in competitive learning. He and I spent the next several months working on competitive learning. I started working with him and put aside this X-OR stuff for a while and worked on competitive learning. We worked on that for while, and then in '83, there was a meeting in Pittsburgh.

Hinton was at Pittsburgh. He had spent the summer working with Sejnowski, and they devised the Boltzmann machine. That summer Jerry Feldman had a meeting at Rochester, in which John Hopfield came and presented his work on the Hopfield nets. Immediately, Hinton and Sejnowski realized that you could use stochastic elements instead of discrete elements and built what they called the Boltzmann machine.

Geoffrey called up one day and said, "You know, about this book, I really don't want to be involved in it anymore because I'm really into the Boltzmann machine, and we've got all these great ideas, and we're going to work on that." So he and Sejnowski, who he had met, by the way, at the conference that he and Jim organized, were working on Boltzmann machines.

In the meantime, Paul Smolensky, also a physicist, had the idea for what he called "Harmony Theory," which was closely related to the Boltzmann machine. These are the ordinary physics ways of looking at things, I guess. But, anyway, there was this somewhat independent pathway that Smolensky was taking, working on things that turned out to be closely related to Boltzmann machines. He had a very different view of it from what Sejnowski and Hinton were doing.

In any case, Geoffrey decided that he didn't want to be involved in the book, so Jay and I thought, "Well, we'll do the book." Of course, it was falling further and further behind as we kept writing more papers. At first we were going to just summarize the literature, but we kept thinking, "Well, gee, here's something else," and so we did this and then we did that, and it just kept accumulating. The book kept getting bigger and bigger.

I believe it was in '83 that Geoff and Terry held a meeting in Pittsburgh. I had my choice about two things to talk about. I had done work on what later became backpropagation and work on competitive learning. I remember electing at the last minute to talk about the competitive learning work rather than the backpropagation work. I had my slides all made out to do both of these talks, and I gave that one.

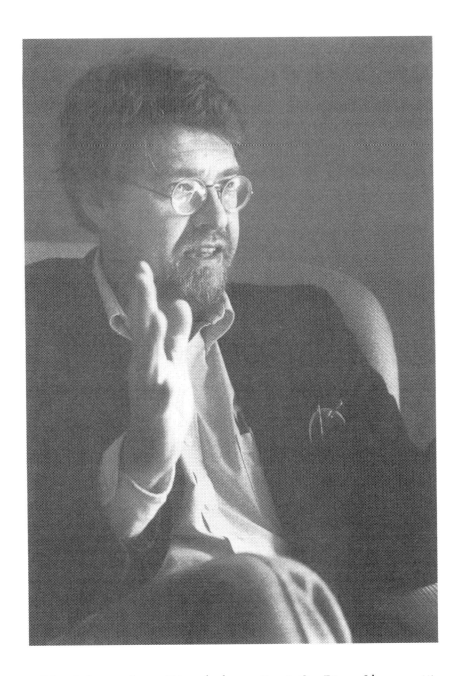

Then in I guess it was '84 we had a meeting in San Diego. I began getting back into this problem of intermediate layers. Paul Smolensky and I were talking about how we could deal with some linguistic information and thought, "You know, we really need these multilayer systems." And so I went back to my old code; by then it was in C [a computer language]. I'd given up on LISP because it was too cranky. By then I reimplemented these things in C.

David E. Rumelhart

I was at the meeting in '84. I explained to Terry Sejnowski about back-propagation and how it worked. Terry immediately understood, and he and Charlie Rosenberg went off and trained up the first really large problem, probably the first one other than toy problems, using the backpropagation.

About this time Hinton realized that this system was a lot like the Boltzmann system and, in fact, maybe would be faster. Boltzmann machines were painful. You had to wait for them to relax in order to do learning. He implemented a version of backpropagation in January, or thereabouts, of '85. I was then working with Ron Williams, who was a postdoc. We had pretty much sorted this out and were working on how to do backpropagation in time.

Geoff and I decided we really should write this up, so we started writing our paper and did a whole bunch of experiments in order to have something to say in this paper. The paper was really written in the spring of '85. I think the *Nature* paper was in the fall of '85. By then I was fairly committed to learning how it might work. I guess I've now spent about another ten years sorting all of this out the best I could.

ER: Multiple five-year plans.

DR: I scrapped the five-year plan. It's now a fifteen-year plan. In the meantime, a sad thing was that McClelland left San Diego and Hinton left San Diego. I had an opportunity to move to Stanford and did in '87.

The other thing was the book. Let's see, for several years—probably from '81 to '85 or '86—I was pretty much a hermit. I was so obsessed that I did absolutely nothing else. I hardly left San Diego except to go to meetings on PDP models or connectionist models or neural nets, or whatever you want to call them.

I was so obsessed that I never went out and gave talks for about five years, except when I had to go to contractors' meetings. I was just totally obsessed with working on this book, and it kept getting bigger and bigger. We kept saying, "Oh, here's another great idea. Let's do this." Jay is more organized than I, and he was trying to manage things and keep us from producing gigantic books. We thought it was important stuff.

In our negotiations with the publisher it looked like it was going to cost $100 or $150 maybe, $75 a volume, or something. They were big fat books. They figured, "Well, we'll sell about two thousand maybe, maybe three if we're really lucky." They estimated how much it would cost. We said, "Look, that's ridiculous. We're not going to sell any books if we charge $100 and $150 for a two-volume set."

We decided to do something. We said, "Look, if we can save money in the production of the book, would you cut the price down?" Of course, the more you cut the price down, the higher the estimate of sales is, and the more you can cut the price. It's a crazy business.

So we agreed to do all the typesetting on the book ourselves. They asked early on if we would do that. I said, "No, we don't want to get involved with that." But finally we decided "Yes." We would do the typesetting and all the proofreading and all the copyediting. Everything. We would send them camera-ready copy. Finished pages. Fortunately, by then the SDF [System Development Foundation] was funding the work.

They said it was OK for us to use their money to produce the book. We hired people to do all the copyediting, to do all the work of producing camera-ready copy. We felt that it would be worth it to be able to charge an affordable price. We got it out of the door for about $45 for two volumes. We made sure it was in our contract that we didn't want extra royalties; we wanted them to sell the book at a lower price.

It turned out that, as it happened, the first printing was already committed before it was actually printed, so they immediately went into the second printing before release, and they've done very well with it. I don't know how many sales there've been, but maybe forty thousand. That's a lot of books. It was July of '86 that the book came out.

Anyway, we felt that it was very important to make the book accessible to people. I mean, you won't buy if it cost $150 for those two volumes. How many people would have gone out and bought at that price? How would you have felt about requiring those as books for your classes? One of the best decisions we ever made was to put in the extra effort. Fortunately, the System Development Foundation [SDF] was willing to pay for the cost, really subsidizing the cost of production.

ER: Was there was any one person who went from Sloan to SDF?

DR: No. I don't know how much you know about the history of all of these things, but the Sloan Foundation came and seeded a number of places, us included. That's what started our postdoctoral program. They then had a competition for larger centers. We applied, but we didn't get one, for who knows what reasons. We didn't get a cognitive science center or institute, even though we worked very hard trying to get one at San Diego. Other places—Berkeley and Irvine, I think, and MIT and Stanford—got some support; we didn't.

Some people thought that was too bad. In particular, the people at SDF approached us and said, "Look, you can continue your program." They agreed to continue the funding of our cognitive science program over the next five years after the Sloan money went away. That's what kept us going.

Most of the money for the PDP work came from SDF, as it turned out. They were funding other things as well. The PDP work was my direction, and Don Norman went off in a different direction. He went off toward human computer interactions. SDF was funding that work too. But in any case, the budget was such that it was possible for us to hire somebody to do this work on the book, which is what we did.

ER: When did you go to Stanford?

DR: '87.

ER: The following year you won the McArthur Foundation Award...

DR: No, it was that same year. The McArthur was in June. I had already agreed to go to Stanford, but then the McArthur Award was given to me in '87 also.

It wasn't an easy decision to go to Stanford because things were quite good at San Diego, but I'd been there a long time, twenty years, and I felt that I was very entrenched. I had a position there, and we had a large staff. The SDF money was going away because they had a close date at SDF. Going out and raising money to keep people on staff was a big job, and I felt that in starting over and going to a new place, my committments were less. And of course I had been a graduate student at Stanford, and I liked it. Marilyn, my wife, had been an undergraduate there. It's a pleasant place.

It was a hard decision because of the people I had worked with for many, many years, Don Norman in particular, and all the other people that I worked with, staff and so on. But it was also a kind of a renewal because it was a matter of, "Here, I'm going to a new place. I don't have all these millions of commitments anymore." So we decided to do it. I've been there for six years now. It seems like less than that.

ER: Could you say something about your work over the last six years and what you've been focusing on?

DR: I've always been interested in everything, very broad interests. I work on things ranging from perception and motor control to memory, language, and attention. When I began to get more and more interested in brainlike systems, I began to expand my horizons and found out I really needed to know more about the nervous system, how it works, and so on.

My work now is in about four different programs of research. They range from what I call neural modeling or biological modeling, where I'm trying to use networks as models of real biological systems as closely as I can, to what I think of as cognitive modeling or psychological modeling, where I work on trying to model things like memory, perception, learning.

In the first case, in biological modeling, the goal is to describe the behavior of the biological system. The second case, cognitive modeling, is to describe the behavior of the organism. The third area that I've spent a lot of effort on is what I call theory, the mathematical underpinings of neural networks and the like. I've more or less accepted the word neural networks now, though I resisted fairly strongly for a variety of reasons. But be that as it may, events have overtaken me, and so I use the term now. In the third area, the area of theory, I'm trying to do the mathematics and trying to develop architectures. A lot of that is statistics. The fourth area is engineering applications or AI applications, where I've been doing quite a bit of work on building systems that solve real-world problems—things like medical diagnosis, things like cursive handwriting recognition, speech recognition, motor control. We did work on mass spectrum recognition. Things that I think are important or useful for pushing on the system and saying, "Gee, how do we solve this problem?"

My basic program of research is the following. I have this image of the mind-brain; I'm still trying to solve the philosopher's problem. I have this image of the mind and the brain as being two views of the same object. We can view it as a physical object, or we can view it as a mental thing. But I think of it as two sides of the same coin. The problem is that when you look at the two sides, they don't look at all alike. One side has all this intro-spection, all this mental stuff going on, behavior and all this. And the other side has all this wet stuff. The way I see my program of research is to say, "How could it possibly be that these two things are the same?"

What can I do? Well, what tools do I have? I'm a computer hacker. The tools I have are modeling tools, so I'll try to link these two things together by making a model, and the model is going to either be more like this, the brain, or behave more like that, the mind. I think there are a whole series of models where I try to link the two. Some of them are more abstract, more loosely connected to the brain and more tightly connected to explaining be-havior. Others are more tightly connected to what we observe in the brain and more loosely connected to behavior. I have this idea that if we have this kind of series of overlapping models, all of which have some common struc-ture, eventually, maybe, we can figure out how to bridge this enormous gap.

So that's the overall program that I see myself doing. I think, along the way I have to learn about the models; I have to know what their properties are. That's where the theory part comes in, developing and learning their properties. How can we make this enormous leap?

I feel we can't know too much about the brain, and we can't know too much about the mind, and we need to find out as much as we can about each. A lot of biologists are critical of neural networks. They say they are not realistic. They're right, of course. We have to abstract. We have to say, "Look, of course you know many, many things about the brain that are not in my models."

The psychologists are the same. They know many, many things about the mind that aren't in my model. But I have to ask, what's the key? What are the most important features that I can bring in? I'd love to have all of them, the problem is that the biologists, (a) know a lot of things that I don't know what to do with, and (b) don't know a lot of the things that I'd love to know. It's a matter of having to make up some things, to say, "Gee, let's suppose it's like this," and at the same time, ignore other things. That's something that neurobiology hasn't figured out how to deal with.

JA: Neuroscientists are very bad at thinking about implications, especially as one starts to go beyond biology.

DR: Right. So here's my general program: to find out more about the brain, to find out more about the mind, and to try to link them with models.

One area that I've started working on recently, which has taken a great deal of energy, has been the area of functional magnetic resonance imaging [fMRI]. We've been doing lots of experiments, looking at brain activity in living humans while they are acting. I see this as a neat way of beginning to make these links between mind and brain because here we can look at the brain—we can see, essentially, what it's doing—while we know what the behavior is, we know what the person is doing. We can observe both at once to a first approximation.

ER: I know you have done some speech-recognition work in conjunction with SRI and ICSI [International Computer Science Institute, Berkeley, CA] as part of the DARPA-funded effort. And the cursive handwriting recognition is ...

DR: I got some money from a gift from Hewlett Packard [HP] to pay for collecting data. I had a postdoc who had his own funds, and I have computers. So the cursive handwriting didn't have a separate funding source.

For a long time I've had this vision of how to do cursive handwriting recognition. HP loaned me a writing pad, and they gave me money to hire somebody to run subjects and collect data. So I collected about a hundred thousand words of handwriting data, which we then used to train a network and devised a network architecture and algorithms for learning. In fact, one of my students and a postdoc went off and started a little company, Lexicus.

ER: And are you involved commercially with that?

DR: No. I've avoided being involved commercially with any companies, other than as advisor.

ER: Is the architecture that you developed different from Lexicus's architecture?

DR: It depends on the level of description. They definitely started out with the architecture that I developed. What they have done since, I couldn't tell you. I don't know. I've made suggestions at times as to things they might do. Whether they've done those or not, I don't know. My interaction has been really as a kind of advisor.

ER: And how do you feel about working on something from a resarch point of view and then seeing it be commercialized?

DR: I love it.

ER: You like it, even if you're not financially rewarded?

DR: I get paid. Stanford pays me.

ER: Suppose some company turned one of your ideas into something, and you didn't know ...

DR: I'd love it. Look, my goal in all of this has been to keep all this stuff in the public domain. When I first was developing the backpropagation stuff, for about two hours I considered the idea of trying to get some kind of device that could be patented. I thought, "That's ridiculous. I don't want to do that."

I want this stuff to be out in the public domain. Why shouldn't everybody use it? That's been my attitude in general. I publish everything. The only issues that are slightly tricky are when I'm literally a consultant to a company. In those cases, the ideas that I have when I'm being paid by them belong to them. I think of myself as a problem solver. I think, "OK, you guys, you have a problem. I have a lot of experience here. Tell me your problem. I probably have an idea about how to solve it."

I've done a number of things that I like that don't belong to me anymore, but I got paid for them. You know, when I'm a consultant, I get paid, and I'm happy. And when I'm doing basic research, I make sure that the ideas get published, so that anybody can use them. If some company uses them, that's great, and some other company can use them too.

ER: That's the thorny issue when you work with commercial entities, the short life span of any competitive advantage.

DR: That's why it doesn't matter so much. That's why the only thing patents are good for is trading them with other people. They're out of date very, very soon.

JA: The stuff academics do, the deep models, the big ideas, when you try to patent those, it doesn't work. The details are what you keep proprietary.

DR: Right, exactly. I just think that I want to get these ideas out there. I want people to use them. I love it when people use them, and I don't feel cheated. I have had what I consider agreements, which have been in the form of, well, if this stuff works out, maybe gifts to the laboratory would be a nice thing. Hewlett Packard has given me several gifts. That's to keep the information channels flowing.

ER: I want to bring up the whole issue of backpropagation and who discovered backpropagation and how.

DR: I don't know if it's a controversy, but as far as I know it's been discovered at least three times, maybe more. Paul Werbos apparently discovered it and wrote about it in his dissertation. David Parker apparently discovered it, and we discovered it. As far as I know, those were all entirely independent discoveries, and there were precursors to all of those. What's surprising is that it hasn't been discovered more often because it's such a simple idea. The reason it caught on is because it is so simple. There's no complexity there. I mean, it's so easy to understand once you look at it.

ER: Has controversy or anything having to do with these multiple discoveries had any kind of impact on your career or your thinking?

DR: No, I don't think so. Our discovery of it was the most publicized with a paper in *Nature.* I think that pretty clearly has been the focus for a lot of the work that's been done using the algorithm. I haven't felt any controversy. I had no idea that Paul Werbos had done work on it. I had never heard of him. I had never heard of his work. There are other examples of work in the control literature in the '60s. If you look at it, they were doing backpropagation going back even earlier than that, but the ideas were never really implemented. It wasn't that there weren't these ideas; it's just no one had really done anything with them.

My view is that we not only discovered them, but we realized what we could do with them and did a lot of different things. I consider them independent discoveries, at least three and maybe more. Amari, I think, suggests that he had another discovery, and you know, I believe that. You can look at his paper. He had, but he didn't do anything with it. I think that was in the late '60s. I don't feel any problem. You know, maybe we should have done better scholarship and searched out all of the precursors to it, but we didn't know there were any.

ER: As you look out at the neural net area today, whose work is exciting and interesting and provocative to you?

DR: Well, it really depends on the dimension that we're talking about. I mentioned those four different categories, and I think there's exciting work in each. I'm very interested in attempts to do biological models. Here's my feeling about them so far. They have not done as well as I had wanted. I had a vision that we would be able to have a stronger connection to biology than we have. I still think there are some examples of biological modeling that are important and interesting. I've thought that the work that Andersen and Zipser did was very nice. Sejnowski and others have done some interesting work with VOR [vestibulo-ocular reflex]. Modeling hasn't been accepted as a real part of neurobiology. Neurobiology is an experimental field primarily, and experimentalists don't know what to do with theory.

JA: They're resistant to it.

DR: Very resistant. I'm afraid that in psychology there's a similar story to be told, although psychologists and cognitive scientists are more open to modeling work. I think there've been some interesting and useful pieces of work, but again, I think we haven't really met the promise that I had envisioned. Maybe I was too hopeful, or maybe it's turned out to be harder—harder than I would have wanted. But on the whole modeling has changed attitudes in psychology and cognitive science, and that's good. There haven't been as many successful models as I would have hoped. I don't know your feelings, Jim.

JA: Very similar.

DR: I think we changed attitudes, and that's a big thing. We haven't changed attitudes yet in biology.

JA: I'm personally most disappointed about neurobiology. They are still so resistant, so anti-theory.

DR: I'm hopeful. I'm not as disappointed. The most successful area has been, I think, in the domain of theory. We've come so far. You know, it was possible in 1986 for people to make absolutely outrageous claims about neural networks, and many of them did. But it's now a concrete thing and largely because we understand the underpinnings tremendously better than we did then. To me, it's like night and day.

The other area where there's no doubt that we have made progress is the area of applications. You look out there, and there are hundreds and hundreds of applications, and they're successful. When the PDP volumes came out, and we talked about the work on back propagation, what did we talk about? We talked about X-OR; we talked about the symmetry problem.

Minsky and others talked about the scaling problem, scaled by a factor of a hundred thousand, and the scaling has not been bad. When I first did the X-OR problem, it took a thousand iterations to solve it. If we thought that was the way it was going to go and that we were going to scale up to a hundred thousand input patterns, my God, we wouldn't live long enough to see the results. But that's not the way it's gone. That problem turned out to be an anomaly. The scaling is about linear. We haven't hit any exponential curves yet. If you make a bigger problem, it's about a linear increase in training time. So OK, we get bigger and bigger problems, but hey, we're not going to beat linearity.

ER: Do you see any architectures that you think have the same kind of potential that backprop displays?

DR: Learning architectures? Well, I don't know. I guess my take on that is I don't know of any, right now. There are conjugate gradient methods. There are all kinds of variations, but they're all hill climbing. By now I've framed backpropagation at such a level of generality that it's hard for me to imagine a system that isn't a backpropagation system. In particular, virtually every learning algorithm that exists can be framed as a gradient search of some kind. Sometimes they use second-order methods, sometimes they use first-order methods, but they're almost all gradient searches.

The only ones that maybe aren't are the methods that involve adding units and things like that. Aesthetically, I find that displeasing. I just don't like it. Don't ask me why. I'd much rather have systems that evolve, starting out with plenty of stuff and then figuring out what to do. My own feelings are that there are different architectures—for example, the society of experts' architecture—but they're all fundamentally gradient search. That's all backpropagation is.

You take things like the Kohonen algorithm, which isn't literally a gradient search, but all you do is smooth the curves, and then you can do a gradient search, and you get the same kind of results. Every time I find a system that isn't a gradient search, I insert a smooth curve; then I can cast it in the general form of a gradient search. In fact, that's about all there is to neural networks. In the relaxation methods, there's nothing there but a gradient search. That's what you're doing, except you're doing your gradient in another dimension; you're doing it in the activation domain.

JA: I think there is also interesting stuff in the temporal dynamics of these nonlinear dynamical systems and how it relates to learning.

DR: But they're doing gradient. It's just that the energy space is unstable; it's changing.

JA: They're doing energy minimization, but the dynamics of the search may allow you to make the contact with the dynamics of the nervous system.

DR: Conceivably so. And that's possibly where the linkage between behavior and the nervous system will come.

JA: I agree, this linkage is what we're all after. That's a place I can see it happen because you have dynamical systems, and they behave quite simply, though they're actually very complex.

DR: That's true.

JA: That simplicity out of complexity ... One of the things that makes psychology so intriguing is that many behaviors are quite simple and lawful, and yet the nervous system is so complex. Things are simpler than perhaps they ought to be. Maybe the only way to link the two together is through these dynamical systems.

DR: I think statistical phenomena are what's really going on here. Some people I talk to think that we have to get complexity out of simplicity. They think the nervous system has these very simple principles of interaction, and the big problem is getting the complexity out.

JA: That's where they're wrong.

DR: I absolutely agree. We can get chaotic patterns and so on. My own view is that's the last thing the nervous system wants. The big change that happened in evolution is that once we got a respiratory system capable of supporting lots of neurons, we could go to a statistical methodology and bank on the law of large numbers.

I should say that one of the things I've been working on lately is trying to factor neurochemistry into my models, neuromodulators and things like that, which I take to be much more important than we've realized. I have a paper on the role of neuromodulators. It's a generalization of our conventional networks, but which have neuromodulators included. If you are interested in dynamics, it turns out that there's a whole host of timescales involved. Different neuromodulators have different temporal properties; the neurons have different temporal properties, and learning has still others. In the nervous system, these things are all overlapping timescales, not independent ones like in physics.

JA: In the nervous system, the timescales of the biological events are relatively close to the timescales of the events they are controlling or responding to. Neural network research has had real difficulty handling time domain problems.

DR: I agree with you.

JA: Part of the reason must be that the nervous system uses lots of special purpose tricks involving conduction times, network settling times, and neurotransmitter actions that build temporal dynamics right into the hardware in a way that's very hard to analyze.

DR: Let me say a little bit about the future. My feeling is that the generic neural network person or the generic neural network conference is probably a short-lived thing. The real interests of biologists, psychologists, engineers, and so on are divergent. There are only a few people who want to link them together. I believe that there will be a field and which will be called the neural network field and which will be the residual, really, the theory. Somebody will continue doing it, and it will get more and more esoteric, as always happens.

But I see a diverging of the fields. I think that biologists really don't care that much about commercial applications. They don't have any reason to care. Commercial people, they don't actually care about biology per se. They like it that you can give the argument that neural networks are biological, but what they want is something that works, very pragmatic. Once these tools are proved—and I think they are being proved—they won't have an interest anymore. In psychology, the same. Some people are interested in psychology, but they're not interested in psychology vis-à-vis neural networks. Neural networks are their own thing. There're not many of those people left whose work spans this generic field. There isn't that much reason for it.

Some of us probably will maintain an interest just for historical reasons and as a practical matter will find it useful and interesting to work in all these areas. But it's incredibly difficult to try to keep up in all these areas. I imagine that there will be a divergence because I don't see a fundamental convergence of interests. I think the real goals are different in the subareas. That's a kind of pessimism. I imagine that the neural network journals that have been started will eventually specialize in various ways on particular subtopics, and some of them will go away.

JA: They already are specializing.

DR: I was opposed to the starting of all these journals for the very reason that my goal was to get these ideas in the public domain. I don't like specialized journals. I think that we should publish our work in standard journals, and they should be interested in it. If you have a choice of publishing a piece of work that could be published either in the star journal of your discipline or in a special neural network journal, you'll probably want to publish in the star journal. The problem was that at first, before the field became established, those star journals wouldn't accept articles on neural nets. But that's changed as we've gotten more and more solid. We want this work to be mainstream, not a little trickling off to the side.

As that happens, there will be less and less of a core remaining for neural networks per se and more of, "Here's a person doing good work in their field, and they're using neural networks as a tool."

That's the way I think. I would like to publish my work in neuroscience journals. My feeling is that we want to establish our work as real, as doing science. This is the way we do science now, and we do it by using these models. I believe they're tools. I believe they are ways of thinking.

JA: It's like mathematical psychology.

DR: Yes, exactly. That was also a tool. When I was a student, everybody published in the *Journal of Mathematical Psychology*. But then, *Psych. Review* said, "Hey, you can publish this stuff in our journal."

So we said, "OK, we'll publish in *Psych. Review*." Now who's left in the *Journal of Mathematical Psychology?* People doing esoteric mathematics. Most scientists want other people in their field to be their readers.

I don't know which journals will go away and which ones will stay. Journals have a lot of tenacity once they get going. There's a lot of inertia. I was opposed to Terry starting *Neural Computation,* although I think it's a fine journal. I think all of the different journals have to find a niche and a readership. The future, I think, is bright. I think we've had an impact.

ER: The more impact, the more it will disappear.

DR: Exactly. Disappear as an identifiable separate thing. It will be part of doing science or doing engineering. And to me, that's not bad. I don't like being a neural network guru. That's not the way I view myself. I think of myself as a scientist trying to solve problems of one kind or another. Now, it happens that the tools that I've been using, conceptually, are good tools. I like them. I want to promote them, but I want to promote them because I think they're . . .

ER: Efficacious.

DR: They're good. But I don't want people to stop all their other approaches. Because it's still only one approach. I want those people still plunking their electrodes in brains, and I want people doing psychology experiments, and I want people inventing new algorithms.

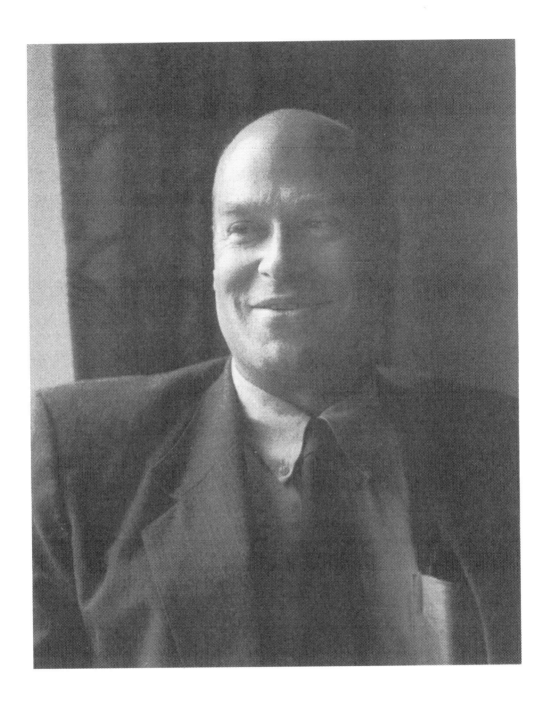

13 Robert Hecht-Nielsen

Robert Hecht-Nielsen is Founder of HNC Software Inc., San Diego, California. He is also Adjunct Professor, Department of Electrical and Computer Engineering, University of California, San Diego, La Jolla, California. He is the author of the 1991 book Neuro-computing, *Addison-Wesley, a good source for more information about his work.*

July 1993, Portland, Oregon

ER: I usually begin by asking people to state their date of birth and to tell us something about their parents, upbringing, and their childhood.

HN: I was born in San Francisco, California on 18 July 1947. My father was an immigrant from Denmark who was born in 1894, and his parents, Anna Hecht and Johannes Nielsen, had decided to put their names together and give it to the children. However, neither of them changed their names, so that's where my hyphenated name came from.

My Dad moved here in 1922, lived in New York briefly, and then lived in Chicago and then San Francisco. My mother is originally from Iowa; she is a musician, and my father was an interior decorator. Neither of them had as great an influence on me as my grandmother. My maternal grandmother graduated from Northwestern in 1906, was a very well-educated, very intelligent, very philosophical person.

My father had a policy of not telling us anything about his past. He had had some incredible adventures growing up in Denmark and then living in Germany just before World War I working as an apprentice. As war approached he left Germany, having no love for the Kaiser. He spent World War I in North Africa, then went back to Germany, and lived in the Weimar Republic. He lived in Chicago during the gangster years and wouldn't tell us a word about it. So he wasn't that useful, and my mother was always working, so she wasn't that influential. That is sort of a summary of my background.

ER: Well, I'm curious to know what your childhood was like, how you grew up. You said your grandmother was very influential. Was she living at home with you.

HN: We actually moved to her house. My father had medical problems when I was about eight years old. So we moved from San Francisco to

Denver, where she lived, and we lived with her for the rest of my childhood. That's how she came to be so influential.

ER: Do you have brothers and sisters?

HN: I have one younger brother. My upbringing was pretty much centered around work. I began working when I was ten, delivering newspapers, and have been working ever since.

ER: Was that your idea, to begin working, or was this from the family?

HN: It was my idea. It was a way of financing my projects and activities. My hobby during those years was flying airplanes.

ER: Flying model airplanes or real airplanes?

HN: No, real airplanes. I began at age fourteen and that consumed all my time and interest. I didn't have the time or interest for school. I eventually got into college on probation and discovered that I was actually interested in intellectual things. I had previously known that I was interested in things, but really became aware at the university that I could do well in terms of studying, and went on from there.

When I was a freshman, I learned I could read technical books the way most people read novels. Because I came into college on probation, I had to take a basic calculus class that was stretched out for those who weren't quite as intellectually capable. Just before the winter break, I asked the professor I was taking the dummy math class from, what a tensor was because I'd heard this term, and I didn't understand it. He said. "Well, I don't remember, but I have a book." He loaned me a book, and then we went on winter holiday vacation.

I took the book home, read it, and worked all the problems. When school resumed I brought it back and gave it to him with my notebook and had him check some of the problems. He responded, "It was a joke! You were supposed to take it home, crack it open, and then about halfway down the first page, give up." It was at that point I realized that I could read these things, so I then went in and devoured the library. Basically, I didn't take any more undergraduate courses.

ER: I want to back up a little bit ·because I'm struck by the fact that at ten years old you wanted to finance your own projects and started your working career. When you were ten years old, were you thinking that you wanted to be an aircraft pilot?

HN: No, no. I had only one interest. That was to fly spacecraft, which didn't exist at that point. This was pre-Sputnik! But, nonetheless, I had this strong feeling that it was going to happen.

ER: Do you remember Sputnik? That was 1957, when you were ten years old.

HN: Very much so.

ER: And what was going on at school? You were saying you got into college on probation ...

HN: Right. I didn't have much time for studying and for those sorts of things, so I spent all my time after school working, which precluded doing homework problems, and then the weekends were spent out at the airport.

ER: You started flying at fourteen?

HN: Yes.

ER: As an apprentice, or ...?

HN: Well, I joined a glider club and learned to fly. It took them a few weeks to get used to the idea that they were going to entrust the club's only aircraft to this young pilot, but they got used to it, and it worked out all right. Flying was, and still is, a passion. I was never troubled by conformity, so it didn't bother me that I wasn't like the other children. I had a strong desire to read things, and so I would read voraciously. I didn't feel I was missing out on much at school.

ER: And were you reading about spacecraft and about aircraft?

HN: I was reading about everything. I read everything I could get my hands on, practically. But, yes, I read extensively on that and anything having to do with science, mathematics, and space.

ER: So it was the interest in space that led you first to science?

HN: Actually, I think that interest began back much earlier, when I was about six or seven. My grandmother bought me a book on astronomy and that's probably what launched that interest. I went, "Gee, it's interesting to read about this, but I'd rather go there." That was the thought process. And then our neighbor would give me magazines; he had *Popular Science* and *Popular Mechanics*. There were articles there about artificial satellites that might some day be constructed. I found all that very inspirational, and that interest continued for a long time. When I got to college, I found that I could learn much more rapidly than my peers, so I did. I just consumed as much information as I could and began taking graduate courses.

ER: Where did you go to undergraduate school?

HN: Mostly at Arizona State University. I started at the University of Colorado, but then I went to ASU, and that's also where I went to graduate school.

ER: When you started at the University of Colorado, it was because you were living in Colorado?

HN: In Denver, that's right.

ER: So it was just the natural geographic place to go?

HN: It's a funny story. The East High School college counselor had refused to advise me because of my performance in high school. He said, "It's absolutely a waste of time for you to go to college. You should become an aircraft mechanic." He had it all figured out. He knew exactly how my life story was going to read.

ER: And he was basing this on your grades, or ...?

HN: A number of things. That was his strong conclusion. He literally refused to provide any advisement about going to college because he thought it would be a big mistake. So I went in to see the Colorado State Employment Service representative, who visited the high school for those of us who weren't worthy of university education. He was telling me about all the marvelous opportunities in dishwashing, things that were out there waiting for me, and then he said, "It doesn't seem to me as if you're interested in any of these opportunities, what do you really want to do?"

And I said, "I'd like to go to college." He had a friend who taught a course called, "How to Study in College," and so when I was a senior in high school, I went down to the University of Colorado Denver Center and took this course. It demystified the whole thing. The course made it seem as if any schmuck could go to college. It wasn't that big a deal. From then on, it was a piece of cake. I just went down and registered, and that was that.

ER: And what made you switch from Colorado to ASU?

HN: That's a very long story. I got married in the interim. My first wife and I were basically very immature when we married, and by the time we were divorced seven and a half years later we'd grown up a lot, and it was very amicable, so it wasn't at all a negative experience. But it was seven years out of an otherwise normal progression. She was my childhood sweetheart. She had moved to Arizona, so I went down there, and we decided to get married down there and live there. I stayed at ASU for graduate school because I had a mentor who was very effective, very useful—a fellow named David Hestenes, who is still a friend.

In retrospect, I probably could have gone to any school and done well, but I don't regret having gone to ASU. It provided an excellent education, and it provided me with a perspective which to this day is extremely useful. There's a certain objectivity that I think I gained that I think a lot of students at other schools didn't gain.

The tensor book was instrumental in helping me understand that I didn't have to go through this lengthy sequence of courses to understand something. I could just jump to the end, read the book, and be done with it, so I did that in a vast array of subjects. I studied all of undergraduate physics on my own. However, I did take the entire graduate physics program because I found that so fascinating, and that occupied a lot of my undergraduate time.

JA: Did you take any psychology or neurobiology?

HN: No, I didn't. The schools I went to had little in these areas worth taking. I simply read things about that. The available courses didn't seem interesting to me. Not even engineering. I never took an engineering course, although that's all I've done in my career.

ER: And what about biology?

HN: I took a year of botany, which was fascinating, but I studied biology extensively. I read books.

ER: And what was your undergraduate major?

HN: Mathematics and a minor in anthropology, and in grad school I majored in math again. Although, as an undergraduate I took a lot of physics, a lot more physics than anthropology, physics didn't seem that big a deal to me.

ER: And did you get a Ph.D. at ASU in mathematics?

HN: Yes, in 1974, in functional analysis.

ER: That's what your thesis was about?

HN: That's right. But I did work in other areas, like differential geometry. Eventually, I did a thesis, a dissertation, on functional analysis. Now, it was in fact while I was an undergraduate at ASU that I first took a serious interest in neural networks. In 1968, we had this beautiful little reading library where current issues, the last three or four issues, of a significant number of journals were kept, and this was just down a few floors from my office, so I would spend lots and lots of time in there reading journals. And one day I bumped into a Steve Grossberg article about systems of differential equations that could be thought of as a model for a neural network. It was real interesting—learning spatial patterns, spatiotemporal patterns, and so forth. Then I began reading the literature more widely—began encountering articles by people like Jim Anderson and a lot of other people, and very quickly became serious about following the literature. And in fact, I was even doing a little bit of research myself. It was absolutely worthless, but it was fascinating and instructive. It was valuable for me personally, and I become convinced that this was going to be a big deal some day.

ER: Had you read any of the older cybernetics work as part of your reading? Did the Grossberg article resonate with other reading?

HN: I had read a few little things on perceptrons but hadn't really thought of them as significant. I understood what a perceptron was, but it hadn't excited me. Encountering this Grossberg article and many others that followed shortly thereafter, I became excited and attuned to neural net theory, so of course I sought it out. And that's what happened. It became the starting point for this career path that I eventually followed. I would constantly read all the relevant journals to find articles because they were sprinkled around across an extremely wide range of literature. And I would go meet people occasionally who were doing work in this field. Nobody of prominence. By the late '70s, say '78, I was spending some of my time actually working on ideas.

ER: Were you working at this point?

HN: Oh yes. After I got out of school, in 1974 I took about a year and a half off to just decompress. I had gone through a divorce. I had been paying for my education by flying airplanes. In fact, because I had been married, I had acquired tastes that a graduate teaching associate couldn't afford. I had to have supplementary income, so I worked as a consultant in heat engine modeling, and I also had a job flying airplanes for a commuter airline.

After decompressing and completing a few relatively short-term engineering jobs, I had concluded in 1978 that neural networks were going to be a big thing shortly, primarily because of the fact that the microprocessor had been invented a few years earlier. There were now capabilities being developed that would allow the implementation of neural network ideas. I mean, I'm sure you were frustrated, Jim, at the time because so many of the ideas you had couldn't really be tried out on any kind of a scale.

JA: That's exactly right.

HN: I had done some experiments with neural networks back in 1968, and my experience was very disappointing. I ran these on a General Electric computer, and none of my experimental runs ever finished. They didn't even come close to finishing. I concluded there wasn't any point in doing research in this area because there wasn't any way to practically apply it. But by the mid-seventies, and particularly as you got into 1978–79, I became convinced that the capability to apply these ideas would soon be upon us.

So in 1979, I decided, "Now is the time. It's time to go off and do neural networks." And so I went to Motorola, which was of course a very appropriate place, and the division's Chief Engineer Russ Yost had built a learning machine back in the '50s. This was all hand designed and then built by hand. It was a simple logic machine, a state machine that could modify its program. He had developed a little game for it to learn. This was an iterative process. The machine would learn a game by playing it against human opponents. Yost had been, throughout his career, an exponent of this idea of learning machines. I approached him with some specific ideas of what I thought we could accomplish with neural networks and asked him if he'd be willing to hire me there and provide some research money to try something.

ER: And how did you know about him?

HN: I didn't know him. I went over to Motorola and just walked in the employment office and effectively said, "I want to build neural networks, and I want you to pay for it. All involved will benefit." That's my style.

ER: And they connected you with him?

HN: Yes. Immediately. He was my first interviewer.

ER: Very perspicacious of a large company like that to be able to make that connection. I'm surprised.

HN: Yes. That's right. Well, it wasn't quite as intentional as you're making it sound; there was obviously a lot of luck involved. They knew that Russ Yost would be able to judge the value of my idea. By 1982, I had been there for three years, and we'd made considerable progress. We had a number of systems running. We'd demonstrated some learning capabilities and some abilities to do associations.

This was the Motorola Government Electronics Division, so these were military applications—things like electronic warfare and radar. They were all very simple applications, as you can imagine, but, nonetheless, they represented interesting capabilities. By '82, we had gotten DARPA [the U.S. government's Defense Advanced Research Projects Agency] very interested, and they were putting together funding for a project to actually build something that would work on a real-world problem.

Right about then, TRW in San Diego began hiring people for a very large ramp up that they were going through. They had some new business activities that they were expanding, and they needed people. It just turned out that one of my friends at Motorola went over there, and of course his first assignment was to recruit more people. I kept getting these calls saying, "No, no, no, don't make any peremptory decisions. Just come over here and check it out."

So I went over, and the strangest thing was that I immediately met yet another senior technical leader, Don Spencer, who had been interested in neural networks earlier in his career and actually had formally studied them at UCLA. He had tremendous interest in doing more work in the area, or at least in having someone on his staff doing more work in the area. He promised all sorts of wonderful things—including startup support and assistance with further marketing.

Since I was a native of California, it was a very interesting concept to move back there. In the meantime, my son and I had both become interested in surfing. We had a little artificial surf reef/wave tank in Arizona. Some people called them toilet waves because there was this huge tank that would fill up and then flush, and then that would create the wave.

We had vacationed in San Diego and knew it quite well. Anyway, we went to San Diego, and sure enough, what Spencer had promised came true. In any event, we did in fact go forward with support from DARPA. This was extremely helpful, allowing us to build some fast neurocomputers, to get enough horsepower so that we could really do some experiments and prove some things.

A young fellow named Todd Gutschow, who had just graduated from Harvard with a degree in physics—had also joined TRW in 1983 and had become interested in neural networks. He and I had become friends and decided that we really should consider commercial applications. Even though we were doing nothing but defense projects at TRW, we thought that the commercial applications of this technology would be really big. So we put together a business plan in 1986, and we tried it out on TRW management. They took it seriously.

They assigned the president of a TRW subsidiary, a small company, to come see us and go over the business plan. He spent about three days with us, TRW ultimately concluded that it was probably a reasonable plan, but that they didn't have any place to fit it into the company. There wasn't a place that had a charter to do this sort of thing. We shopped the business plan around to some venture capitalists and modified it to be a venture-backed company plan, and we were successful.

In September of '86, we started. Todd and I resigned at TRW—it was an amicable separation—and began HNC Software Inc. [Originally called Hecht-Nielsen Neurocomputer Corporation]. At about that same time, in mid-1986, I had gone to the Snowbird meeting, which was actually the second of the first two fairly large neural network meetings. There had been one at Santa Barbara in '85, and then Snowbird was the one that followed.

The Snowbird meeting had been run by Larry Jackel [of then-AT&T Bell Labs] and some others. They had created this obnoxious conference registration form, where you wrote a little paragraph justifying why you should be invited to this meeting, and then underneath there were two boxes that they could check. One was "accept" and one was "reject." And as I understand the numbers, there were approximately five hundred of these forms returned, and something on the order of 125 of them were accepted. The others got them back saying "rejected." To say the least, there were a lot of angry, disenfranchised people.

Anyway, having come back from Snowbird, I had lunch with a friend of mine, Bart Kosko [now at the University of Southern California], a fellow who had worked in the San Diego area. We'd been collaborating on projects, and we actually had a joint project going at that time. He and I had lunch, and we were lamenting the fact that this meeting had been closed, limited to 125 people carefully selected by Bell Labs, and that there was probably—given the sudden enthusiasm for this field—a vast number of people who wanted to participate in the meeting. We saw that having a major meeting with unrestricted attendance was an absolute prerequisite for further growth and progress in the neural net field.

At that lunch, in June of '86, we devised a plan for a new conference, and of course that became the IEEE ICNN [International Conference on Neural Networks] and later the IJCNN [International Joint Conference on Neural Networks]. We went ahead and got the plan formally put together and presented it to the IEEE San Diego section, and with all sorts of tribulations and fights and battles, it all happened.

At HNC we developed our first product by the middle of '87. We did that on a seed round of venture-capital [VC] financing. Then after the product was out and was selling, the company started growing. Then we had a first full-fledged round of VC funding. The company began to grow, and business began to go forward. The overall plan at HNC was very simple: to explore a variety of application areas, looking for some that had the potential of growing to a large size.

Our strategy from the beginning was to have a very high-quality team and to eventually grow the company to a very large size. From the very beginning we had the intent of someday employing hundreds of thousands of people. And by setting our sights on that kind of strategy, we had the opportunity then to evaluate opportunities, to explore them far enough to know whether or not they had a large market associated with them. Eventually, we found a set of businesses that had the right characteristics, and then we began to specialize in those.

Perhaps the best expression of that approach was last fall when our optical character-recognition [OCR] division was divested. We sold it to Mitech Corporation for multiple millions of dollars. That was part of this focusing process that we had planned from the beginning. The OCR business was different from everything else we were doing. It required different management, different marketing, different sales, and the customers were very different, so it wasn't really a compatible business. That brings us up to the present.

My personal involvement has also included teaching a graduate education course at night at UCSD [University of California, San Diego]. I just finished the seventh year of that course. Every single year, it's been the most popular graduate course in the electrical and computer engineering department. I have a number of graduates who are now illustrious participants in the neural network field. It's been just a joy to do this class. It's been of great value to me personally.

JA: Could you briefly discuss the '87 ICNN meeting? It was very important in the history of neural networks.

HN: Well, that was a very difficult period because this was something that had never occurred before. There was already a very large clash under way between people who had been in the field for a long time and who had really prepared the foundation in the field and had all the good ideas, and new people who had come along and really didn't add much to the field, if anything, except perhaps an infectious enthusiasm and a following.

In particular, John Hopfield was an irritant for many people because of the fact that he had published some very elegant papers, which it turned out were obviously based on outstanding, well-known earlier work by Shun-ichi Amari that wasn't cited. I don't know exactly his academic research style, but obviously it doesn't include searching the literature. This was a point of real difficulty for the field because Hopfield had an enormous following of people. He was a very effective lecturer. He would go around the world getting people whipped into a frenzy about this field, and they would, of course, go out and start proselytizing. There was this very broad base of misunderstanding that Hopfield had created this field.

There was this body of individuals who really had created the field and really had all the original ideas at that point, who didn't even exist as far as maybe a majority of the new people interested in the field were concerned. So one of the roles of the 1987 meeting, which Bart and I were very committed to, was to firmly and unequivocally establish the history of the field in people's minds in a more correct sequence of events.

And so we made a point of emphasizing all of the ideas, the good ideas, that existed from people in this field, including John Hopfields's. He wasn't excluded; he gave a lecture, and he was there. But anyway, that was a very important part of it. I think another aspect of the meeting that was really important was that many of the people who had been working in the field had personal difficulties with others who had been working in the field. There were a lot of personal animosities. It took us a while to figure out how we were going to overcome that and have everyone show up.

The technical program was easy. There were so many good people and so many ideas that had never really been adequately aired, that it was just a joy, but the hardest part was the problem of getting people to actually show up.

With a list of plenary speakers, tutorial presenters, session chairs, and special invited talks from that conference, you would have a pretty good list of the pioneers of the field. Now, we didn't get everybody. There were a lot of people who had made good contributions to this field that weren't there.

ER: You couldn't do it all at one meeting.

HN: That's right, but the list that we ended up with was pretty darn good. For us, we felt that we had succeeded well beyond our expectations.

Many IEEE leaders were against our conference plan from the beginning. By the time a couple of organizational meetings had passed, the forces that were arrayed against us had had a chance to regroup and redouble, and they were absolutely committed to the idea that they were going to kill this thing. It was not going to ever happen again. The plan had been born, but now it was time to kill it before it grew up.

The efforts against us the first year were strong, but by the second year they were immense. But then again, we had learned a lot, and we had formed some very powerful allies, like the Executive Director of the IEEE, who was very, very clever and politically astute.

ER: Were you surprised at the attendance at that first ICNN meeting?

HN: It was higher than we expected.

I also wanted to say a few more things about DARPA and ARPA [the names DARPA and ARPA refer to the same agency whose official name changes sporadically] and its role in the history of neural nets. ARPA was begun in 1958. As you know, President Eisenhower had this very real fear that there was a military-industrial complex being formed. He saw a perversion of the defense activity, which is a proper activity for a government to have, becoming some sort of self-serving beast that would become its own self-contained entity. DARPA was created over his objections, in a sense, and it was a product of the perceived Sputnik deficiency. It was specifically set up to allow the Department of Defense to efficiently conduct research and tap the scientific talent of America for defense purposes.

The important thing is that ARPA, from the beginning, was run by very strong-willed people who had very definite ideas of what they wanted to do and who demanded autonomy. That was the key thing. From the very beginning, the directors of DARPA demanded that they be really separated from the rest of the Department of Defense. They answered directly to the Deputy Director for Research and Engineering. They basically went right up to the Secretary of Defense. They still have that same autonomy.

DARPA began funding neural network research somewhere in the neighborhood of 1960, and, if I'm not mistaken, they were funding Cornell Aeronautical Labs and some of the perceptron work.

ARPA had been involved in some of that. However, one of the things that they did from the very beginning was try to operate on the basis of seeking advice from people in academia who were in fashion. I don't want to make it sound like that's negative. But they've always had this practice of identifying a group of people, typically senior academics, and depending upon them as fashion evaluators, if you will. Then periodically these things go through upheaval and revolution, and they have new people come in, and some of the old people get canceled out; this is very healthy for the nation.

Today [in 1993], DARPA probably has somewhere in the neighborhood of 120 personnel—including everybody, the secretaries, the phone receptionist—and they dole out about $1.5 billion dollars. DARPA operates with a very, very tiny bureaucracy and just shoots from the hip. That shapes the organization. They became interested again in neural nets in 1982, and they began funding some work.

But they were doing it tentatively. They had some very selective projects, and they were looking at it and exploring it. They tend to be remarkably objective and unencumbered by conventional wisdom. Even though they depend upon fashionable advisors, and even though they have a tendency to go a little bit overboard in the support of their favorites, they are absolutely open to new ideas. They will take researchers coming in with new ideas and listen to them, and really listen to what they have to say, and evaluate it fairly. I think, I've really hardly ever heard of anyone who went to DARPA with a good idea who didn't get funding, or who felt they were treated unfairly. Now, a lot of people with bad ideas who go there get kicked out on their face, and that's probably the way it should be.

In the early 1960s DARPA and other research sponsors began significant funding of neural network research. However, much of this work turned out to be of rather low quality and some of it was little more than wishful thinking or alchemy. Further, after about 1963, the flow of good new ideas seemed to dry up.

During this era of the early 1960s, a significant group of researchers with a less "biological" and more computer science-oriented approach to what they called "artificial intelligence" [AI], found themselves out of fashion and could not get the large levels of funding they felt their approach warranted, although, as it turned out, this approach never amounted to much—a realization which it took two decades and billions of dollars to establish and which did yield a handful of valuable accidental discoveries. Further, at least some of these researchers on the outs found it emotionally intolerable that some of what they saw as "lightweight" research on neural networks was

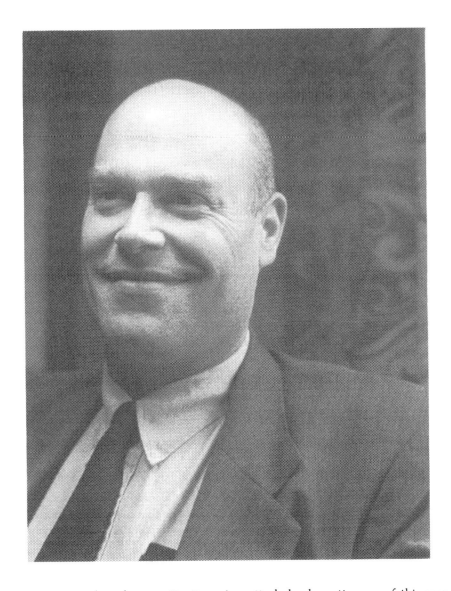

receiving a lot of press attention. A particularly dramatic case of this was Marvin Minsky. Minsky had gone to the same New York "science" high school as Frank Rosenblatt, a Cornell psychology Ph.D. whose "perceptron" neural network pattern recognition machine was receiving significant media attention. The wall-to-wall media coverage of Rosenblatt and his machine irked Minsky. One reason was that although Rosenblatt's training was in "soft science," his perceptron work was quite mathematical and quite sound—turf that Minsky, with his "hard science" Princeton mathematics Ph.D. didn't feel Rosenblatt belonged on. Perhaps an even greater problem was the fact that the heart of the perceptron machine was a clever motor-driven-potentiometer adaptive element that had been pioneered in the world's first neurocomputer—the "snark," which had been designed and built by Minsky several years earlier! [In some ways, Minsky's early career was like that of

Darth Vader. He started out as one of the earliest pioneers in neural networks, but was then turned to the dark side of the force (AI) and became the strongest and most effective foe of his original community. This view of his career history is not unknown to him. When he was invited to give the keynote address at a large neural network conference in the late 1980s to an absolutely rapt audience he began with the words: "I am not the Devil!"——R. H-N.]

By the mid-1970s Minsky and his colleagues (notably Seymour Papert) began to take actions designed to root out neural networks and ensure large and, in their view, richly deserved funding for AI research by getting the money currently being "wasted" on neural networks, and more to boot, redirected. They did two things. First, Minsky and Papert began work on a manuscript designed to discredit neural network research. Second, they attended neural network and "bionics" conferences and presented their ever-growing body of mathematical results being compiled in their manuscript to what they later referred to as "the doleful responses" of members of their audiences.

At the heart of this effort was Minsky and Papert's growing manuscript, which they privately circulated for comments. The technical approach they took in the manuscript was based on a mathematical theorem discovered and proven some years earlier—ironically, by a strong supporter of Rosenblatt—that the perceptron was incapable of ever implementing the "exclusive-OR" [X-OR] logic function. What Minsky and Papert and their colleagues did was elaborate and bulk up this idea to book length by devising many variants of this theorem. Some, such as a theorem showing that single-layer perceptrons, of many varied types, cannot compute topological connectedness, are quite clever. To this technical fabric they wove in what amounted to a personal attack on Rosenblatt. This was the early form of their crusade manifesto.

Later, on the strong and wise advice of colleagues, they expunged the vitriol. They didn't quite get it all, as a careful reading will show. They did a complete flip-flop, *dedicating the book to Rosenblatt!* As their colleagues sensed it would, this apparently "objective" evaluation of perceptrons had a much more powerful impact than the original manuscript with its unseemly personal attack would have. Of course, in reality, the whole thing was intended, from the outset, as a book-length damnation of Rosenblatt's work and many of its variants in particular, and, by implication, all other neural network research in general.

Minsky and Papert's book, *Perceptrons*, worked. The field of neural networks was discredited and destroyed. The book and the associated conference presentations created a new conventional wisdom at DARPA and almost all other research sponsorship organizations that some MIT professors have proven mathematically that neural networks cannot ever do anything interesting. The chilling effect of this episode on neural network research lasted almost twenty years.

It was this powerfully negative conventional wisdom that those of us attempting the work in the field encountered almost continuously and had to overcome. We did overcome, and eventually this conventional wisdom was itself discredited, but not without many fierce battles.

By the mid-1980s, DARPA, which had played a central role in establishment of the Minsky and Papert conventional wisdom, had strongly reversed its position on the subject. This was mostly due to the efforts of two DARPA people, initially, Ira Skurnick, and later, Barbara Yoon. They faced significant and visceral opposition, but prevailed. Since DARPA is one of the world's chief arbiters of technological fashion, ONR being another, the world's opinion of neural networks soon changed. The rest is history.

One byproduct of this episode is a healthy caution that infuses the field. Many people are concerned about checking their work for correctness and insisting on significance of results before publication, to try and avoid a repeat of this scenario.

There was at least one exception to the calamity that struck in the late 1960s, and that was the Adaptronics Corporation, a company with a most amazing story. They had started about 1960 with what later we thought of as polynomial neural networks—the idea that you build layer after layer of polynomial networks, and you train each unit. Let's say you have multiple real number inputs and one real output, and you're trying to approximate a fixed mapping for which you have examples. So what you do is have each unit try to yield the final output that you want. That's the training method. Then you put in a whole bunch of units, each of which gets a pair of inputs from whatever previous layer you have, and then whichever ones of these turn out to be pretty good at approximating the desired output, you let them stay, and you throw away the others. Then you build another layer. That's the scheme, anyway.

Adaptronics had invented this themselves, even before a similar approach emerged later in the decade from Ivakhnenko in the Ukraine. Adaptronics had done all sorts of interesting and successful projects, and DARPA had funded them, and they had this little company. That company existed and was profitable from 1960 all the way through the dark years up until about 1984, when they sold the company. Roger Barron and Lewey Gilstrap were the principals of that company. Anyway, besides Adaptronics and maybe a few little sprinklings of things that were sort of neurobiological, ARPA had quietly funded a tiny bit of neural network research here and there, but other than that, they really hadn't done anything. So in 1982 I began talking to them, specifically to a new fellow, Ira Skurnick, who had just joined DARPA and was very openminded. He paved the way. He brought influential DARPA people to meetings. He allowed me to have my say. I would review the arguments in well-established papers—such as yours, Jim—and even though these were things that they should have known about, they weren't aware of them because of this drought.

I could stand up and present things that were well known in the field and would be considered old stuff; yet to those at ARPA, it was all new. It was marvelous—like, "Wow, you mean, that really works, that will really learn?" It was interesting because it was so easy. I didn't have to do anything new, really, except look at applications, which was the whole emphasis, and implementation, how we build hardware to do this learning in a human lifetime.

What happened was that as this process went on and John Hopfield emerged and then we had this [ICNN] meeting and things began to accelerate, the scale of DARPA funding went up to certain point, but then they began to hit significant barriers. DARPA is divided into offices, and some of these offices were going to maintain the faith that Minsky and Papert had begun. They weren't going to question the faith: "The common wisdom is in fact correct; this is garbage." So for a period of time there was a bit of controversy. Then pretty soon that all went away, and now the original supreme defender of the faith, that office at DARPA, is having a neural net conference this spring [1994], so the controversy's over; that's completely gone.

ER: And is Ira Skurnick still at DARPA?

HN: Yes, he is, but his role as leader ended when Barbara Yoon joined them, and that was intentional. I mean, she was hired into the same office that he was in specifically to become the program manager for neural networks. He was never doing neural nets as his full-time activity; that was only part of his activity. He turned that over to her. So he's still there, and he's doing other things, but not neural networks.

ER: Do you know if Craig Fields [director of DARPA during this period] was a champion of neural networks?

HN: Oh, I know for sure. When I first met Craig, which was in '81, he was someone who was significantly open to these ideas. He had not acquired the conventional wisdom. Part of the reason was that he went to school with Steve Grossberg, at Rockefeller. So he had been already indoctrinated, if you will. Although he wasn't enough aware of the details to be a rabid champion, he was never negative, and as he became familiar with the arguments, he became more positive. When he went down to MCC [Microelectronics and Computer Consortium], this was one of the areas that he pushed. As you know, they have had a lot of successful neural network activity.

ER: Right, they have spin-off companies, and so forth.

HN: Exactly. Right. When Craig Fields was the director, Barbara Yoon was appointed director of the DARPA ANN (Artificial Neural Networks) Program. Fields had a very definite role in that. By then, he was a convinced person; he was converted.

ER: Thanks for sharing that history.

Are you mostly interested in engineering applications? I noticed that most of the conference tutorials and the sessions that you're involved with are basically application oriented, but you've talked about your wide spectrum of interests in the field. How does that balance itself in your view—the engineering side as opposed to the more scientific questions about understanding the brain and mind?

HN: Applications are my job. I make my living by applying this technology successfully and growing a business in this area—hopefully, growing the nucleus of a huge business that can someday employ hundreds of thousands of people. That's my job. Now aside from that, I have a personal interest which is much broader and where I'm interested more in the fundamental understanding of things, the deeper issues. I spend at least a certain amount of time continuing to read the literature to understand the advances that are made, and every once in a while, I have the pleasure of doing a little tiny, tiny bit of research, but that's not very much because there isn't much time.

ER: Well, I wanted to ask you about some of your own ideas and some of the things that you've developed.

HN: Well, I would characterize my contributions as nil. I mean I have made very few contributions, and all of them have been minor, in terms of actually creating new ideas. That's my view.

ER: I was thinking of counter propagation and . . .

HN: Yeah, well, that's OK. That's not a bad contribution, but it's minor. It's better for others to judge, but I see it as something which is useful and worthwhile, but minor. Actually, a piece of work that I've just completed with two grad students may be something that will be perhaps graded above minor somewhere, but that's not published yet. That's coming out.

It has to do with the geometry of error surfaces for multilayer perceptions—understanding just what the surfaces look like. What we've discovered is that the surfaces basically look like this: there's a certain place in the weight space where you can take a little slice and look at the surface that lies above that little tiny slice of the weight space, and the whole rest of the surface is just copies of that. It's just replicated over and over and over again a vast number of times. And we've figured out exactly what slice that is. We've written it down, and the equations are remarkably simple. That's all. Is that valuable? I don't know.

ER: Are there other minor contributions that you'd like to at least put on the record?

HN: I guess the ideas that I think were really important only a few other people think about. I noticed back a long time ago that Kolmagorov's theorem could be reinterpreted as a statement that neural networks can really approximate arbitrary continuous functions. That was before all of these universal approximation theorems.

In fact, Hal White [a professor of economics at UCSD] very kindly attributes that work as the thing that got him interested in proving universal approximation theorems, which he's done in abundance.

ER: How would you characterize the reception of your ideas by your peers?

HN: Oh, I think it's been generously handled, generously accepted.

ER: Have you been surprised at anything? Have you been surprised that one idea was lauded and another perhaps not paid as much attention to?

HN: Well, as I say, I've never thought of myself as having produced anything of real significance, at least not yet. I have hopes. I'm trying, but nothing so far. In fact, I've been flattered on numerous occasions. I mean, I remember when this counter propagation thing came out, enough people liked it that I was actually asked to write a paper on it for the journal *Neural Networks*. There were a few things like that that kind of shocked me. My textbook has been useful. It's been translated now into Japanese, Chinese, and Russian; it's used a great deal and has been adopted at many universities. So that's been a reasonably satisfactory experience. I feel like that made a contribution. But is it the greatest book on neural networks ever written? No. You guys wrote that. I mean, your collection of papers is classic.

ER: At least it has a wonderful title. [Both Robert Hecht-Nielsen and James A. Anderson and Edward Rosenfeld published books with the same title: *Neurocomputing.*]

HN: Now, that's interesting you mention that because you just triggered a remembrance. The question is, who invented the term "neurocomputing." And you know, I don't remember. I know people who claim I invented it. I know people who claim you invented it. Maybe not, but it was the title of your book.

ER: I thought it came out of the air, and we didn't want to call it neural networks.

HN: So you did invent it.

ER: We didn't have long conversations about this, and I don't know that we invented it.

HN: But the bottom line is that everything that I've done has been really just kind of having fun and on a light basis. I don't take anything I've done very seriously. If it's been useful, that makes me happy because that was the intent.

ER: Are there other people whose work you think is specifically important, and you are very excited by it?

HN: I think we're at a really interesting time, when we're about to see an entire phase change in neuroscience, in particular in neurophysiology, where virtually all of the dominant ideas are going to be trashed in the next five years. Of course, Wolf Singer is one of the main causes of this. I don't know if you caught his talk [at the meeting where the interview took place]?

JA: Could you just mention what that talk was about?

HN: I think the experimental work Wolf Singer has done is going to be explained in ways that he isn't currently thinking of. In fact, Judy Dayhoff had an excellent talk today about the learning of delays. My vision is that within five years we're going to see a whole new world where people are thinking of synapses as delay elements and that some learning is the learning of delay. That nerve cells, at least in some of their roles, function as matched filters, where you have these large number of pulses coming in, arriving, and then being delayed by different amounts at different synapses, and then having all of those effects hit the soma at once, causing a spike. And that individual spikes, the timing of individual spikes, is a code. This was originally Christoph von der Malsburg's idea and Singer's results support this. That's the information code: it's the relative timing of spikes coming from different cells and having influence at other cells by arriving simultaneously, or at least by being given corrections by the synapses.

ER: When people come to you in business or as a professor and ask you about how to start out in this field, what advice do you give them?

HN: Well, first of all, the most important advice is to not get discouraged because, like any field that's really hot and which is still at a fairly early stage, we're still in the process of attracting and recruiting the best people in related fields. What that means is that all the resources that are available are being sought by people of significant talent and accomplishment. That really makes it hard for new young people to join the field.

The main advice is, "Don't get discouraged. It's true, you're up against these very formidable individuals, but there's plenty of room here." The other thing that I try to get them focused on are realistic career paths because if they're going to be in academia, they better be thinking very early on about what field they're going to be in, what it takes to be employed in that field, and what kind of preparation they should be doing, day after day to prepare for a realistic possibility of being employed. If they're going to go into business, same thing. There really aren't that many different kinds of opportunities available, and they can do the right things to help ensure their getting a job.

ER: People often ask me, "Where is the neural network killer app [application]? Where is the thing that neural networks can do that nothing else could do that's going to break the field wide open toward universal acceptance?" I'm sure you've been asked that question or some analog of it.

HN: I have to argue a little bit that I think the premise is not quite right. I think we've already achieved universal acceptance, in some sense, or at least we're in the process of achieving that, and we're probably going to do it without the killer app. Today, there are well-publicized applications of neural networks that almost nobody knows about. They work, they're being used; it's not a stunt, it's not a press event, it's a real thing.

ER: A couple of examples, please ...

HN: Well, for example, our handprinted character OCR systems. By the way, if you ask three-fourths of the academics here, they'll tell you that's an unsolved problem. Yet, the state of Wyoming does all their tax forms using this system. The Avon Corporation reads all their order forms. But it's an unsolved problem!

That's the problem. There are applications like that in use all over the world that are largely unknown and unappreciated. They've been publicized; there's plenty of magazine articles; we could bring in a stack of them. And yet they haven't become widely known, maybe because they're not multi-billion-dollar applications.

And those larger applications will probably emerge, and then there will be this big parade of apps. What we're really seeking is permanence and a rational level of research activity and the ability to feel as if this is a subject that's going to in fact meet its destiny, its correct destiny. That is really what a lot of people have fought for for so long: to see this field actually go somewhere over a long period of time. I think that is happening now. That's almost assured. That's not something we have to work towards or fret about; it's a fait accompli.

ER: There's another question I want to ask. I consider HNC a small company in the broader business sense, and HNC, from what I know, is a healthy company ...

HN: Oh, sure. It started with two people. Small enough.

ER: Well, but you have sixty people now, or ...

HN: About seventy.

ER: ... and you would like to have hundreds of thousands.

HN: Right. We're still a tiny company in my view ...

ER: ... and in most people's view in the general world of business. I wonder if you're disappointed in the economic growth of the field and disappointed at what's been happening with some of the other smaller companies? Some of them have already gone by the wayside, and others are certainly struggling. I wonder if you'd discuss that?

HN: There are two perspectives. I am disappointed because it seemed at the beginning that there would be scope for a lot of success stories—a lot of small companies succeeding in this field and growing and becoming large companies. But, on the other hand, there's another perspective, which I think is OK also, and that is that this is a technology that has now penetrated all large businesses, effectively. The resistance to it and all those problems we had at the beginning are all gone. People are now treating it as just any other technology and weighing the use of it on a rational basis.

There's also always the fact that, statistically, small businesses fail, particularly nonventure-backed businesses. Venture-backed businesses have a 60 percent probability of being around five years after foundation. Nonventure-backed businesses have a much lower probability, much lower, probably no more than 10 percent under the best of circumstances. So you're talking about a population which I think you yourself ranked as being roughly 250 or 300 companies. Of those, assuming that the vast majority are not venture backed, we're only going to see ten or twenty even make it five years. And I'm not talking about big financial success; I mean just survival.

In the venture world, about one in ten of the companies really is successful. That is to say, it grows, it goes public—it does something that ensures its ongoing growth and success. In the nonventure world, it's probably down around one tenth of a percent. It's very low; it's under 1 percent. And so out of three hundred companies, as you quantified them, we can expect at most three to succeed. Well, if HNC is one, there's only two left, and they haven't been invented yet. I don't know ... Statistically, it's the expected outcome.

This will be not just the decade, but the millennium of the brain. There isn't any question that our society has been transformed by information processing already to the point where we can't go back. I mean, if this doesn't work, we're going to be back in those caves because that's the next step. We have become inexorably and irrevocably dependent upon information processing.

I think as we go forward, we're going to see the evergrowing capabilities of machines take over more and more activities that humans themselves perform. Hopefully, there'll be some rational selection of those activities, but probably not. And we will see this technology that we all know and love really become the last human technology because what will happen is that by a few hundred years from now, there won't be any human technologists. The machines will in fact be intelligent, and they will take on the role of building machines and designing machines and taking our orders and carrying them out.

I don't think that's going to happen soon. I think we are at least three hundred years away from an intelligent machine. Not so much because it couldn't be done earlier, it's just because I can't envision a scenario in the future, even war, that is going to be so dire that we would put the resources into building such a device. It could be done—not that far in the future, probably—but I don't think it ever will be. It will happen on a much more gradual basis, transforming society as it goes.

Soon our whole species is going to have a lifestyle and a manner of life that depends upon these machines. It's already happened. So I think it will be a long time, not necessarily because it has to be a long time. I think there are going to be a lot of problems understanding how brains work. It's like anything else, but it's much more difficult because there are so many specialized tricks; there are so many different brain areas.

JA: There's not going to be a single brain theory.

HN: No. There's going to have to be a hundred brain theories or a thousand brain theories. It will take three hundred years to understand how the brain works, and then we'll find out you can't really do a lot of those things except with meat and chemicals.

ER: Wetwear.

HN: Yes, exactly. The far future is impossible to predict. I think we've done something good here, in summary. I would say that the efforts that you've put in and the efforts that many of the others of us have put in are coming to something. This is not a flash in the pan. It's not something that becomes a small part of something larger. This IS that large thing, and we made it happen. Maybe it would have happened anyway. Historians will certainly chalk it up to that, but I don't think so. History has a way of bifurcating and going in strange directions, and at least in this instance we made sure that it didn't and that it went in a rational direction. So someday people are going to owe us a lot. I just hope we're around to collect.

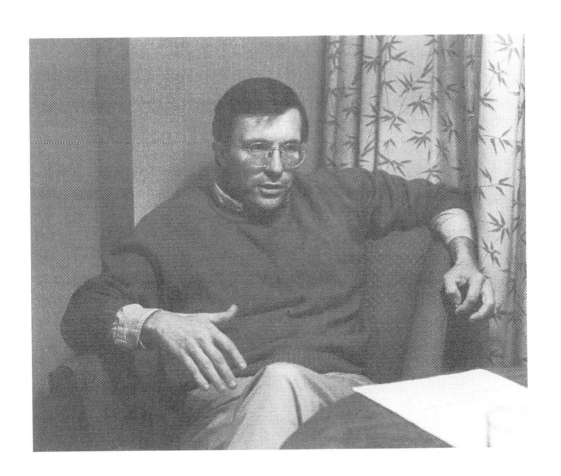

14   Terrence J. Sejnowski

Terrence Sejnowski is Professor of Biology at the University of California, San Diego and is also Investigator in the Howard Hughes Medical Institute Research Laboratories, Computational Neurobiology Laboratory, Salk Institute for Biological Studies, both in La Jolla, California. Some of his recent research can be found in "Bee Foraging in Uncerain Environments Using Predictive Hebbian Learning," Nature, vol. 377, pp. 725–728, 1995.

December 1993, Denver, Colorado

ER: Maybe we could start with general biographical material—your date of birth, where you are from, how you grew up, your early education, your parents . . .

TS: You want to go back that far?

ER: Absolutely.

TS: Well, I was born in Cleveland in 1947 and went to college in Cleveland, Case Western Reserve. I graduated from there in '68.

ER: Maybe we could back up a little bit. One of the things we're interested in is trying to find out how people became interested in the brain . . .

TS: OK.

ER: What influence their parents had on this, how their growing up affected their interests . . .

TS: There were many intangible influences. I grew up in a family where science was in the air. My father was an engineer, so I had lots of motors and electrical things to put together in the basement. If you want an interesting historical document, take a look at my high school literary magazine. I wrote a short story about a government computer project meant to simulate a brain. It was about the experiences of somebody who was talking about this blackout experience he had where he didn't remember this one period in his life. This person is actually the computer project. All his experiences are being piped in from the outside. All his internal feelings and everything else were being simulated inside the computer. He didn't know that his world was the computer.

One of my motivating interests was to understand enough about the brain to be able to build one.

ER: So you were obviously thinking about things like that before you wrote the story?

ER: That's something that had been in my mind for a long time. Everybody is curious about what makes their brains tick. I learned a little bit about brain cells, not very much, but enough to know that there was some sort of pattern of activity. So the natural question is, "Can you build one?" If it's just a machine, you should be able to build one. But at the time, back in the '60s, the standard of computing was prehistoric compared to what we have today. I imagined it would take the whole surface of a moon or a planet. Can you imagine vacuum tubes as far as you can see? The technology has changed, but it is basically the same idea.

ER: So you went to Case Western. What did you major in?

TS: I was a physics major. I finished top of the class in physics. I went on to Princeton for graduate school because I wanted to work with John Wheeler in relativity. I was part of his group working on projects during the period in which black holes became a major scientific enterprise. Wheeler had coined the term. Before that, a black hole was considered a singularity in the equations, which was unphysical. John Wheeler has a very physical imagination and said, "Well, what if they exist in the universe? What would they look like?" So we were doing calculations about what would happen if the black hole was in the middle of a galaxy. What would happen if there were little black holes in the middle of the earth? What are the astrophysical consequences of this very esoteric, mathematical result?

ER: What had led you to choose physics to begin with?

TS: I had always been interested in science, and physics seemed to me to be the most basic area of science that all other areas grew from. And I was good at it. When I had to choose my major as a sophomore I asked a friend "Well, why did you pick physics?"

And he said, "Well, what other choice is there?" And that convinced me.

Physics was very attractive, very intellectually exciting. Physics was also a wonderful education for neuroscience. For what I'm trying to do now, which is to marry basic neurobiology with neural networks, physics helps both with the experimental side and with the mathematics that you need to understand networks. Physics was an ideal background. If I'd planned it, I couldn't have planned it better.

ER: So you said you were in Wheeler's group for a couple of years and working on the black holes.

TS: They have general exams at Princeton where you are required to master all areas of physics and demonstrate that in a week long test. It's just one exam after the other for a week.

The summer before, instead of studying for these exams, I went to the library, and I read the *Josiah Macy Conference Proceedings*, on the early days of cybernetics. It was more than that because Margaret Mead, Norbert Wiener,

Gregory Bateson, and other really interesting people were there. What was interesting was the excitement that they were on the verge of understanding something basic about the brain, about how the control systems in the body work, and how it could be related to psychological phenomena.

Those meetings were from the '50s, and I followed the thread from one conference proceedings to the next. There was *Organization of the Mind*, the Teddington conference. The British had meetings, and there were big American meetings. Self-organization was big.

After an interesting summer reading these books I realized that nothing ever came of it. That is, there was all this excitement, but it seemed to peter out. Cybernetics became splintered into a lot of mainstream fields like control theory and signal processing that became standard engineering discipline, but all the exciting parts died out. That was at least the impression I got from reading the literature, without talking to anybody.

I did ask someone in biology what had happened since then on the brain. I don't know who it was, but somebody, a postdoc probably, said, "Oh, Hubel and Wiesel have done some interesting things. Why don't you go and look up some of their papers?"

At the time, I desperately wanted to know the answer to one question: "Do neural cells fire in a regular sort of clocklike fashion, at a fixed clock rate? Or is it more random? Is there a stochastic component to it?"

The postdoc said if I read Hubel and Wiesel's papers I would find the answer to that question, so I went to the library and looked up one of their papers in the *Journal of Physiology*. I think in retrospect it was probably the '62 paper because that's one of the few papers you can go to where they actually give raw data. And lo and behold, sure enough, the firing was random. [This classic paper is one of the most cited papers in science. D. H. Hubel and T. N. Wiesel. 1962. "Receptive fields, binocular interaction, and functional architecture in the cat's visual cortex." *Journal of Physiology* 160:106–64.]

Then I started taking some courses in the psychology department. Charlie Gross was giving a graduate seminar in vision; he had recorded from different parts of the visual cortex, à la Hubel and Wiesel, but much farther up. That was fascinating because I got a chance to catch up on all the work that had been done in vision since the early '60s. This was back in the early 1970s. Discovering the classical vision literature had a big impact on me.

JA: Was there anyone at Princeton you talked to about these issues?

TS: I had a few really wonderful mentors at Princeton. I spent a summer in Charlie Gross's lab participating in experiments. This hands-on experience verified my surmise from the literatures that there was an enormous amount of random component in the firing patterns of cortical neurons in the visual cortex, especially in the inferotemporal cortex, where Charlie Gross was looking at higher-order visual neurons.

Another person who had a big impact was Alan Gelperin, who works on garden slugs. I did a year postdoc in his lab after getting my degree in physics.

ER: So you passed the week of exams?

TS: I passed the exams, but at that point I realized that my interests were already departing from physics. One doesn't really know why one decides to do things, but I was a little frustrated with the prospect of working in a field where it was very unlikely in my lifetime that anyone could verify any prediction I could make. In gravitational radiation, which is the area that I was expecting to do my thesis, you can't do an earth-based experiment; you have to wait for a supernova. That's not something that happens every day. The techniques for recording from gravity waves were just being developed. They are still being developed. We're still far from having any experimental data at all.

What was very attractive to me about the brain was the fact that you could hold it in your own hands.

ER: It was local.

TS: It was local in space and time, it was every bit as much a mystery as quasars, and there was the prospect that within my lifetime we could make some progress. Furthermore, from my contacts with the biologists at Princeton, I became interested in experimental work.

At that time, I was writing neural network–modeling papers, theoretical papers. Taking courses in the biology department and getting research experience were influential. I was beginning to realize that just writing down and solving equations, by itself wasn't enough to really give key insights into the basics, the fundamentals of the brain.

As I learned more in the courses I was taking, I began to realize that there's a much richer depth to the brain. It's not just spiking that's important. There are intracellular variables. There are other complexities. If you really want to understand the basic principles of how the brain works, you first have to understand those variables. This was after many years of theoretical physics and then theoretical neural network modeling.

By the way, the network modeling that I did grew directly out of Charlie Gross's lab. I took a classical network model that Jack Cowan and others had worked on, and I injected noise into it and tried to analyze the stochastic differential equations. I came to the conclusion that correlations should be important. Unfortunately, there was very little data on correlations at the time. It's now a big industry to record from pairs of cells and measure correlations. My early intuitions about temporal coding were on the right track.

ER: So had Charlie Gross led you to Cowan's work?

TS: During that summer, I discovered that Jack Cowan had taken a similar path, so I read all of his papers. I was a little disappointed by the fact that he never followed up on some of his early exciting work. He started developing a statistical mechanics of networks but then stopped publishing it. He still hasn't published anything more. Who knows when he'll publish? But in any case, I saw myself in that tradition in my modeling work. It was about that time that John Hopfield started getting interested in the brain.

ER: He was at Princeton?

TS: He was at Princeton, before moving to Caltech. [In 1997 John Hopfield moved back to Princeton where he is a Professor in the Department of Molecular Biology.] It became clear that I wasn't going to complete a thesis in relativity because I wasn't spending any time working on it anymore. I was spending most of my time talking to biologists. Fortunately, John had gotten hooked up with the NRP [Neuroscience Research Program, a group first at MIT that later moved to Rockefeller University]. He was going to their meetings and listening to talks from neurobiologists, and he had a sympathetic ear. Furthermore, he was just at the point of making a transition into that field himself, so he was a natural mentor for me.

ER: Jack Cowan told us that Hopfield had gone to some of the conferences in the mid-seventies.

TS: It was helpful to me to be able to talk to him about things that he had heard at those meetings. John was extremely supportive of what I was trying to do, and without his help I would have been lost. John also had an old friend at Rockefeller, Bruce Knight, who I had met earlier. So John said, "Look, why don't you go and talk to Bruce Knight? Bruce Knight would be a good person to give you some feedback."

Bruce was extremely helpful. He read through the papers and gave me realistic advice about the likelihood of experimentally verifying prediction from the model, but said it looked very promising anyway. It was wonderful to have someone like Bruce, who was an expert modeler and a mathematician, read through my papers with that care.

During that period of my life, every few years I would make a transition, thinking, "Gee, this isn't going to work the way I thought it would work." The move to neurobiology was the real shift in my career, where I drew a dividing line. Everything I did up to this point was basically physics and extensions of physics. What I was doing in my thesis was a physicist's approach to neurobiology—writing down some equations and analyzing the equations.

But as I talked more to neurobiologists, I began to understand the deep complexities that you have to grapple with. If I were serious about understanding the brain, I had to get my hands on real neurons and real data and to get a better intuition for what was going on, then later come back to modeling. At that point I decided to immmerse myself in the biology.

I had good fortune. I took a course at Woods Hole at the Marine Biological Laboratory in 1978 just after getting my doctorate in physics. I took the neurobiology course, and that changed the way I thought about everything in terms of both the brain and the human enterprise that's involved in understanding it. Physicists approach problems a little differently, I think, because in physics there's a tradition of a single brilliant idea or a single experimental breakthrough. In other words, it's something that involves singularities, whereas it became clear that biology had a different tradition. Yes, there were also exceptionally good people in biology, but there weren't many singularities. There's such a fantastic complexity, that no matter what system you pick, you have your hands full. You're never going to solve that system. No one's ever going to solve anything in biology in the same sense that physics solves a problem like magnetism. Even the simplest neural circuits are far beyond what any one lab can work out, so you have communities of labs working on them.

Take one simple circuit, the lobster stomatogastric ganglion, which has only a handful of neurons. They've worked out all the connections, and they know most of the properties of most of the neurons, but they still don't understand how that ganglion works. They're getting there. In the process of uncovering all of these details, they've uncovered many important principles. For example, neuromodulators can change and reconfigure the network, which is going to have important implications for mammalian brains. They've run into very important nonlinear membrane properties, which are going to be essential for the mammalian brain as well. To discover the basics in a little circuit like that has probably involved a community of twenty labs over a period of twenty years. That's a unit of biological advance.

There are leaders, and there are followers, and there are people who are good at technical things, and people good at synthesizing. You need all those different talents focused on one system, but there are probably a hundred systems like that and a hundred communities studying different parts of the brain.

For me, it meant going back to the ABCs and really learning new techniques. During the neurobiology course I learned how to record from single neurons and how to use the freeze-fracture technique to look at single synapses.

I was particularly fascinated with the hair cell sensory receptors in the ampullae of Lorenzini in a skate. Skate brains have very, very acute electrosensitivity, down to the microvolts per centimeter range. I was fascinated and wanted to know what kind of receptor could possibly pick that up, given that neurons work on millivolt ranges, not microvolts. So we did the first study ever that summer on the skate electroreceptors. No one had ever done freeze-fracture on it before. That amazed me. It seemed that no matter what you picked up in biology, no one ever did it before.

We had the world's leading experts teaching us. We had skates that were brought in off a boat, and we dissected out the ampullae, which itself is an exciting thing—to see the actual little sock with the electroreceptors on it. We then processed it and put it in a machine that freezes it to liquid nitrogen temperature, fractured it, got a replica, put it in a electron microscope, and zoomed in on the ultrastructure of the synapses and the vesicles. It was exciting.

I remember that experience vividly. For each fracture, the electron microscope gives you a three-dimensional landscape. It's almost as if you could zoom down into the moon and go into a crater and see all the little rocks down there. And the little rocks turn out to be molecular, receptors, in the membrane that were exposed in the fracture. That changed my whole life. After that I wasn't interested anymore in just abstract understanding of the brain. I really wanted to understand how it was made. I was committed to the idea that you had to understand the actual substance that the brain was made from if you're going to understand how it works.

That was '78. I went back to Princeton to start the postdoc with Alan Gelperin. One day I got a phone call from Steve Kuffler from Harvard Medical School, who was the preeminent neurobiologist of his era. He said that he had a position in his lab and was wondering if I could come to Harvard. That was practically like getting a call from heaven. It was a wonderful experience because the neurobiology department during that era was a special place. The research ranged from uncovering the cytochrome oxidase blobs in the visual cortex—that was David Hubel, Marge Livingstone, and Johnathan Horton—to the molecular basis of development. Steve Kuffler and I were working on peptidergic synaptic transmission in bullfrog sympathetic ganglia. The whole gamut from molecules up to systems was represented in that department.

The three years that I was at Harvard made a deep impression; in forming my own lab I've recapitulated a lot of their traditions. I have a tea room, which is a miniature version of the lunch room at Harvard. I have daily teas, which is something that they did. There is the larger social part of doing science, as well as the scientific part.

During those three years I refused to touch a computer. When I left Princeton, I wrote my thesis using nroff with a box of punch cards because it was a batch system. When I left Harvard Medical School to take my first job at Johns Hopkins, it was the age of the micro. I bought a PDP 11/23, and I sat down and learned Unix. I felt like Rip van Winkle. During that period, which was not that long, perhaps only five years, things changed completely from big computer center-dominated computing to lab-style computing, to individual workstation-style computing.

Although I was completely committed to the biological side, at the same time I realized the limitations of a purely biological approach. In the biology, there's an enormous amount to know before principles emerge. You first need to understand the basics before you can understand the systems-level issues. This pure bottom-up approach has the limitation that there's an infinite number of details, and you don't know a priori what's going to be important.

At the same time that all this was going on I attended a meeting in San Diego in '79 that was also a turning point. Geoff Hinton and Jim [Anderson] organized a meeting that later resulted in the book *Parallel Models of Associative Memory*. It was an exciting meeting. Based on reading the literature, I had concluded that network modeling was in decline. There were a few people in little pockets where the torch was still burning, but there was no heart. Here at this meeting was the heart, a group of people who still believed that we needed to understand how networks work, that there are important principles and fundamental phenomena that could be understood at the network level.

Jay McClelland and David Rumelhart were there. The meeting included a rich tradition of statistics with Stu Geman. Jim and I represented biology. There was also AI and computer science, represented with Scott Fahlman and Jerry Feldman. Teuvo Kohonen, a legendary Finnish engineer, also attended.

Although we came from all of these different fields, there was a common belief that networks of simple processing units could be used to solve difficult computational problems. Cooperation was needed, and here was a group of cooperative people who were able to talk to each other despite different backgrounds.

Out of that meeting came long friendships. Geoff Hinton is still my closest friend, a friendship that started at that '79 meeting and developed over the course of many years. Whenever he was coming through Boston, he would stay with me, and when I was in California, I would stay with him.

There was also a highly influential series of followup meetings held at Rochester that Jerry Feldman and Dana Ballard organized, that was primarily in the area of vision, a vision focus group from a network perspective. I trace many advances, like the Boltzmann machine, directly to discussions at these meetings. Geoff and I thought that networks could be used to solve a lot of difficult unsolved problems in vision. We thought that if we had the right representation, we could bootstrap from the work that was done on the visual cortex. We had a reasonable algorithm for relaxation, and we developed methods for constraint satisfaction and figure-ground segregation, but we didn't have any good convergence proof.

Dana Ballard also handcrafted algorithms during that era. He would take a conventional computer vision problem, like finding lines in an image. He would use Hough transforms and put little units together to make lines support each other. The idea was that units were hypotheses about the objects in the three-dimensional world.

I remember John Hopfield was invited to one of these Rochester meetings. For the first time, we heard his energy formulation. Both Geoff and I within seconds realized that this was the convergence proof we needed to show that our constraint-satisfaction schemes in vision could actually be implemented with hardware. That's how the Boltzmann machine was born. It was the result of a week of solid thinking about what would happen if we had a noisy Hopfield network.

We realized immediately how a Hopfield network could be used for global optimization. The way to jump out of local minima was to add noise. I had just read an article in *Physics Today* where Scott Kirkpatrick described simulated annealing. So we immediately started simulating the idea, and sure enough—it was slow, but it would work. It would, in a rigorous way, implement all the things that we wanted done. Little did we know, however, that constraint satisfaction was really just an entrance to the part of the Boltzmann machine that had the biggest impact, the learning algorithm. Once you have a thermodynamic framework that allows you to analyze the probability of any state, you can begin to ask, "Well, how can I alter the probabilities?" Then you need to deal with how to sculpt the landscape—not how to search it, but how to change it. That became the Boltzmann machine learning algorithm.

Geoff was the one who really appreciated the importance of learning. He calculated the information-gain measure. I remember him calling me and saying, "You know, all the bad terms cancel." We were convinced this was the solution. Something that simple had to be important. It was the first in a long line of learning algorithms that broke the logjam. Sometimes you really don't know what's the most important when you're working on something since you're deeply involved in it. It's not until much later that you realize what's going to prove to be important in the long run.

ER: When you had figured out the Boltzmann machine, where were you? Were you already at Hopkins?

TS: It was on my way between Harvard and Hopkins; during the summer, in '82 we worked out a lot of the applications to vision and inference and started working on little networks that would do symmetry and exclusive-OR. It took about a year though before the learning algorithm was firmly established.

Geoff was going to be a coauthor on the PDP [parallel distributed processing] books but because the Boltzmann machine looked so exciting, he felt that it would be more important just to focus our energies on working it out. He has as many chapters as anyone else, so he should probably have been coauthor. He deserves a lot of credit for spearheading that San Diego group. He was the seed that led to PDP, as well as a lot of other important contributions. Jay McClelland was fantastic for pushing forward and writing the book, and Dave Rumelhart kept coming up with new ideas, and back-propagation occurred during that era. That was a very special time too, that whole era in San Diego.

ER: How did you get to Hopkins?

TS: There weren't that many jobs that a physicist with biology training could get at that time—jobs where I could use my skills. I would have been out of place in a pure biology department, and I would have been out of place in a pure physics department. But I found a wonderful home, the bio-physics department at Hopkins, which had a long tradition in neuroscience. The colleagues I had were terrifically supportive. They understood what I was doing. They understood the importance of computational biology and made it possible for me to build a strong group. That's what was great about the environment. I wasn't isolated because I was in direct contact with all of the major researchers who were contributing to network research. Also, at that time email was just becoming a major way to do research, so Geoff and I would send email on problems we were working on.

This sense of community was also extended to students. Geoff and I organized the first Connectionist Summer School in '86 at Carnegie Mellon University. That was before the PDP books came out, and very few people knew what was happening from word of mouth. When we put out the announcement for the Connectionist Summer School, somebody at MIT put out a spoof advertising a connectionist cooking summer school.

The people who turned up at the summer school came from every-where—it was pretty uniform in terms of geography. The students were fantastically enthusiastic. Many of those students are now the people giving major talks at meetings. We also had a summer school at CMU in '88, and there was one in San Diego in '91. In each of those classes there were students who went on to do brilliant work.

ER: Was it around then that you started with NETtalk?

TS: NETtalk was a project that grew out of a talk on the Boltzmann machine I had given at Princeton in the spring of '85. Charlie Rosenberg, who was a student of George Miller in the psychology department, came up to me afterwards and said he'd like to come and work in my lab over the summer. I said, "Well, what do you want to work on?" And he said, "Language."

I said, "Well, OK, we'll try to think of a project."

At that time, I was still working on the Boltzmann machine and was beginning to do simulations using backprop. I discovered very rapidly that backprop was about an order of magnitude faster than anything you could do with the Boltzmann machine. And if you let it run longer, it was more accurate, so you could get better solutions.

When Charlie showed up, backprop was up and running. We also had lots of horsepower. I had another stroke of luck in receiving a Presidential Young Investigator award from NSF [National Science Foundation]. I had picked up a Ridge computer, made by a company that is now defunct, but it had the power of a VAX 11/780 which at that time was the standard candle of computer power. I had one in my lab, but at that time the whole computer science department only had a 780, so I had as much computer power as the computer science department, for a while at least.

We had a real computer, and we had a real algorithm, and we looked for a do-able project in language. Often in science, the most important decision you make is the first one, the project. If you pick one that's too easy, then so what? And if you pick one that's too hard, that you can't solve, then so what? It's always the cases that are on the borderline that are the most inter-esting. We were fortunate to find just such a problem in phonology.

I went to the library and found a book on text-to-speech that had prob-ably one thousand rules in it. It was just lists of rules and exceptions. After

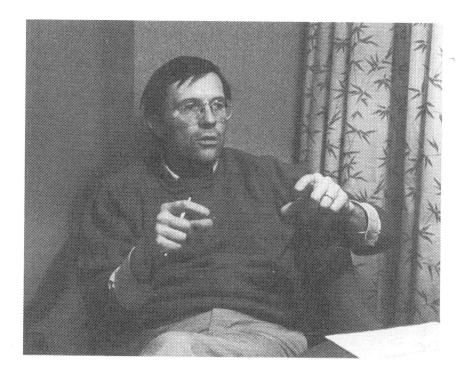

every rule, there were dozens of exceptions. I figured that either they're doing it the wrong way, or this is a really tough problem. We considered finding something that was simpler—after consulting the experts in linguistics. They said, "Chomsky worked on the problem, and it is well beyond the capability of anything that you could imagine trying to do."

Even Geoff Hinton, who visited that summer, thought it was an ambitious problem. He suggested starting with a children's book with simple three- and four-letter words. So we went to the library and checked out a child's book and coded it up by hand. We figured out all the phonemes, and we assigned them to each of the letters. That book probably had about one hundred words in it. We were prepared to start out with three words and then work our way up to ten words, and then by the end of the summer we might get up to one hundred words. That's a lot of words for a small network since it added up to over five hundred letter-to-sound correspondences.

Charlie was a very good programmer, so he was able to get a simulator up and running very rapidly. When Charlie turned the network on, it started out very slowly—it wasn't doing very well. Then it began making some progress, and we kept coming back and looking at it, and it kept making more progress and more progress and more progress. By the end of the day, it was perfect. It had absorbed this children's book; no problem at all.

It was now August; we had discovered that text-to-speech was a much better match to a network than the rule-based approach. Now the question was, "Is the network up to real language?"

Terrence J. Sejnowski

We came across a book of transcriptions of children at various ages. The advantage of this corpus was that it had the words on the left side, and on the right side were all the phonemic sounds that the child actually made on the tape, transcribed by a phonologist. So here we had a training set. We had the whole book. We had many thousands of words. But taking that book and converting it into a computer-readable format took weeks and weeks because we had to sit there, align the letters and sounds, and proofread it.

The childrens' transcriptions seems wildly ambitious in retrospect because we didn't just have dictionary definitions and pronunciations, but full-blown, real-life speech, which includes a lot of sounds that are "wrong," that are missing, or elided. It was difficult. In linguistics there is a distinction between competence and performance—that is, the theoretical grammar, which is what the linguists work with, and what people actually say in practice.

The third corpus was a twenty-thousand-word dictionary. That required a lot of work because the dictionary wasn't aligned. That corpus is still being used today as a a standard database, a twenty-thousand-word dictionary. That's a lot of words.

I am amazed at what we accomplished that summer. In addition to the phonemes, we also did stress, word boundaries, and syllable boundaries. We naively just coded them into the database and came up with some representations for the output. The network accepted whatever we gave it. It took a day for the network to learn a two-thousand-word corpus of first graders' speech. By the time we got around to using the dictionary, it was the end of August. I went off to a meeting at Woods Hole. I had a Ridge there, and we had a DECtalk speech synthesizer, so it was the first time we actually heard NETtalk speak. It was amazing to hear it for the first time. We started from scratch and built a working system in just three months. But now we had to analyze it. That took three years; Charlie's thesis was an analysis of how NETtalk represented the hard "c" in "cat" and the soft "c" in "city".

ER: When I met you in 1986, I didn't know you were doing NETtalk. And next time I saw you, you were on the *Today* show.

TS: That was another experience.

ER: That's when I thought neural networks were real. I saw you on the *Today* show. That made a major impact.

TS: We had no idea how well it would work or that it would make an impact. In retrospect it was an ideal choice for a problem. It was difficult with conventional techniques, and it was not clear that the network could handle it. For that era, it was a big network; with thirty thousand weights and several hundred units. But it is tiny by today's standards.

An important lesson from that era was the importance of representation. You need to have a powerful learning algorithm, but you also need to have good representations, both for the inputs and outputs, that are compatible with the learning algorithm.

A good example is Dean Pomerleau's car driving neural network, ALVINN. It was exciting to watch a car going down the road without a driver. There's nothing more real than seeing the car try to take that turn or go through that intersection. That's real life. But if you look into the steering network, there are only four hidden units. Who could have guessed that driving a car on a highway would only take four hidden units? That's a discovery. It was an easy problem once you had the right representation. The intuitive representations that you would think of for the car-driving problem, which is a visual motor control problem, don't necessarily work. The natural features to use are local ones like road stripes, but these come in many forms, or are sometimes absent. Dean Pomerleau's network uses global features. The hidden units see the whole visual field. They integrate a lot of small pieces of information from all over the road.

The same type of internal representation was discovered by NETtalk. There's some very crude distinctions that it makes, like that between vowels and consonants. But then it used nonintuitive statistics on how to represent all the rest of the so-called rules. The network picked up higher-order correlations and organized all of that information in a correlational structure with nonlinear hidden units.

We knew back then there were many local minima in the network, and we knew we were getting trapped. The surprise was that this did not prevent the network from finding good solutions. There are two approaches that are extremes. One is to start out with something that works, and try to analyze it and figure out why, which is what happened to us. The other approach is to start out with a completely mathematically analyzed system and try to get it to work. That turned out to be more difficult. A mixture of empirical and analytic approaches has proved to be most effective.

ER: I know there's a tremendous amount of other work that comes after NETtalk. Can we talk about your sonar work with Paul Gorman?

TS: Each one of those projects was an exploration into another domain. The name of the game was database. Whoever had the data could be the first to see what that data really looked like using networks. It was like a child in a candy shop. Anything you touched was interesting. Paul Gorman was at Allied Bendix, which has since become Allied Signal, and had been working on a sonar classification project for several years as a master's project, using classical linear discriminants. Paul came around asking whether this was something that networks might tackle, and I said, "Well, let's give it a try."

They had collected sonar echos from mines and rocks. They went around systematically every ten degrees or so and took a complete set of sonar reflection data. Most of the time you only get a few smatterings of data. It's very expensive to get data. In speech, there are now some standard labeled databases, like the TIMIT database, but in the early days, starting with NETtalk, 90 percent of the battle was getting the database together and figuring out what the input representation should be. After training a network on sonar echos from mines and rocks, Paul Gorman showed that the network could generalize to new echos and correctly classify them—a lot better than humans could.

Another problem we looked at was protein folding, predicting secondary structure. After a talk I gave, someone from the audience said, "Look, instead of using letters, you could use amino acids, and then you can predict secondary protein structure."

We were fortunate because Brookhaven had a crystallographic database of protein structures, which included as a subset the secondary structure assignments. We were able to pull out the data and started training the network. I had a very good graduate student, Ning Qian, now on the faculty at Columbia, who really pushed that problem forward. It still is the best existing method for predicting secondary structure. We improved the performance from 55 percent up to 64 percent and estimated that with more tweeks, you could probably get it up to about 70 percent. A paper I saw recently came pretty close to that by improving on the original network. That's exciting to have the world's best secondary structure prediction for nonhomologous proteins.

That was a do-able project because I was in a biophysics department, where everyone was familiar with molecular structures, and we had a good crystallographer in the department who gave us advice about the database, Warner Love. The combination of a powerful tool, a good question, and a large database is a good place to start. The question was, "Can the network extract the answer from the database?" In many cases, you don't know until you try.

ER: Were there ones you worked on that weren't good?

TS: There were only a few aborted projects. But it's hard to say whether it was the project or the people who sort of lost interest in it. A lot depends on how persistent you are—like Charlie Rosenberg, who's incredibly energetic and will just keep working at a problem until he solves it. That's what you need to get anything to work.

I am still working on problem in the visual system. Unfortunately, vision is such a difficult domain that we haven't really made that much progress. Even now, we are just beginning to recognize some of the enormous problems that vision poses. It's not just a recognition problem. It's a representation problem. How do you represent complex objects? No one has a clue.

Geoff Hinton probably has the best insight right now into how to use distributed representations to represent complex objects componentially. But we're far, far from being able to solve real-world problems in vision. Geoff has a knack for picking small test problems, like the shifter problem, which is a test problem for stereo vision. I'm still looking for problems like that, which are challenging but not so difficult that finding a solution's going to be impossible.

It's ironic because back in the '70s when we started, we were inspired by the visual cortex. We thought that if we only had the right algorithm for doing constraint satisfaction, we'd be able to solve a difficult problem like separating an object from the background.

It's a difficult problem partly because the number of units you need and the amount of processing you have to do just to look at an image are enormous. The classical work on computer vision at the University of Maryland was done on a PDP 11/34, the equivalent to a little PC, like a 386. That made it very difficult even to store all the images.

ER:　Could you say a little bit about moving to the West Coast?

TS:　After being at Hopkins for six years and building up a group there, I began spending more and more time on the West Coast. I was a visiting professor at Caltech in '87 and had an opportunity to interact with the San Diego group. It was a wonderful community.

Getting an opportunity to work at the Salk Institute was a perfect match to my interests. I had close ties with Francis Crick and Pat Churchland, and we were already collaborating on book chapters. My interests now are primarily in neuroscience and using techniques and tools from network modeling to understand different pieces of the brain.

The community in San Diego is very special. I said earlier that a major advance in biology involves a team. To understand something as complex as a psychological or biological system, you need to have expertise in many different areas, and the people in these areas have to talk to each other. There has to be a common language. San Diego was at least five years ahead of any other place that I had come across, mainly because of Dave Rumelhart, Jay McClelland, Geoff Hinton, and the others in that community.

ER:　Is your lab at UCSD?

TS:　I have a faculty position at UCSD and I teach there, but my lab is physically in the Salk Institute. I have a joint appointment at both places.

There are several other community and institutional groups that I am involved in which I think are very important. One of them is a workshop that I founded at Woods Hole in 1984—the first workshop on computational neuroscience. I had taken a neurobiology course at MBL [Marine Biological Laboratory] there in '78, and went back as a researcher for several summers with Steve Kuffler.

Steve Zucker and I were stuck at the Denver airport one day coming back from some meeting. The flight was delayed, and we had hot cocoa in a little restaurant. It turned out that Steve was really excited about Woods Hole, too. "Well, let's have a meeting there."

I also was very fortunate that at that time the Sloan Foundation was just starting to fund computational neuroscience. I submitted a grant, and they gave me three years of support for running a workshop at MBL. It was a fantastic group because unlike most big meetings where people bounce off each other, there were only twenty young researchers and intense discussions. Many invited to the very first workshop have come back year after year so there has been some continuity. This includes Richard Andersen, Bob Desimone, John Allman, Dana Ballard, and Steve Zucker. There was a balance of physiologists and computer vision people. Friendships developed and common projects blossomed. In terms of getting networks and biology together, those meetings were a key development.

Another group I'm involved in is the Helmholtz Club, which is a coming together of psychophysics, physiology, and theoretical analysis with a focus on vision. It was founded in '83 by V. S. Ramachandran and Francis Crick, meets once a month at UC Irvine and comprises about thirty people at Caltech, San Diego, UCLA, and other places. It's like Woods Hole, except that it happens once a month.

My guess is that history will tell, many years from now, that a lot of the key, seminal ideas in the area of vision primarily, but about other parts of the brain too, came out of discussions held at Helmholtz meetings. That's something you probably won't hear about because the meetings aren't published. New ideas happen in small groups, not in big meetings. Big meetings are where the results of ideas are presented.

ER: It underscores what you were saying before about the social component of doing science.

TS: The seminal meeting in '79 that was held in San Diego marked the beginning of a cooperative venture of a community of researchers, who shared some common assumptions but had a lot of differences too. At the outset they had more differences than they had things in common, but at least they were willing to sit down and talk and argue with each other, and to understand the other person's language.

This also happened on a much larger scale at the early NIPS [Neural Information Processing] meetings. When someone gave a talk, no one in any other field would understand what was said because the terminology and jargon was not understandable to anyone outside their particular fields. The mathematicians had various detailed concerns like convergence. The biologists couldn't even understand that these should be concerns. The brain works. Why should you worry about it converging? What's gradually emerged at NIPS is a larger community of people who are beginning to understand the concerns of other groups and are beginning to realize that those concerns may have some impact on their concerns. Some of the new ideas are getting incorporated into their research.

There are timescales for everything and for creating a new field the average timescale is probably a decade. It's not going to happen in a year; it's not going to happen even in five years. Probably it needs a decade for a field to get to a point where there are standards and there's an understanding of what the difficult problems are. The danger, though, is that after a certain period you may get boxed in if you don't renew and grow and reach out into other directions. You may end up going in circles on the same issues and topics.

ER: Where do you see the neural network field going in the future?

TS: The field is healthy to the extent that we are working with real-world data, not toy problems. Toy problems are nice for theorists to play with, but if you don't test them against the world, then I doubt that they're going to amount to much.

AI went awry by taking toy worlds too seriously. We should be figuring out what the real-world problems are, which may be different from the ones that we imagine them to be. The real world tells you that immediately. When you drive the car, you've got the steering wheel in front of you, and you can't rely on some symbolic buffer to save your data for you. You have to deal with it as it flows in, in real time.

Carver Mead had a big influence in convincing me that you really need to study real time systems. All the simulations are fine as far as they go, but unless you can get the information flowing through and understand how you're going to deal with it in real time, you really haven't understood the essence of the computation. You're just doing off-line stuff. So I see the real problem in the next five, ten years is coming to grips with real time signals, and imperfections. You don't have sixteen bits of accuracy in real neural circuits. You have only a few bits of accuracy. There have to be ways to adapt around that, to take advantage of a limited dynamic range.

It's going to be a long time before we create anything that is autonomous. Truly autonomous. You can create something in a very artificial environment that will continue to work autonomously, but as soon as you have uncertainty, variability, something that you didn't anticipate, you have trouble. We have to deal with uncertainty all the time—different lighting conditions, something that you trip on, something that someone says that you didn't anticipate. Unless we build a system that can anticipate surprises and take advantage of new things happening, then I don't think we're going to appreciate what the real problems are.

In twenty-five years we should have hardware that can do the enormous computation needed for real-time vision. We have to have new ways of putting together all of the chips. It's not enough just to have a retina chip; we have to have a retina chip that is integrated with the motion chip. The motion chip has to be connected to the motor chip.

In other words, you have to have a way of putting it all together so it works as a whole, as a system. We need an arbitrator to figure out which networks control the motor system. But what if there's no arbitrator? You then have an anarchy of hundreds of networks, all competing for attention and control. Somehow it's organized in such a seamless way so that control's passed over from one part of the brain to the next, depending on the context and what's needed at that moment.

ER: Do you think there will ever be a single brain theory?

TS: What we see now as a lot of isolated results and pieces that don't fit together perfectly could at some future date be seen to be limiting cases of a much broader and far-reaching framework. But it's just as likely that it's going to go the other way. If you look in the brain, you don't see one system, one network. What you see instead are hundreds, perhaps thousands, of subnetworks that have been honed by evolution to perform particular tasks, interacting with lots of other pieces that are specialized for other tasks. And then there is some sort of overall organizational scheme so that they don't trip over each other's feet, so to speak. There may be a dozen theories up there dealing with different problems that have to be solved.

At some future date there may be a way of seeing how all the pieces fit together: Given that you have this type of representation in the cortex, then it follows that you must use this kind of motor controller to move limbs. In other words, there may not be independent solutions, and there may be evolutionary strategies—parallel evolution of strategies in different parts of the brain—and we'll see a commonality. Maybe it's being obscured by the fact that the neurons look different. But there may be a commonality that will emerge in the long run. But so far, we don't see it.

We know that across species there's fantastic diversity—all the different invertebrate plans, with creatures that crawl, swim, and fly. There may be at least two or three different theories, different solutions to the same class of problems.

ER: Is there anything special you wanted to say about the role or influence of government and government funding on the field?

TS: I've been fortunate to have support through government and also private foundations. My first grant was from the Systems Development Foundation, which helped get the field started. Some inspired funding is coming from places like the Air Force, and the Office of Naval Research.

One of the advantages of a system that offers a large variety of places for people to go for funding is that a lot of ideas are explored in parallel. The $500 million that was spent by DARPA's Strategic Computing Initiative on the Autonomous Land Vehicle seems in retrospect to be a fantastic waste of resources, fantastic beyond anything we can even imagine. $500 million is real money even by government standards. But a lot of other factors were involved there. Perhaps other approaches couldn't have gotten as far as they did because they wouldn't have developed the infrastructure and the experience. The future is difficult to predict and often it is difficult to judge the value of a project until you get there.

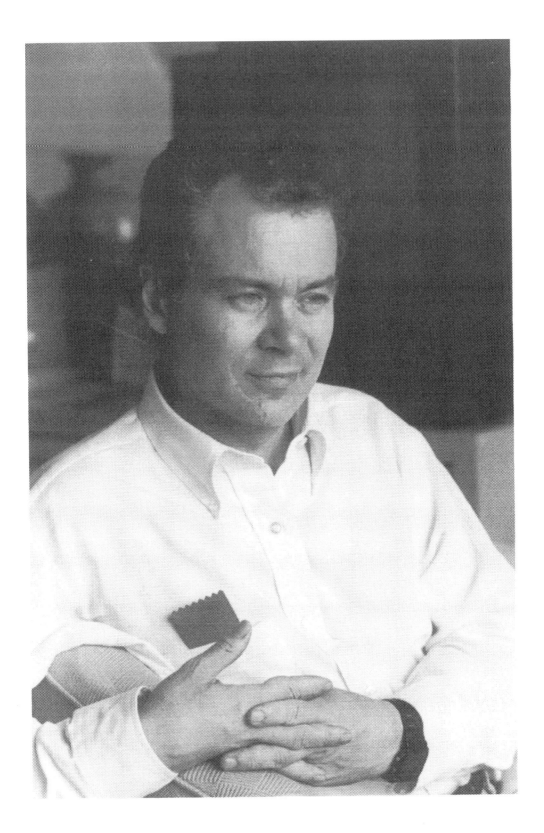

15 Paul J. Werbos

Paul Werbos is Program Director of the Knowledge Modelling and Computational Intelligence program at the National Science Foundation, Arlington, Virginia. The best source for further reading is his article, "Optimization: A Foundation for Understanding Consciousness," in D. Levine and W. Elsberry, Editors, Optimality in Biological and Artificial Networks?, Lawrence Erlbaum Associates, 1996.

June 1993, Baltimore, Maryland

ER: Paul, can you tell us something about your growing up and early childhood?

PW: I was born on September 4, 1947, in the suburbs of Philadelphia. When I was very young, I was interested in mathematics. I remember getting a book when I was about eight, *All about the Stars*, from my parents. Then I went out and weeded lawns to earn money to buy books by Hoyle and Gamow, people like that.

The book that influenced me most was Fred Hoyle's paperback book. The title was *The Nature of the Universe* [Harper, 1951] and I remember reading it when I was eight, in 1955. I remember it because my family was very strongly Catholic, staunch Catholics. They originated, at least on my father's side, from the same neighborhood where von Neumann originated, around Timmesfarb, a German enclave in Romania. They were staunch Catholics, and my mother was a staunch Irish Catholic. I can remember when I read the first chapter of Hoyle's book, I was thinking to myself something really obnoxious like, "Oh, the glories of God's universe." And I got to the second chapter, and it got even better. Then I got to the last chapter, where it says there is this little planet full of these walking robots, and they had this incredibly arrogant idea that the universe was formed by a walking robot. They have these meaningless things called communism and capitalism that they shoot each other about, and they think they're important. And all of that is total illusion. All we have are the laws of physics.

My initial reaction to that was, "My God, this is what they've been telling me is evil. This is terrible. This is horrible."

And then I started thinking it over. How do I know? What is the basis for my knowledge? And the more I thought about it, I started saying, "Gee, my source of knowledge for Catholicism is what the nuns told me. This guy Hoyle probably knows more than those nuns do anyway." And so that was the end of Catholicism for me.

Independently, I became interested in mathematics. Obviously, mathematics fit into what Hoyle was talking about. I found in the attic one of my mother's old algebra books, and I snuck it away. When I told my elementary school people that I was already studying algebra, they laughed. But then somewhere around the fifth grade they decided, "Why don't we check? He does seem to know his multiplication tables pretty well." So they checked, and I did know algebra.

I finished the calculus course by the end of sixth grade. They sent me to the University of Pennsylvania to take the junior honors calculus course, complex variables and such, when I was in the seventh grade. My parents sent me to Lawrenceville in New Jersey so that I could go to Princeton. I had the equivalent of an undergraduate math major with a graduate course or two before I graduated at fourteen or fifteen from Lawrenceville.

During that time I took some summer courses in computing. This was one of the good things that NSF [National Science Foundation] did back then, but you couldn't easily measure results from it. It has since been discontinued because you couldn't measure it. I took one of those summer courses at Temple where I learned how to do computer programming. Then, the Moore School of Electrical Engineering at Penn. had an advanced version of the same thing, which I took. I guess I was fifteen at the time.

I worked for a summer before I went to Harvard. I worked at the University of Pennsylvania Hospital, Jefferson Hospital. We were supposed to be studying the circulatory system. The guy I was working for handed me D. O. Hebb's *The Organization of Behavior* [Wiley, 1949; a classic in the behavioral sciences]. I thought that was neat. I was supposed to give a talk back at the Moore School, to inspire the next generation of high school students. So I said, "How about I program this thing up [Hebbian learning], and I'll give a report on it."

We scheduled a date. But I looked at it, and I said, "Wait a minute, this is not clear." I tried different ways of looking at it, and I said, "This won't work."

It was obvious to me from a statistical point of view that Hebbian learning was going to be measuring correlation coefficients, and for multivariate problems it would not work. I never gave the talk. I said, "Now I'm going to figure out something with the same flavor that does work."

At that time, I guess I was sixteen. There were some other things that influenced me. I'd read the *Foundation Trilogy* [by Isaac Asimov, science fiction classics]. It had some ideas about organizations and thinking. I had forgotten that book, but when I reread it later, it was like a blueprint for my life. I didn't consciously remember it, but the impact of that book was incredible. I'd also read Feigenbaum and Feldman's *Computers and Thought* [McGraw-Hill, 1963]—a beautiful simple book. Ironically, Minsky's chapter was one of the things that got me most excited and turned me on. Minsky was one of my major influences. Well, Minsky and Hebb and Asimov and Freud.

I decided I wanted to do this. This will help us understand the human mind; it will help human beings understand themselves. Therefore, they will make better political decisions, and better political decisions are vital for the future of humanity. I remember explicitly thinking about how developing this mathematics could help us make better political decisions.

I got to Harvard and I was still interested, but there were no courses in it [brain theory]. There were math courses, but I already had them. There were computer courses, and I felt I already had them. Even the graduate courses didn't look as if they had anything that was really new. So what could I do? I took the one and only neurophysiology course they had. It was a course for premeds. You were supposed to spend a lot of time memorizing various hormones. I didn't do what I was supposed to do, so I got only a C+ in the course.

I spent a lot of the time reading Rosenblith's *Sensory Communication* [MIT Press, 1961], reading Morgan and Stellar [*Physiological Psychology*] and getting that vocabulary down straight and thinking about modeling. I spent a lot of my college career not doing what I was supposed to do but instead thinking about neural networks. I wound up majoring in economics.

You may ask, "What does economics have to do with it?" Well, by that time I'd decided reinforcement learning was the paradigm I wanted to pursue. I really felt reinforcement learning was the right way to think about it. I was still frustrated by the fact that I knew Hebb wouldn't work, and I wanted to find something that would work. Before you start fine-tuning it, you need a first-order thing that works. That's what we're still doing today. I feel as if I'm actually past that stage, but I feel the profession still has not reached the stage of having things that work.

I suspect if you take people in the audience here [the interview was held in Baltimore at an International Neural Network Society meeting], they're still doing supervised learning. They haven't really grasped reinforcement learning and what it means. I wanted to do reinforcement learning, and I knew it had something to do with distributed optimization because a neural net is a distributed system.

In economics, some people had spent years and years trying to figure out how to build an optimal, decentralized decision-making system. I was interested in that problem for its own sake, and it had larger political and social implications, which I still care about. I figured it's the same mathematics you need for neural nets. I wound up learning about linear programming, how that interfaces with economic systems, marginal thises and marginal thats, how you get nonlinear optimization out of a distributed system. My real goal was to build a mathematics to help you understand the human mind.

In senior year, one of my suitemates was Dan Levine. We all had single rooms on the gold coast in Adams House at Harvard, but he was the closest thing I had to a roommate. He and I spent hours and hours discussing neural nets. I'm the one who got him interested in them, and afterward he went to work for Grossberg in part because we had fun conversations. We used to debate optimization. He's going to be coming out with a new book [D. Levine and W. Elsberry, 1997. *Optimality in Biological and Artificial Networks.*" Hillsdale, NJ: Erlbaum]. He says his real goal was to recreate our old discussions at Adams House about optimization and the human mind.

I wanted to publish some of this because even though I didn't have a working system, I felt as though this was a start toward a working system. Trying to publish the start of a new concept is very, very hard, especially if you're a mere student.

I was in London the year after Harvard, more for R and R than for anything else. I got a master's degree in London. That year I sent in a paper to *Cybernetica*, which was published in 1968. It was not a coherent thing, but it had the germs of all the later ideas. If somebody had ever had the mathematical ability and had pursued those ideas, a lot of this stuff would have been in the literature sooner than it was. Being published is not the whole thing. Maybe it was the wrong journal.

I talk in there about the concept of translating Freud into mathematics. This is what took me to backpropagation, so the basic ideas that took me to backpropagation were in this journal article in '68. I talked a lot about what was wrong with the existing [two state] McCulloch-Pitts neuron model, and how it was only "1" and "0." I wanted to make that neuron probabilistic. I was going to apply Freudian notions to an upper-level, associative drive reinforcement system. When I look at what Grossberg is talking about now, it's very, very similar because his gated dipole system basically is measuring a matrix. That's what I put in this paper. This paper showed how if you had that kind of matrix arrangement, you could derive a secondary reinforcement system that would allow you to do optimization over time. There's a link between the concepts in there and Grossberg's current concepts. In order to make it work from an engineering point of view, I later shifted to a different approach altogether, but it's possible that original approach could work. It's possible that what Grossberg and Levine are talking about could work. Nobody has yet applied the necessary engineering mathematics horsepower to find out if that kind of architecture could work because the engineers basically won't listen to what Grossberg writes.

ER: Where did you go to school in London?

PW: London School of Economics. To describe it as recreation may be a slight exaggeration, but Harvard was a problem-set kind of environment. There was a little bit of the treadmill, and, frankly, there was also a little bit of the monk, being an undergraduate at Harvard. If you wanted to spend half your time doing neural nets and still pass your courses, you wound up in a very monkish style of existence. Going to the London School of Economics was great for my sanity because they had a totally different style of education. It was a seminar-based system, not a lot of grades, and you learned a lot in class. We were doing international political systems. I wanted to understand these systems and see if that understanding could help do useful things in the world. That still is one of my major concerns.

We can complain about credit assignment in the neural network world, but in the political world it is ten thousand times as bad. [The "credit assignment" problem in artificial intelligence refers to the notorious difficulty of assigning credit or blame to the appropriate parts of a complex interacting system.] To get a good idea through the system, you have to abandon any pretense of credit, and then after you do that, you won't be able to continue on with the same endeavor. It's hard to apply systems theory to political systems—not for intellectual reasons, but for social organization reasons.

Then I went back to Harvard to get a Ph.D. in applied math. Having been fortified with humanity from London, I then descended into the bowels of the machine, stopping off at the RAND Corporation for the summer of 1968 along the way.

I was excited about working at RAND because I heard they were good in two things: U.S.-Soviet relations, and cybernetics and dynamic programming. I said, "My God, that's the right mix for me." Then I got there, and they told me I was going to work on the Vietnam War. I said, "Gee, it's not that I'm opposed to it; I have no moral inhibitions about it. It's just that you're going to get zero product from me because I don't know anything about Asia. I know lots about Europe, the Soviet Union, I know lots about mathematics, but if you give me work on the Vietnam War, it's just going to be crap. I'll do the best I can, but I want to warn you, the product isn't going to be good."

They interpreted that to mean that I was an evil war protestor. A guy named Ikle who later became director of ACDA [Arms Control and Disarmament Ageney] and then number three in the Pentagon personally threatened me that if I did not work on this Vietnam project and stop giving them caveats, I would be blackballed and would never have another job for the rest of my life.

At that point I said, "All right, all right, you want it, you get it."

Actually, I did learn a thing that summer that surprised me. It turned out one of their problems was coming up with a measure of success in the Vietnam War. A lot of people were using a measure called the body count. The body count was a total disaster. It came from a very highly classified paper, presumably declassified by now, which was total nonsense in any event. Niskanen, who later became head of the President's Council of Economic Advisors, made a very thorough, econometric study of the Vietnam War. Basically, he used factor analysis, which is a stupid method for this purpose. People then said, "Gee, enemy deaths are correlated with American deaths." They didn't say exactly that, but that's what drove the factor analysis. The prime factor therefore turned out to involve deaths of American soldiers. They didn't quite want to say it in these terms because basically it said the more soldiers you got killed, the better you were doing.

I looked at this, and I said, "OK, not only is this silly from a substantive point of view, but from a methodological point of view. Knowing something about systems design and control, I know why this is crazy. This is not a good measure of success."

So I immediately went into doing a dynamic system identification kind of thing, causal analysis, which was part of the adaptive critic design that I was into, that I even talked about some in *Cybernetica*—model-based optimization designs over time. I used all that to come up with an argument for better measures of success.

I looked for stable invariants, and they were things like Vietcong attacks on Americans. That was the best stable invariant underlying measure. I used that as a success measure and came to the conclusion that we should radically change our policy and do things like small-unit actions instead of these large sweeps.

They sent the paper to the Pentagon. The guy who was theoretically the principal investigator didn't discover it until very late in the game because of security and because he wasn't physically on site. So in September of that year, on my birthday, I wound up flying to the Pentagon, talking to the number three guy in the Pentagon. His name was something like Einthoven.

It was a strange conversation, because they walked in, and the number six man in the Pentagon said, "Uh, Mr. Einthoven, these guys have come up with an interesting result based on a statistical analysis of this data."

His first reponse was, "Bullshit." He just sat there. Meanwhile, everybody was shaking. He turned around and uttered two sentences. He said, "It's all the Marines, false correlation. It's I Corps."

Scurry around, scurry around, then number six guy said, "They did a separate split-sample study, and they excluded I Corps. They got the same results."

And Einthoven said, "Really? Well, we'd better look into it."

Of course, it was all classified, and I read it on the front page of the *New York Times* two weeks later, which immediately made me very cynical about American security. The minute it's useful, it's on the front page of the *New York Times*. That made me very cynical—that event plus a few other things that happened at the RAND Corporation. They were very diligent about checking your suitcases and having you show up to work at 9 point 00 point 00. When it came to major fundamental strategic matters, of course, that goes on the front page of the *Times*. What else do you do with important, critical things?

I went on to Harvard graduate school and descended into webs of problem sets. Mainly what I studied at the graduate school was mathematical physics and quantum theory. I minored in decision and control. I took Bryson and Ho's course and learned more about dynamic programming. After I had done the basic course work, I was torn because I wanted to do something very fundamental in science. There were two or three areas I was interested in. One had to do with the foundations of physics. But that was further out than backprop. Another area was models of intelligence. Another was models of motivation because you have to figure out where the reinforcement function comes from. I spent time thinking about all three areas.

I had passed all my course requirements. It seemed dumb to me that I had to sign up for four courses when I was supposed to be working on a thesis, but that was Harvard's rule. I decided to take a course where you get free computer time and do a computer project. Initially, I was going to do something on quantum physics. I learned something about partial differential equations, but not enough. I couldn't produce a really useful product at the end of x number of months.

So I went back to the committee, and I said, "Gee I can't do that, but I have this little method for adapting multilayer perceptrons. It's really pretty trivial. It's just a by-product of this model of intelligence I developed. And I'd like to do it for my paper for this computer course."

They said, "Why don't you go talk about it to Larry Ho?"

I said, "Look, I've got a problem with this course. I can't solve the problem of reality in a course of six months, and so now I want to do a fallback. I've got this method for training multilayer perceptrons. I'm convinced it would work, and I know it's not a big thing, but at least I'll get credit for the course."

Ho's position was, "I understand you had this idea, and we were kind of openminded. But look, at this point you've worked in this course for three months, admittedly on something else. I'm sorry, you're just going to have to take an incomplete in the course."

And I said, "You mean I can't do it?"

"No, no, you'll have to take an incomplete because, basically, the first thing didn't work. We're very skeptical this new thing is going to work."

"But look, the mathematics is straightforward."

"Yeah, yeah, but you know, we're not convinced it's so straightforward. You got to prove some theorems first."

So they wouldn't let me do it. One of the reasons that is amusing to me is that there are now some people who are saying backprop was invented by Bryson and Ho. They don't realize it was the same Larry Ho, who was on my committee and who said this wasn't going to work. Ho was right to be skeptical because I was flying by intuition. If he couldn't reproduce my intuition in his head, it was entirely legitimate for him to be skeptical. I do think they should have given me permission, however.

By the time my orals came around, it was clear to me that the nature of reality is a hard problem, that I'd better work on that one later and finish my Ph.D. thesis on something small—something I can finish by the end of a few years, like a complete mathematical model of human intelligence.

So I defended before my thesis committee a mathematical model of intelligence and motivation. I said, "These are the things that I'm interested in. But I think intelligence is the one I'm going to do for the thesis."

I can remember those orals very well. It turned out the committee was more interested in motivation than they were in intelligence. I had a one-page prospectus that talked about each problem. Somewhere in that page, I think I made a statement that there might be parameters affecting utility functions in the brain, parameters that vary from person to person. You could actually get a significant amount of adaptation in ten generations' time. I was speculating that maybe the rise and fall of human civilizations, as per Toynbee and Spengler, might correlate with these kind of things. The political scientist on the committee, Karl Deutsch, raised his hand. I'd worked for him, by the way, in previous summers. He wrote *The Nerves of Government* [Free Press of Glencoe, 1963], arguing that the political system is a neural network system. He became president of the International Political Science Association. His book, *The Nerves of Government*, which compares governments to neural networks, is one of the classic, accepted, authoritative books in political science.

He raised his hand and he said, "Wait a minute, you can't get significant genetic change in ten generations. That cannot be a factor in the rise and fall of civilizations. That's crazy."

Next to him was a mathematical biologist by the name of Bossert, who was one of the world's authorities on population biology. He raised his hand and said, "What do you mean? In our experiments we get it in seven generations. This guy is understating it. Let me show you the experiments."

And Deutsch said, "What do you mean, it's common knowledge? All of our political theories are based on the assumption this cannot happen."

And Bossert said, "Well, it happens. Here's the data."

What happened was my oral defense became a discussion between the political science department and the applied mathematics and biology guys. I could scarcely get a word in edgewise. I passed the orals having said about two sentences and not having discussed models of intelligence.

I said, "OK, now I can do what I want to do because I passed with flying colors, even though I didn't say anything."

Then I got started. At some point, I had to write a prospectus on the model of intelligence. I did, and it was with an adaptive critic, and backpropagation was part of it. But the backpropagation was not used to adapt a supervised learning system; it was to translate Freud's ideas into mathematics, to implement a flow of what Freud called "psychic energy" through the system. I translated that into derivative equations, and I had an adaptive critic backpropagated to a critic, the whole thing, in '71 or '72. I actually mailed out copies of that paper to some people out at Stanford and certain people around Harvard.

The thesis committee said, "We were skeptical before, but this is just unacceptable. This is crazy, this is megalomaniac, this is nutzoid. So you have to do one of several things. You have to find a patron. You must find a patron anyway to get a Ph.D. That's the way Ph.D.s work."

I was under the illusion that getting a Ph.D. was your own creative piece of work. I'd read that. I believed democratic theory. I thought we were in a completely free country. I had lots of illusions back then.

"OK, I've gotta find a patron." They suggested that I go to MIT, and there were a few people the committee would accept. One of them was Grossberg. One of them was Minsky. One of them was Lettvin. I spoke to all three of them in a search for a patron. The committee didn't like the neural network area generally, but they said, "Look, you find a patron for your thesis, and we'll let you graduate in this area."

I went to speak to Steve Grossberg, who was an assistant professor at MIT. I remember this very wooden office. I walked in, handed him the papers, came back, and he said, "Well, you're going to have to sit down. Academia is a tough business, and you have to develop a tough stomach to survive in it. I'm sure you can pull through in the end, but you're going to have to do some adaptation. So I want you to sit down and hold your stomach, maybe have an antacid. The bottom line is, this stuff you've done, it's already been done before. Or else it's wrong. I'm not sure which of the two, but I know it's one of the two."

Well, if he'd said one or the other, I might have felt bad, but when he said, "I know it's one of the two, and I don't know which," I thought, "Gee, there might be a loophole in here somewhere."

Then he handed me some of his papers, and he said, "See, I have theorems to prove that it's already been done. So either you have replicated my work, or your work is wrong. I don't know which. But based on these theorems, I know that my work is the solution to those problems. So if you're willing to work within this approach, there might be something to do."

But I didn't hear that part, frankly because I was doing something else, and maybe there was a little pain in my stomach because clearly I had a problem. How was I ever going to graduate at this rate?

So he handed me his papers. I can honestly say, based on those papers—this was really early, like '71, '72—I know that he was talking about what we now call Hopfield nets because that's what was in these papers. He was having trouble getting it published. It may be that what happened with Grossberg is in part what happened with me—namely, we had the exact same idea in the exact same form, but people weren't willing to publish it. He had to dance it through and change it and modify it and screw it up before people would allow it to get through the system. And then after the screwed-up version got through, then people would allow the full form of it to come in from places that they trusted. We were not people they trusted, neither Steve nor I.

At any rate, what I heard from Steve was not encouraging. He did say, "You know, it might be nice if you had found an elegant thing like a LaGrangian formalism from which you rederive what I've got. That might be intellectually interesting if you found a way to rederive what I've got from a more general perspective."

I confess at that time I did not know LaGrangian mechanics. The funny thing was that the first course I'd ever taken in physics was quantum mechanics, and that was the only physics I knew.

I spoke to Minsky. I remember I had my Rosenblith, and I said, "You know, I've got a way now to adapt multilayer perceptrons, and the key is that they're not Heaviside functions; they are differentiable. And I know that action potentials, nerve spikes, are 1 or 0, as in McCulloch-Pitts neurons, but here in this book that I had for my first course in neurophysiology are some actual tracings. If you look at these tracings in Rosenblith, they show volleys of spikes, and volleys are the unit of analysis. This is an argument for treating this activity as differentiable, at least as piecewise linear. If you look at that, I can show you how to differentiate through it."

I went to Minsky for help, but Minsky would not offer help. Minsky basically said, "Look, everybody knows a neuron is a 1-0 spike generator. That is the official model from the biologists. Now, you and I are not biologists. If you and I come out and say the biologists are wrong, and this thing is not producing 1s and 0s, nobody is going to believe us. It's totally crazy. I can't get involved in anything like this."

He was probably right, I guess, but he was clearly very worried about his reputation and his credibility in his community.

Minsky also said, "You know, I used to believe in all this kind of stuff with reinforcement learning because I knew reinforcement learning would work. I knew how to implement it. I had a nice guy named Oliver Selfridge who came in and acted as my patron and gave me permission to do it. We co-authored a paper, but it was really my idea, and he was just acting as patron on the Jitters machine. I'll hand you the tech report, which we have deliberately never published."

It was his bad experience with the Jitters machine that turned him off on reinforcement learning and all the neural net ideas. It just didn't work. I later looked at that paper, and it was transparently obvious to me that what was wrong was that he didn't understand numerical analysis. He didn't understand the concept of numerical efficiency. We still have people in the learning business today who do not understand the concept of numerical or statistical efficiency. He had a system that was highly multivariate with a single reinforcement signal. The system can't learn efficiently with that. At any rate, he was totally turned off. That was the end of Minsky.

So I decided, "All right, now I'll try Lettvin." It was funny. I walked in, and he said, "Oh yeah, well, you're saying that there's motive and purpose in the human brain."

He said, "That's not a good way to look at brains. I've been telling people, 'You cannot take an anthropomorphic view of the human brain.' In fact, people have screwed up the frog because they're taking bachtriomorphic views of the frog. If you really want to understand the frog, you must learn to be objective and scientific. And besides which, even in physics, you know you can show the physical universe maximizes a utility function, but that doesn't prove it's an anthropomorphic entity. People have just got to get out of this whole style of thinking."

Besides, he said, "We will never understand the brain. It is too impossibly complex and ad hoc."

I recently ran across Lettvin, just this past year. He has mellowed in many ways. He recognizes that plasticity is what's really exciting about the brain. I'm an extremist about plasticity. He's even more extreme. I believe that within any layer of the nervous system, you have the same learning rule. Everything is produced by learning at the higher levels. The lower-level systems are so complex that we'll never get a total mathematical handle on them, but they're inherently boring anyway. At the higher levels, I would argue, there is an inherent modularity in the learning, which means that it is inherently understandable. A relatively simple set of learning rules explain the whole diversity of what we observe after the fact.

I believe it's just like the physical universe. You can't know everything in the physical universe, but you can understand the laws of dynamics, the laws of change. I would argue you can understand the laws of the learning that underlies the interesting stuff in intelligence. The cortex and the cerebellum, the olive—the fun places that provide higher intelligence. Lettvin is so extreme he even argues that one neuron can take over from another neuron, so it's really general and really modular. I don't think it's quite that general, but in terms of the learning mechanism, there may be histological development mechanisms that provide some additional flexibility.

I might add that when I was an undergraduate, I had a few conversations with McCulloch that influenced me a lot but had nothing to do with my Ph.D. thesis. Maybe the conversations with McCulloch changed my view of what neural nets were. I really got along with him. He was a really neat guy even though it was his model of the neuron I was challenging. Maybe if I'd talked to him about this model, I would have saved my career.

McCulloch changed my view of the human mind a little bit. I guess I should be totally honest, given the obscure nature of what we're about here. OK? This is a personal, not a scientific, sort of a thing. From age eight, I believed that when we understand the brain and we have the mathematics down pat, we'll get rid of a whole lot of mystical crap that has confused people and distorted their decisions and made them do bad things. As a result of some things that followed from conversations with Warren McCulloch, I eventually was convinced that maybe there are attributes of the human mind that we can't reduce down to neurons. I got so far off the deep end that I now go to Quaker meetings.

I think there is something out there beyond what our models of the brain are going to give us. It's ironic. The main thing Warren McCulloch did to my head was to send me into that orbit. But I still believe the mathematics is important because I believe that mathematics is a universal, just like the Pythogoreans used to say. I believe all forms of intelligence that we can possibly conceive of have to be governed by mathematics. Whether these forms are physical neural nets or not, I still think that mathematics is relevant. These days, if people ask me what my religion is, first I say Quaker Universalist, and if that doesn't work, I tell them to read Bernard Shaw's *Back to Methusalah*, which is the next best approximation. And then I actually discuss what I think is going on if they're intelligent enough to be interested in my idiosyncratic views of the mind. That's what Warren McCulloch did.

I didn't find a patron. Nobody would support this crazy stuff. It was very depressing. I tried to simplify it. I said, "Look, I'll pull out the backprop part and the multilayer perceptron part."

I wrote a paper that was just that—that was, I felt, childishly obvious. I didn't even use a sigmoid [non-linearity]. I used piecewise linear. I could really rationalize that to the point where it looked obvious. I handed that to my thesis committee. I had really worked hard to write it up. They said, "Look, this will work, but this is too trivial and simple to be worthy of a Harvard Ph.D. thesis." I might add, at that point they had discontinued support because they were not interested, so I had no money.

Approximately at the same time there were scandals about welfare fraud, about how students were getting food. They cut off all that kind of nonsense, so basically I had no money. NO money. Not even money to buy food.

A generous guy, who was sort of a Seventh Day Adventist and a Harvard Ph.D. candidate in ethnobotany, had a slum apartment that rented for about $40 a month in Roxbury in the ghetto. He let me share a room in his suite, in his suite with the plaster falling off, and didn't ask for rent in advance. I had no money at that time for food. There was a period of three months when I was living there in the slums. To conserve the little bit of money I had, I remember eating soybean soup and chicken neck soup. I remember getting the shakes from inadequate nutrition.

As for applying for jobs, this was in the days of the great aerospace layoffs. People were called overqualified, you know. I remember getting one very short-term job doing a computer program for an astrophysicist at MIT.

It was really terrible. I was a mile from the Harvard Medical School Library, where I would walk to keep my sanity every day. Past tons and tons of dog shit. They never cleaned the streets. And through the gangs. So I guess I was starving for my convictions.

Finally, they said, "Look, you know, we're not going to allow this." There was this meeting where we sat around the table. The chairman of the applied math department at that time was a numerical analyst, D. G. M. Anderson. He said, "We can't even allow you to stay as a student unless you do something. You've got to come up with a thesis, and it can't be in this area."

Karl Deutsch was the political scientist I had worked for, and he wanted to be helpful. He had a funny feeling something bad was happening here. Ideas like this shouldn't be totally destroyed. He didn't have the math, but he had a feeling something was going on here. He knew that I had done very good work for him in previous summers.

So Deutsch said, "You're saying we need an application to believe this stuff? I have an application that we could believe. I have a political-forecasting problem. I have this model, this theory of nationalism and social communications? What causes war and peace between nations? I have used up ten graduate students who've tried to implement this model on real-world data I've collected, and they've never been able to make it work. Now, do you think your model of intelligence could solve this problem and help us predict war and peace?"

I had actually seen that model and some of the earlier results. It was my conclusion at that time that some of the problems with that model were due to subtle stochastic effects, which I had worried about in a neural net context, but which also had conventional statistical aspects to them. I felt that the cutting-edge statistics that really relates to the neural nets—ARMA modeling—could do the job. My response to the mathematicians was to say what I just said. I said, "I can do it. It's not exactly a model of intelligence, but I believe I can handle this problem."

They nodded their heads, and they said, "All right. If you can use this new model of intelligence, and it actually works in predicting models of conflict—if you succeed, yeah, we'll give you the degree."

My impression was that half the guys felt, "Boy, this is a good way to get rid of him." And one or two felt, "Well, he'll do the statistical thing, but it will be legitimate, and it won't be any of this funny neural stuff."

So they said, "OK, go ahead."

The next thing, I went back to my Box and Jenkins and said, "Of course. The multivariate generalization is trivial; I'll go ahead and do it." And I went to the algorithm that was in the book by Box and Jenkins to implement it. I got computer time from the MIT Cambridge Project, which Deutsch was connected to. It was a joint MIT-Harvard project at that time. I said "I'll just code this up."

And then I looked at the algorithm, and suddenly, pain in my stomach because the cost of estimating multivariate ARMA processes, with the good, standard algorithm published by statisticians, increased like n^6. Even though n was small, that would be enough to blow the computer budget. Suddenly, I felt very, very sick to my stomach. My God, I'm not going to graduate after all. I remember those days of sheer agony. It did hurt in my stomach a lot. And I'm not being figurative.

I remember pounding the walls with my mind and thinking, "Dammit, I can build a brain in order n. How come I can't do this faster than order n^6?" And I thought, "Wait a minute, wait a minute. Why can't I go back and use this little backpropagation algorithm and solve this statistics problem?"

Then I generalized backpropagation to handle time-varying processes— what people would now call recurrent or time-lag recurrent systems. I showed that I could use that to solve the statistical estimation problem within the allowed computer budget. So I went ahead.

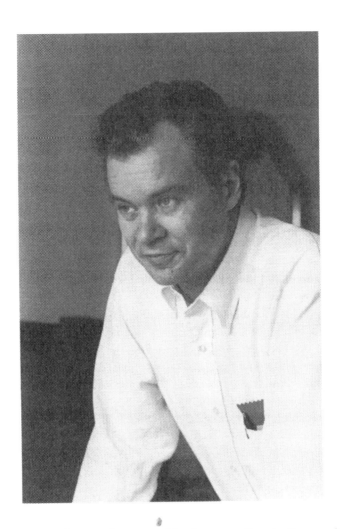

The first application of backpropagation in the world in a generalized sense was a command that was put into the TSP [Time Series Processor] at MIT, available to the whole MIT community as part of their standard software. It was published as part of MIT's report to the DOD [the Department of Defense] and part of the DOD's report to the world. It was part of the computer manual, so the first publication of backpropagation was in a computer manual from MIT for a working command for people to use in statistical analysis. I was a second author of that manual. It was Brode, Werbos, and Dunn.

That manual went out. It said, "We're using this funny method," which I called dynamic feedback. One of the funny things was that we discovered that ARMA modeling was not the way to solve that statistical estimation problem. I'd gotten an idea for another way to solve the problem that did work, fortunately. The other method is something that the neural net community has not grabbed onto. I did a lot of nonneural tests of this alternate estimation method, which I called the pure robust method.

But, you know, you have to go one step at a time, and that's what I didn't understand. I got a lot of bad advice from people who said, "You know, you shouldn't have your next publications all be just your Ph.D. thesis. You've got to go on to do something new."

Well, that was bad advice because my Ph.D. thesis had enough for about five careers in it. What I needed to do was to publish one idea at a time, but it was so hard to get published that I tried to cram a lot into individual papers. I think that's one of the reasons they weren't widely recognized. Also, I felt very insecure about my access to journals because of the way people dumped on me in the past and the lack of encouragement, and that probably is why, like Grossberg, I have these early papers in the seventies that have twenty ideas—you know, two paragraphs on each, each of which will work—but that wasn't enough to really catch the eye of the community.

That's a digression. The new method worked. I did forecast nationalism and political assimilation. At that point, the Department of Defense became interested. In fact, when you can predict conflict twenty, fifty years in advance, it's amazing who can become interested. I had a prior track record from the Vietnam War that the community as a whole didn't know about, but they knew that "My God, this is the guy who told us how to get out of Vietnam," which was essentially true because that change in strategy led to a doubling in efficiency, which was what was behind our ability to remove troops from Vietnam to a great extent, although there are many other aspects to that story.

OK, so I had some brownie points at that time with the Department of Defense. I had two job offers after Harvard. I didn't know that the way the system works is your thesis advisor gets you a job. My advisor was Karl Deutsch, so my job had to deal with political science. There was no choice.

I went to the University of Maryland in what was supposed to be a public policy program. The provost had approved that. After I arrived, the approval had disappeared, so instead of being the quantitative guy in applied math and public policy, I instead found myself in a political science department proper, which was not a totally comfortable fit.

When I got there I also walked into being PI [Principal Investigator] on a major grant from DARPA [Defense Advanced Research Projects Agency]. It wasn't like I had filled out a grant application. It's like the DARPA guys came and spoke to me and said, "Now you are going to head a DARPA grant."

That's where the job came from, too, because the head of the department had been in charge of that office in DARPA—CTO, the Cybernetic Technology Office. It was a three-way grant. I was one-third PI on crisis management and forecasting. It was a three-year grant that bought off two-thirds of my time.

One third of my time was teaching. I would teach quantitative methods, like trying to teach backprop to graduate students in political science.

Two-thirds of my time was working for DARPA. They kept telling me, "Look, we don't want pure theory. You can spend some time on pure theory, maybe half your time. But you've got to do it as crisis warning. And we want a practical application."

I spent a lot of time working on adaptive critics. I already knew how to do heuristic dynamic programming [HDP]. Temporal difference methods are a special case of heuristic dynamic programming. But in the initial proposal to my thesis committee there was a statistical efficiency problem with having a scalar critic.

It was in this early period that I figured out how to get a multivariate vector critic, which I called dual heuristic programming, that solves the essential combinatorial problem. I published it in *The General Systems Yearbook*.

I also published the idea of heuristic dynamic programming. Barto and Sutton's TD [temporal difference] is a special case of HDP. It's fun, but it's not a model of the brain. After I'd done this theoretical work, DARPA was really pushing me for applications. "We need a real-world application of this stuff."

So I said, "OK, they want it real world. What's a real-world forecasting model?"

I found out that DARPA had spent a lot of effort building a worldwide conflict forecasting model for the Joint Chiefs of Staff that was used in the long-range strategy division of the Joint Chiefs. It was based on a worldwide data set that they'd spent millions of dollars on as the basis of global stratagy planning for the U.S. I said, "That sounds like a practical application. What we'll do is we'll take that model, which is based on something, which is sort of the equivalent of a TDNN [time-delay neural network], except classical. We will reestimate it using the pure robust method and the more advanced methods that I've derived since then in the same vein."

So I sent someone to get the database. First of all, the database was secret. Secondly, I was able to get it anyway. Third, it turns out that the data was grossly misleading. I think that is the right way of putting it. The fact of the matter is that it was largely interpolated data based on relatively unreliable sources. To make statistical causal inferences based upon this kind of data is highly improper in my view. I wound up sending a couple of graduate students to create a really good database of Latin America.

I said, "You want variance, high variance. Something hard to predict." I thought conflict in Latin America would be the most beautiful case. I figured there were enough cultural homogeneities that it would be a single stochastic process, but with lots and lots of variance in that process. So we got truly annual data going back, I don't know, twenty or thirty years for all the countries in Latin America and then reestimated the Joint Chief's model on it. It had an r^2 of about .0016 at forecasting conflict. By jiggling and jiggling we could raise it to about .05. It could predict GNP and economic things decently. Conflict prediction we couldn't improve, though; it was hopeless.

DARPA wasn't happy when I published that result. They wanted me to do something real and practical and useful for the United States. This was useful, but it was an exposé. They didn't like that. Therefore, the report, which included backpropagation in detail and other advanced methods, was not even entered into DOCSUB. Every time I tried to enter it into DOCSUB, somebody jiggled influence to say, "No, no, no, we can't publish this. This is too hot."

It was published in the *IEEE SMC [Systems, Man and Cybernetics] Transactions Journal* in '78 anyway because they couldn't block the journals, but it didn't include the appendices. So that paper in 1978 said, "We've got this great thing called dynamic feedback, which lets you estimate these things. It calculates derivatives in a single swoop, and you can use it for lots of things, like AI."

That was all in the paper, but the appendix on how to do it was not there because of page limits for a journal article. The fact that we could get better forecasts than conventional statistical methods was in the *IEEE SMC Transactions Journal* in '78.

At that point, DARPA was no longer happy. Things were getting uncomfortable at Maryland. Marxists wanted to take over the department and hated DOD people. I was not on the top of DARPA's list. I began to feel uncomfortable. Nobody was in my camp. I was just a lone, middle-of-the-roader surrounded by Marxists and military contractors and really traditional kind of political scientists. So, somebody offered me a chance to work for a year at the Census Bureau developing these ideas. I wouldn't commit myself to leave Maryland, but I spent a year at the Census Bureau.

We had reports for the Farmers' Home Administration that were just adaptive critics translated into policy language. The USDA was just about ready to put $1 million into using adaptive critics to allocate $20 billion a year of agriculture loans. They might have done it if I had accepted the job to stay on at the Census Bureau.

The Department of Energy [DOE] offered me a job. They said, "How would you like to be the person evaluating our global long-range forecasting models to tell us what is really true in the whole global energy policy area in order to advise the U.S. government?"

I said, "Gee, that sounds like an important job. Based on what is useful to the United States, maybe I ought to take that job." They wanted me to do the quantitative stuff too—maybe not as much as Farmers' Home Administration, but some. To this day, I don't know if I made a mistake. I accepted the job.

The guy who made me the offer is this wild guy, Charles Smith. He's a real personality. You may remember how *Alice in Wonderland* was based upon high-level people in the British establishment. There's a certain style that book tried to convey, and Charlie had much of that kind of style. At one point, he was a clubby at Princeton. He had good degrees. I think he had taught for Mosteller or Tukey [well-known statisticians]. He had a mathematical background, but he also had a unique personality as well—definitely the opposite of what you find in bureaucracy. Too far in the other direction, many people believe.

So Charlie hired me, and my job was to evaluate these models. I was sincerely concerned about energy. I had some credibility in that part of DOE because I wasn't just a guy trying to sell a methodology. They really, really wanted a sensitivity analysis of their very large long-range energy forecasting model, the official model used for long-range forecasting. They wanted to know how the inputs depend on the outputs.

They had a million dollar contract at Oak Ridge [National Laboratory] to study that model. They wanted me for several things. One, they wanted me to be a translator between engineering and economics. Two, they wanted a critique. They wanted exposés. They wanted me to rip apart the models of the Department of Energy in a very scientific, objective way that didn't look like I was trying to rip them apart, but was anyway. That's exactly what they wanted to hire me for, and I didn't really know that was the motive. These particular people didn't like modeling very much.

So at some point they wanted sensitivity analysis. And I said, "You know, I know a little bit about calculating derivatives."

Now the Oak Ridge model was not really a time series model, so they used their own sensitivity analysis methods, which they called adjoint methods. Historically, if you wanted to find roots outside of neural nets for backprop, you know, where I got it from was Freud, and maybe dynamic programming to a lesser extent. Another possible root, if you're looking for historical roots of things, would be the adjoint methods and people like Jacob Barhen. Jacob used to work at Oak Ridge.

Based on what Oak Ridge sent me, what they were doing was very different. A good way of describing it might be as follows. I had developed a technique to operate through time by way of arbitrary nonlinear sparse systems, dynamic systems. Oak Ridge had a technique for taking what we would call simultaneous recurrent nets and getting derivatives out of them, effectively but without really exploiting sparse structure.

It was about 1981 or '82 that I figured out how you combine time-lag recurrence and simultaneous recurrence and get derivatives efficiently out of both systems. I applied it to a natural gas model at the Department of Energy. In the course of applying it I did indeed discover dirt. They didn't want me to publish it because it was too politically sensitive. It was a real-world application, but the problem was that it was too real. At DOE, you know, you don't have First Amendment rights. That's one of the terrible things sombody's got to fix in this country. The reality of the First Amendment has deteriorated. Nobody's breaking the law, but the spirit of the First Amendment has decayed too far for science. At any rate, they finally gave me permission to publish it around '86 and '87. I sent it to the journal *Neural Nets*—that is, how you do simultaneous recurrent nets and time-lag recurrent nets together. Then the editorial process screwed around with it, made the paper perhaps worse, and it finally got published in '88, which makes me very sad because now I gotta worry about, "Well, gee, didn't Pineda do this in '88?"

So once again I had trouble working with journals. That's always been one of my problems. In fact, there is one case of a paper that I submitted to a journal where the reviews came back and said, "We can't publish this because it is a challenge to good people like Rumelhart."

But the paper wasn't negative. It just simply said, "I did this."

I've had a few other experiences that are much in the same spirit. We're probably better than a lot of other professions, but it's hard to stay objective when you have these experiences.

So that was in '81. I had an interesting opportunity then, when Charlie Smith was going to leave DOE. He was offered a job as director of the System Development Foundation. He told us, "I'm supposed to go out there and figure out how to combine weird things like brains, artificial intelligence, and math. Nobody's done it. Whoever gave us the money said, 'This is what we're going to fund.' You know, people who give money are sometimes a little crazy. So we're going to find legitimate things we can fund, but how can we fund such a weird thing?"

I went up to Charlie, and I said, "Charlie, let me give you a little briefing?"

I said, "Charlie, it's not as crazy as all that. I think there's a way to do it. And let me show you how. First of all, you've got this sensitivity analysis stuff. You know it works. You've seen it work. So why can't we apply it to a differentiable model of the neuron?"

I drew a little flow chart of where I thought the field was going and how this would fill a critical hole. And I said, "Charlie, this is what I think is do-able. You don't have to throw away the money. It can be done. And what's more, I'd like to participate in doing it."

To substantiate that I showed him a paper. Now, he was actually the reviewing authority for me. I couldn't publish anything without it going through the chain of command. You remember what I was saying about the First Amendment? In order for me to publish a nonenergy paper, it had to be reviewed only at the lower level, like a number two guy in the agency. If it was an energy paper, it had to go up to the highest level. Charlie Smith had signed off on a conference paper and on a tech report. Both of them, conference paper and tech report, described backpropagation in general terms for first and second derivatives, for sensitivity analysis, and for eigenvalues and applied it to energy models with substantial pages on applications to artificial intelligence and neural nets.

I said, "Charlie, you signed off on this. You understand the mathematics" —he certainly did—"so therefore you know that this could be applied. If you approved this paper, presumably the concept is reasonable."

He thought about it. He came back, and we had another conversation. I remember very vividly being in Charlie's office where he basically said, "Yeah, these are fine ideas and good directions to go, but if you want to do this stuff ... You are a civil servant. If you want to consider losing your tenure and your salary as a civil servant, and getting one third of the salary you have today for a job that ends in one year, with no security whatsoever beyond that, then I have some friends and I might be able to arrange something. But if you really want to work in this area long term, I mean, really, you are not the right person to do it because in a deal like this, we need to have the best people in the country with reputations. Otherwise, you're not going to be able to change the culture. I think you're not the right person to do this."

I don't know when he moved to California. I do know in the PDP books if you look in the acknowledgements section, there is acknowledgement of Charlie Smith and his critical role. Now, I obviously was not present in any conversations between Charlie Smith and anybody else. I do know I've heard people say, "Oh well, Charlie Smith didn't know any math." I know that much is not true. I mean you don't teach statistics at Harvard and Princeton without having at least some knowledge of math, and he did understand what this was about. But beyond that I don't know.

The other thing is that ideas can spread by nonverbal means. Even with the best intentioned people. When I was working at MIT and doing my thesis at Harvard, I remember attending a party once ...

You know, MIT guaranteed my survival. Once I started doing software for them, they discovered I was pretty good at it. Once I had put backpropagation into a TSP command, they offered me a full-time job at the Harvard Cambridge Project, so I did the Ph.D. thesis while having a full-time job.

While I was doing these things at MIT, I remember going to one party. I didn't go to a lot. And one of the people there said, "We have heard through the grapevine that somebody has developed this thing called continuous feedback that allows you to calculate all the derivatives in a single pass."

And I sat back and thought, "This says something about the grapevine." When you've got an idea that's hard for people to understand, it doesn't move fast. As soon as you've done what the whole world says you should do, which is distill the essence into a few understandable ideas, it spreads like wildfire. The people who have better access to the journals publish it before you do, which is a trap if you are a young person trying to develop good ideas.

After that party I decided that I would be a little closed lip for a while. After that, in 1981 in New York, I presented the conference paper that I mentioned, the one Charlie Smith signed off on. I presented it at the International Federation for Information Processing. IFIP was this gigantic conference. They seemed to know what I was saying. There was lots of applause. It seemed to be finally accepted. I mentioned we have applications, and now we can apply it to neural nets. I published the paper in their proceedings in '82, which became a Springer book. It's not like the usual conference papers, which never see the light of day. It was a real book and a real conference, and I had really talked at length about artificial neural nets and Grossberg and the limbic system and the brain. That's where I had the little diagrams with the circles of the multilayer perceptrons, only with reinforcement learning and backpropagation.

At that point, I thought, "Based on this publication, now my priority is assured, and I will relax a little bit. Now that I know that I've established that I've done it, now I will relax and let the grapevine hear about it. I will give the condensations, and I will send them out all over the world"—you know, even to people who have not heard of me because I knew how to jiggle the system to get the idea out.

I don't think it was a coincidence that shortly after I jiggled the system, all of a sudden things popped up. One place was with the System Development Foundation and California. Another place things popped up was MIT, and that was definitely one of the places I jiggled because I was running a contract at MIT at the National Center for Economic Research. I was contract manager there. I tried to get them to implement backprop. They said, "We'll send it around to the engineers at MIT and see if they are willing to implement this thing as a sensitivity analysis tool." They weren't willing to.

At any rate, the National Center for Economic Research is one of the places where my ideas popped up. I think that I did succeed at jiggling the system there. As contract manager, you know, you can do things like that. It is easier to create heresies from the top, sometimes, than it is from the bottom. One of the reasons I wanted to become a contracting officer was I'd seen how often our present system prevents new ideas from getting through. I wanted to be in a position to do the opposite, to take advantage of a position in the government to encourage what I felt was the best future direction. I think history has vindicated me. It was a legitimate direction to push. There's this incredible conservatism built into the system.

I had a disappointment with Charlie Smith. I stayed at the Department of Energy and got a chance to do a couple of papers. There was one on energy models and studies on the long-range economic modeling system at DOE and how you can use backpropagation to analyze convergence behavior of very large complex systems. That paper got good reviews in the operations research community. At least half the paper dealt with how you can implement backpropagation for complex energy models without using neural nets at all. That was '83. That's when I first had the idea of a dual subroutine, which I think is still crucial to the engineering implementation of these ideas. The guy who did the book that the paper appeared in was going to do something on factory automation, so I wrote a paper for that. He said, "Gee, it isn't real world enough for the factory; it's kind of general."

In that paper, I was putting the reinforcement learning in a new context, so he suggested I submit it to the *IEEE SMC Transactions Journal*. I sent the paper there, and it came out in January '87. That was the paper that Barto and Sutton read in January '87, and they suddenly realized there was a connection between what they had been doing and what I was doing. We got together in '87, very shortly after the paper was published.

I had a long talk with Rich Sutton and Oliver Selfridge at the GTE Research Labs in Waltham, Massachusetts. That conversation didn't work very well because Oliver Selfridge said things like, "I don't believe in any of this kind of crap. You know, I'm a good Anglican, and I believe in the soul."

I tried to reassure him by saying, "No, this is consistent, and I believe in the soul too. I just have a slightly different outlook on it."

That was not the way to handle Oliver. What I should have done was get down to the nitty gritty and show him how to design things. But I made the mistake of responding to the question, so we didn't get into the nitty gritty.

I think there were a lot of results from that discussion, at least with Rich Sutton. Rich was the one who mentioned Dave Parker to me, saying, "This guy has been doing backpropagation."

I got in touch with Dave Parker. Parker and Widrow were the people who invited me to the second ICNN [International Conference on Neural Networks] conference in San Diego in 1988. If it were not for Parker and Widrow, all these things—the advanced adaptive critics, the advanced estimation techniques, the generality of backprop theorems—would not be in the literature. We would be doing pure, simpleminded supervised learning until we quit and died from boredom. The next generation moving into neural control would not have happened if Parker and Widrow, for reasons of conscience, had not given me a chance to exist when a lot of people wanted to treat me as persona non grata.

To this day, there are people who are screwing up the discussion of recurrent nets and confusing people about recurrent nets because they don't want to cite my 1990 paper in the the *Proceedings of the IEEE*, where I describe backprop through time, very explicitly. I think that may be the best tutorial paper around on what backprop is—what backprop is through time and how to implement it. But they don't want to cite it, and so they'll cite the 1986 Rumelhart, Hinton, and Williams paper that deals with simultaneous recurrent nets. Then these poor guys will go out, and they think backprop through time has to do with simultaneous recurrent nets. They get mixed up between time-lag recurrent nets and simultaneous recurrent nets, which are really like night and day.

Widrow and Parker, on the other hand, were helpful. And when they gave me that opportunity, the very first thing I did in '88 was to say, "I thank you for the platform. Now let's talk about the real problem, which is not supervised learning. The real problem is intelligence. Intelligent systems, the mind, that's what I really want to do."

At that point, I was halfway well known, and NSF asked me to be a program director. I've been doing that ever since '88. I've been pushing the attempt to understand intelligence. When I took the job, 90 percent of my motive was to help us understand the human mind. My real ulterior motive was that I think the development of mental, spiritual potential is one of the imperatives in life. I think a better understanding of the mind in universal terms is crucial to that. I think that's the ultimate value of what we're doing. My goal in taking a job at NSF, even though it totally involves engineering applications, is to give me a chance to promote and develop the kind of mathematics that we need to begin to understand the human mind. I don't think a purely bottom-up approach by itself is going to do the job.

I've seen guys like Grossberg and Klopf do random searches through the space of models. It's clear that if you do that kind of random search, you get lost. There's just too much stuff, too many possibilities. You need to have a guideline, a magic trick that will lead you through the maze. Knowing what works and what doesn't is that kind of a guideline. The kind of mathematics we're developing does that. And so while the program is developing the mathematics, I hope eventually we'll come back and make the connection. It's going to be hard with the barriers that exist in our culture to make the connection from the real mathematics, the working mathematics, to the hardcore neurobiology and from there to psychology and from there to a greater appreciation of human nature.

These are hurdles we're going to have to go through on the way to changing the culture. It's clear our culture needs to be changed. It's clear that our understanding of the human mind is wrong in many fundamental ways. Mathematics can correct a lot of the basic fallacies.

Once I started on the job at NSF, it became apparent to me that the engineering applications were not only real, but some of them were truly important. At first I thought, "We'll make a billion dollars here and there for some company. There are a hundred technologies that are not being funded, each one of which could generate a billion dollars of product a year, no sweat. Neural nets are competitive, so they're one of those technologies."

But when I started learning about what some of the applications were, I began to realize, "Hey, these aren't just billion dollar applications. They could affect human history." I began to discover that the ability to achieve things like the human settlement of space required a technology that ultimately falls back to really tough nonlinear control problems.

I found out that greater efficiency in control can lead to major reductions in waste or pollution coming out of chemical plants. I found out that control or system integration is probably the biggest remaining challenge, along with manufacturing process control, in replacing the internal combustion engine with something clean, efficient, and sustainable.

After I learned all that, I began to shift my emphasis somewhat. At the present, I'd say that about half my motivation in the program is to push the kind of mathematical development that will help us understand the brain and the mind, and about half is to make a real and critical contribution to these major technological needs.

[Paul Werbos made the following additional comments in 1995.] Some of these areas have moved forward a whole lot, some seem to be just taking off now, others are still stuck. My greatest frustration is that there is such a huge amount of work still to be done.

The link to brain circuitry and new experiments has also grown stronger. We are talking seriously now about an emerging understanding of how intelligence works in the brain, an understanding that we are replicating in engineering. NSF has initiated two programs in engineering-neuroscience collaboration that open the door to funding this kind of development. NSF is also developing a still larger initiative that would strengthen the links to cognitive science and computer science as well. I have also initiated a small business program at NSF on fuel-cell electric cars, where neural networks have begun to contribute.

On the other hand, on the deep level of fundamental research and basic ideas, we still have lots of problems due to paradigm blinders and the walls between disciplines.

You would be shocked at what people can ignore even when it is staring at them in the face. We already have sketched out all the basic ideas we will need to build a truly brainlike, intelligent system, but filling in the holes will take a rare degree of creativity.

For myself, I've been drifting away from trying to fill in the big holes in the neural network area because I see some areas that are perhaps equally important that are much more in need of an early explorer. Issues involving basic physics hold most of my personal research attention. I have solved some of the problems that I worried about years ago, but a whole lot of follow-through is still needed.

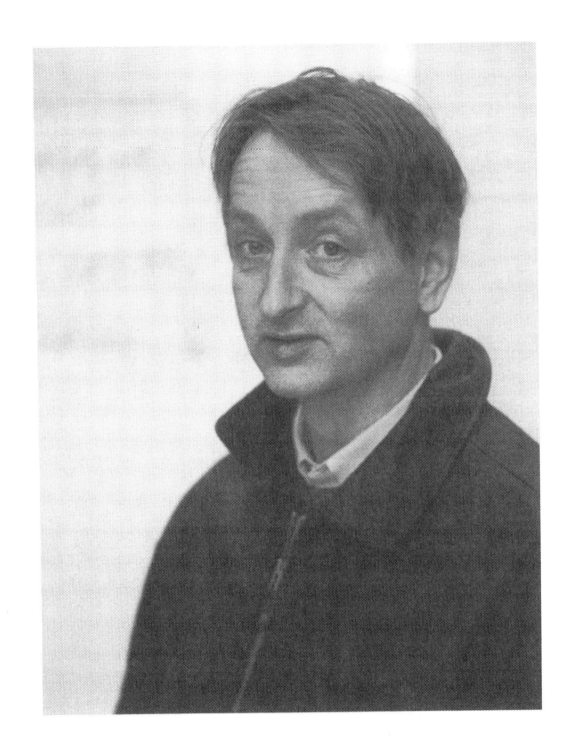

16   Geoffrey E. Hinton

Geoffrey Hinton is Professor of Computer Science and Psychology and Nesbitt-Burns Fellow of the Canadian Institute for Advanced Research at the University of Toronto, Toronto, Ontario, Canada. For further information about his work see his article, "How Neural Networks Learn from Experience," Scientific American, September, 1992.

August 1995 and March 1997, Toronto

ER: Where you were born, and when?

GH: I was born in Wimbledon [UK] in 1947, sixth of December. I didn't actually grow up in Wimbledon. My parents moved to Bristol when I was a year and a half. I grew up in a big house in Bristol. My mother was a school teacher, and my father was an academic. He was a zoologist. He was an entomologist; he studied beetles. He was also a Marxist, a Stalinist.

ER: How many brothers and sisters?

GH: I've got an older brother, an older sister, and a younger sister.

ER: And what do they do now?

GH: My older brother is a historian at Warwick University in Britain. He's the chairman of the history department there.

ER: And your older sister?

GH: She was a headmistress at a school in London, and now she's taken early retirement.

   My parents sent me to a British public school—that is, a private school, the same one that John Cleese [of Monty Python fame] went to. I got Christianity at school and Stalinism at home. I think that was a very good preparation for being a scientist because I got used to the idea that at least half the people are completely wrong.

   I guess that was a very important sort of experience for me—going to school and getting these religious services and having scripture classes and being convinced that it was all complete nonsense. I was convinced throughout my childhood that the whole Christian ideology at school was just complete rubbish. I'm still convinced of that. So I always felt like a bit of an outsider at school.

My number one story, when I first went to public school ... This is when I was about eight. We're having a scripture lesson. The scripture teacher says, "All good things come from God." I realized there was something very suspicious about this remark. The way I would put it now is that she didn't have any independent evidence of this because the only way in which she decided that things came from God was because they were good. So she just assumed that if they were good, they came from God, and actually argued that this showed that God was good because all the good things came from God. I tried to argue about this with the teacher, although I'm sure I didn't put my argument very well. After a while the teacher said, "OK, Hinton, where do you think all good things come from?"

So I thought for a bit and said, "Russia."

ER: And what was her reaction?

GH: She looked a bit bemused; I think she probably wondered how such a kid had got into her school.

ER: Was this a school where you lived there?

GH: Most of the kids lived there, but it was in the same town as I was in, so I lived at home.

ER: So your father was able to exert influence ...

GH: There were some options when you were older. You could do biology, physics and chemistry, or you could do mathematics, physics and chemistry. I wanted to study biology. My father wouldn't let me do biology; he said they'd teach me about genetics, and it was all nonsense, so he wouldn't let me do it for ideological reasons. Anyway, it was much more important to do mathematics, he said, even if I wanted to be a biologist. He was keen I should do more mathematics. It's probably just as well that I did the mathematics. He could never do mathematics at all, so he was very concerned that I should learn to do it.

ER: Did you have hobbies as a child, things that particularly piqued your fancy?

GH: I was very interested in insects. That's what my father studied. I also liked carpentry, and I liked mathematics too.

ER: Are your memories of public school happy ones?

GH: No.

ER: Not at all?

GH: I felt like an outsider there.

ER: For the whole eleven years?

GH: Yes. I was definitely an outsider, which I think set me up for being a sort of revolutionary later. My first reaction when someone tells me something is to try to show that they are wrong.

ER: And when you went to University, was that directly following public school?

GH: Pretty much. I took a year off in between. I actually went to University straight after school for a month, and I dropped out.

ER: Where did you go to University?

GH: To Cambridge, to Kings College.

ER: What did you do on your year off? Were you free from parental constraints?

GH: Yes, I worked in London doing various odd jobs, trying to find myself.

ER: I laugh because that's what my mother said, "Well, one day you'll find yourself."

GH: I didn't succeed.

ER: Did you feel like an outsider in college?

GH: No, much less so there because I went to Cambridge, where everybody was weird.

I started off studying physics and physiology. I planned to end up being a biophysicist. This was the second time around; I'd gone back after a year. I decided I'd never be much of a physicist because the equations were too difficult. When I saw several integral signs next to each other, I felt they were ganging up on me. I was also still interested in finding the meaning of life, so I switched to philosophy. I was actually naive, switching to philosophy in order to discover the meaning of life, but I then did philosophy for a year. I didn't like philosophy because you couldn't tell whether you were right or not. Very unsatisfactory not being able to tell if you were right.

I got more intrigued by the mind. I had a friend from school. He was a very interesting character. He read a lot and was a very clever mathematician—got me interested in neural networks about the time we went to University. I can't remember whether it was before or after.

ER: And was he at Kings College with you?

GH: He was at Trinity. He'd been at the same school as me. I'd known him since I was seven, and he also went to University at the same time as me. He's called Inman Harvey.

GH: And are you still in contact with him?

GH: Yes, I am.

ER: Is he still involved with neural networks, with things related to it?

GH: Well, it's very interesting. He dropped out completely for about twenty years. He became a businessman and imported things from Afghanistan. He was one of the main importers of things to Britain from Afghanistan. And then, I guess in 1986, I sent him a copy of the Rumelhart and McClelland books on parallel distributed processing. His reaction was if that was as far as we'd got, then maybe he should go back into the field. He was unimpressed by them, so he became a graduate student again. Now he works at Sussex University, but he works on evolutionary computation there.

After a year of philosophy, I switched again in my third year—did psychology. I was extremely discontented with psychology. I guess what I was discontented about was they didn't seem to have any good models of anything. I expected them to have models of how the mind worked, but they didn't. Instead of thinking how the mind worked, they did things like study rats in mazes. The closest they had to a decent model were things like signal-detection theory.

I organized the other students to protest about the content of the course. Rats in mazes, signal-detection theory—it wasn't really about the mind at all. I got the other students to join me because the whole psychology course didn't have any mention of psychoanalysis. In the end, the chairman of the department agreed that he would put some psychoanalysis into the course, so then the undergraduate psychology course at Cambridge had one lecture on psychoanalysis in it, and the lecture was entitled, "Freud, Jung, and Adler." They figured they could cover it all in one lecture.

Of course, the stuff I do now, the psychology that it's closest to is like the stuff that goes on in signal-detection theory. It turns out that's the bits of psychology most relevant to what I'm doing right now.

ER: Did you stay with psychology?

GH: No, after that I became a carpenter.

ER: Where were you?

GH: I was in London. I had a lot to learn about carpentry. I met a really good carpenter. He was making a door for a very damp cellar. And what amazed me was that he was figuring out where each piece of wood in the door should go so that when they all warped, all the warps would cancel out because the wood was bound to warp because it was in a damp location. He figured out exactly how everything was going to warp and then put it the right way around so that the warps would all cancel out. I was completely amazed at that level of planning.

After I'd been a carpenter for a year, I got a job as a research assistant on a project in Bristol. It was just before Watergate. The idea was to see what people actually said to small children because linguists like Chomsky had made the assertion that you couldn't possibly learn English grammar from what was said to you because what was said to you was impoverished and incorrect.

So we got some people to agree to be part of the project. Their children wore a little jacket with a radio microphone in it so that everything that the children said or that was said to the children was broadcast.

In the home, we had a recorder and every twenty minutes it would take a two-minute sample of what was said to the children. Unfortunately, the frequency we used could be picked up right at the top of the VHF radio, so basically anybody in the neighborhood could listen to what was going on in the house. We discovered this after a while. We used to go and sit outside the houses just so we could make sure it would all work, see what was going on inside the house. At that time, bugging wasn't seen as a terribly, big crime. It was after Watergate that people thought that bugging was a no-no. So we got a sort of unbiased corpus of what got said to little children, because pretty soon the adults forgot about the fact that it was all being recorded.

All the mothers were meant to be native English speakers, but one of them wasn't. We were looking at tags—things like, "Isn't he?"—because they have a lot of syntax packed into just a few phonemes. One of the children received the following utterance from his mother, "Santa don't give you no toys if you don't talk proper, isn't he?"

One of the other things I had to do on that project was develop a questionnaire to assess the mother's attitude towards their child's language development. I didn't know anything about questionnaires, so question one on my questionnaire was, "What's your attitude towards your child's use of language?"

So I made up this questionnaire, and then I cycled out to a suburb of Bristol and tried out the questionnaire on social class five parents. In Britain, all jobs are divided into different social classes, with an official list of the social classes of different jobs, and the lowest social class is social class five. We wanted to have balanced social classes in our set of families, so I went out to try my questionnaire on a social class five mother. She let me in and made me a cup of tea, and then I said, "OK, now the first question is, 'What's your attitude towards your child's use of language?'"

And the mother said, "Oh, if he uses language, we hit him."

ER: Did you go on from there?

GH: No, that's when I realized I needed to redesign the questionnaire.

GH: When I wanted to do a Ph.D., there was a well-known British psychologist called Broadbent. I knew someone who was a friend of Broadbent's, so through my friend I asked Broadbent where a good place would be to do a Ph.D. on neural networks. Broadbent said that I should either go to Sussex, or I should go to Edinburgh and work with [Christopher] Longuet-Higgins.

ER: What happened when you went to Edinburgh?

GH: Longuet-Higgins was a very good mathematician. He'd done some very interesting work on a simple kind of neural network. A former student of his who was then a postdoc there was David Willshaw, so it was a very good group in Edinburgh. The problem was that by the time I arrived, Longuet-Higgins didn't really believe in neural networks anymore. He believed much more in conventional artificial intelligence [AI], partly because of Winograd's thesis, which had just come out. Winograd had done a very impressive job of natural language understanding, so at that point that's what Longuet-Higgins was really interested in.

I kept working on neural nets anyway. I guess most of what I did was fairly intuitive stuff without a very good mathematical foundation. Because

Longuet-Higgins no longer thought that was a sensible area to be working in, and because what I was doing didn't have a very good mathematical foundation, he was pretty skeptical about it.

ER: Do you remember what problem you were working on?

GH: I wanted to have something that learned to understand natural language.

ER: And he wanted you to put more AI-related material into it?

GH: Yes, he believed in a more, what would now be called classical AI approach. Rather than having learning consist of adjusting weights in a neural network, it would consist of building new symbolic expressions and building on previous symbolic expressions.

ER: So did he change the nature of what you were doing?

GH: Not really, no.

ER: And did you get a good degree from Edinburgh?

GH: I got a degree from Edinburgh in the end, yes. Actually, what was interesting about him was that a lot of the stuff I was doing, he didn't really believe in, but he did feel that I had the right to work on what interested me. So he supported me, even though he didn't believe in what I was doing. That's a very British kind of a system. He was very good about supporting me, and a lot of his criticisms about putting it on a proper mathematical foundation were very useful.

In my second year at graduate school, there were two main issues I was interested in. One was how you do unsupervised learning in neural nets. I became convinced that most of the interesting learning that went on had to be unsupervised. I knew about the perceptron convergence rule. I sort of understood the linear version of that, the Widrow-Hoff rule. I had just started thinking about how you could get something to learn interesting categories with no supervisory signal.

I remember the concept I worried about was a cat. Why was it worth having the concept of a cat? I hit on something that had been discovered many times before and many times since—which is, the reason it's worth having the concept of a cat is that the properties of cats are highly correlated. The chance of coming across something that's furry and has whiskers and goes "meow" is much higher than the product of the chance of coming across something that's furry and the chance of coming across something that says "meow" and so on.

I decided that the criterion for unsupervised learning ought to be to find categories where the joint probability is much higher than the product of the separate probabilities of the properties. Then I started thinking about what particular function to use to measure that difference. Should you just measure the difference between the joint probability and the separate probabilities? Should you measure the ratio? What should you measure?

I had the idea that you have to have some measure and then try to optimize it—that is, change the weights of a network to optimize it. I ended up with an information theory measure that seemed like the right thing. At that same time, I read one of the early information theory books. It might have been by Shannon and Weaver, or it might have been just by Weaver. It was a short little book, and it had the information-gain measure. I realized that was a good measure to use.

I cooked up a learning algorithm. The idea was to make a statistician look as stupid as possible, an idea based on the assumption the statistician would use the naive idea of computing the joint probability by multiplying together the independent probabilities. It wasn't really the statistician that was stupid; it was the independence assumption that was stupid, but it seemed easier to personify that as a statistician. You could compute the probability using the independence assumption, or you could compute the probability using the true joint probabilities.

I used this information theory measure as a measure of how different those probabilities were, and figured out how to get to set the weights. I showed it actually did learn, in little cases. It did interesting unsupervised learning for a single neuron. If you gave it a number of input lines, and you took a subset of them and made them be correlated, it would pick out that subset of the input weights. It would tune itself to those. It was a nonlinear neuron, so it was doing something a bit more interesting than just finding the first principal component.

There were problems with that algorithm. One was I never could see how to make different units do different things. I could cook up heuristics to try and make them be decorrelated from each other, which is the standard way to go about things, but that wasn't really very satisfactory. I wanted some overall objective function that would make them do different things—just like the hidden units in a backpropagation net end up doing different things because that's the way to satisfy the overall objective function.

I never could see how to do it for that kind of unsupervised learning. In fact, I didn't see how to do it properly until last year. Now I know how to do it.

There were other problems with that algorithm. One of the examples I tried it on was an attempt to detect oriented lines. I had a window with some piece of image in it, a synthetic image. I put an oriented edge in there. I wanted it to produce an oriented edge detector. Even though I didn't know how to get different units to be differently oriented, I wanted to produce at least one orientation detector, so what I did was put in bars, oriented bars. This was a problem I'd learned about from Christof von der Malsberg, who visited Edinburgh in, I guess, 1973. I wanted my little unsupervised learning algorithm to pick out these edge detectors.

One of the things I was interested in was that Christof von der Malsberg had a way of modifiying the synapses, which was basically competitive learning. He didn't have an overall objective function for it; he just viewed it in

Geoffrey E. Hinton

terms of an algorithm for changing synapse strengths so the right thing would happen. I was convinced that you had to write down an objective function and differentiate and get the algorithm. Now I had an objective function, and I wanted to show that it would work on his example.

The problem was that whenever I turned it loose on oriented bars, what it would do is produce on-center off-surround fields or off-center on-surround fields. It would produce circularly symmetric fields because I would be showing it bars of many different orientations. Actually, that's the most sensible thing for it to produce. That is what maximizes the information measure I was using. That is the same thing a principal components analysis would do.

That was one of the reasons I didn't pursue the algorithm further. It didn't do what I wanted it to do; it did the right thing instead, so I didn't go back to it until many years later. I never published it.

The other thing I got interested in in my second year at graduate school was why receptive fields are so large in the visual cortex as you go higher up. The standard view is that by being large, they give you translation invariance. I got interested in the idea that by being large, they actually do just the opposite. It's not in order to get translation invariance; it's in order to get more accuracy about where things are. As you go higher up in the visual system, you represent more and more complex entities, but there are fewer and fewer of them present at once. It's getting more and more sparse in terms of how many entities there are at a time. For these complex entities, it pays to have very big, overlapping receptive fields. Then you get much better accuracy about where they are. I was enchanted by the idea that the obvious explanation of big receptive fields was exactly the opposite of the truth. Rather than the big receptive fields causing you to be vague about where things were, they were actually allowing you to be more precise about where things were.

JA: That was the genesis of the ideas about coarse coding?

GH: That was my coarse-coding work, and the mathematics of coarse coding I worked out then. I remember I gave a talk about it to the group, and I'm not sure if they understood a lot about it. Christopher understood what I was all about. I remember, he liked the fact that I finally had produced a paper that had some equations in it. But again, I never published that stuff.

After that I got interested in relaxation approaches for vision. I stopped working on learning and representation, and worked on how to use a parallel network to settle on the interpretation of a visual scene. It was really a search algorithm. In many ways it was lucky I did that because that research came from work in computer vision on things like parallel constraint-satisfaction algorithms. I realized you could do parallel constraint satisfaction in a neural net and developed a version of it that essentially solved integer-programming problems. You're searching for an assignment of ones and zeros to many different hypotheses. Each little part of the scene could be interpreted in a number of different ways. You want to pick the interpretations for each part of the scene so that all those interpretations hang together as some coherent entity. My thesis was on doing constraint satisfaction in a parallel network.

At more or less the same time and independently, Rosenfeld, Hummel, and Zucker developed a relaxation algorithm [1976. "Scene Labeling by Relaxation Algorithms." *IEEE SMC Journal* 6:420–422.]. It wasn't as good, in my opinion. Relaxation in things like neural networks became quite a hot topic at that point. I was interested in how you do constraint satisfaction in neural networks. Later on, I could see the relation between the work that Hopfield had done and this.

After I'd done my thesis, I applied for a job in California, a postdoc job working with Don Norman. I got a very polite letter saying that I hadn't got the job. I'd been offered a job by Azriel Rosenfeld at the University of Maryland, working on relaxation. I didn't really want to go to Maryland. I didn't like the place.

ER: Had you visited?

GH: I'd visited. I'd given a talk there. It was very odd. It was the first talk I'd ever been paid for. I was impressed. They paid me $100 for a talk. I thought that was the big time. I gave a talk about my thesis. I ended up the talk by explaining why my method of doing relaxation was so much better than their method of doing relaxation, and all the things that were wrong with their method. This was to Rosenfeld's research group.

At the end of the talk, I expected there to be a big argument, and nobody asked any questions. Nobody said anything.

Then Rosenfeld said, "I'd like to see you in my office in half an hour." He said it like a school headmaster would say it.

I thought, "Oh my God, he's going tell me I shouldn't be so offensive, and I shouldn't come there and criticize their work."

I talked to a graduate student for half an hour or so and then went to Rosenfeld's office. I walked into his office, and he handed me a contract, and he said, "Sign that." It was a postdoc contract. I didn't really want to go there, so I asked him how long I had to decide. He said I had about a month to decide.

I'd already been turned down by California, so I looked around for other jobs and didn't find any other jobs. It was hard to get jobs in Britain. At the last possible minute, I called him up and said, "OK, I'd like to accept the job."

Then an hour later, I got a call from Oxford, from George Mandler, who was visiting England. Norman and Rumelhart hadn't been able to get in touch with me because of the time difference. Someone had turned down one of their postdoc jobs, and they now wanted me.

I got this offer in California about an hour after I accepted Rosenfeld's job, so I called him right back. I was calling him about two or three hours after I'd accepted the job—to unaccept it. He was absolutely outraged. He said I couldn't do that. I'd accepted the job, and that was that. So I said, "Well, I'm not coming." He's never spoken to me since. I think he's still cross with me. He was furious.

I'm very glad I went to California. California was wonderful. It was completely different from England in that they were very open to ideas. They were far less critical than in England. It was much more of a pluralist society in the sense that people in the States accepted that there simultaneously could be multiple schools of thought about something. You know, if MIT thought about it one way, then Berkeley would think about it some other way. England wasn't quite like that. England was a much smaller, more closed community, where there was a substantive view and there was nonsense. So I felt coming to California was very liberating.

I guess Don Norman—at that point, more Don than Dave [Rumelhart]—was very interested in neural nets. He didn't actually do them himself, but he knew about them. I can't remember the chronology exactly, but I think Jim came out a little after I'd got there, right? I was there for a bit, and then you came out.

JA: About a year after, something like that.

GH: That was a really nice time because I got back into things like learning and representation in neural nets. There was no longer the atmosphere where this research was some sort of naughty activity that I shouldn't really be doing, where it was obviously hopeless and they were only letting me do it because they were willing to suffer people doing silly things. This was an environment in which people thought these subjects were interesting.

Don, in particular, was interested in how you do complex associations in neural nets and how you represent relational structures in a neural network. I did some work on that and more work on coarse coding.

I got to know Jim. I can't remember whether David Willshaw was still in Edinburgh, but he wasn't really working on neural nets anymore. He was getting into the biology. California was very liberating. I had a good couple of years there.

JA: That was 1979, when the conference was held that led to the book *Parallel Models of Associative Memory.*

GH: Oh, I have a good story. Jim and I organized this conference. We started off by rounding up the usual suspects. Then we decided it would be a good idea to try to find some new blood, so we advertised. We sent flyers 'round to a whole bunch of computer science and psychology departments about this conference we were going to have in San Diego and how we were going to pay all the expenses. We got quite a few applications, and one of these applications—I couldn't decide if the guy was a total flake or not. He was a guy who was at Harvard Medical School. He had been a physicist. He had publications in physics. Applicants had to write a little spiel about what they were interested in and why they should come to this conference. He wrote a spiel about the machine code of the brain and how it was stochastic, and so the brain had this stochastic machine code.

It looked like rubbish to me, but the guy obviously had some decent publications and was in a serious place, so I didn't know what to make of him. At that time there was a conference in Austin, Texas. It was also organized by the Sloan Foundation. This was all Sloan Foundation money. I went to this conference in Austin. David Marr was there, who I'd met once before in England. I thought, you know, maybe David Marr knew this guy, so I asked him if he'd ever heard of this guy. He had some kind of unpronounceable name. David Marr said, "Oh yes, I've met him."

I said, "So what did you think of him?"

David Marr said, "Well, he was a bit weird, but he was definitely smart."

So I thought, OK, so we'll invite him. That guy was Terry Sejnowski, of course.

I remember when the people arrived for that conference. Terry arrived, and Stu Geman arrived. I remember them in the little suite of offices that the postdocs shared—Terry and Stu, writing down lots of equations about correlations. I remember thinking, "Gee, those are impressive equations; this must be real science."

ER: So did this conference represent some sort of turning point?

GH: I'm not sure. It did for me personally. I got to know a lot more people. I met Stu, and I met Terry and Scott Fahlman and Kohonen. It wasn't like there was any sort of big insight at the conference. I guess I wouldn't say it represented a big turning point, but I guess the book was one of the first books to come out about neural networks for a long time. It was the beginning of the end of the drought.

ER: That was a turning point.

GH: In that sense, it was a bit of a turning point, but the conference itself didn't seem so much like that.

ER: So there was no sense when you were doing it that this was the first time that all these people were coming together?

JA: Actually, both Dave Rumelhart and Terry said that from their point of view, just getting all these people interested and in the same room was a real legitimizing breakthrough.

GH: I guess. One important thing was that Jerry Feldman came. He was an AI figure, and so was Scott Fahlman. Having AI people talk to people like Terry and Stu Geman was important.

JA: I remember one of the high points of that conference was Jerry Feldman standing up in front of the group and computing how many cells you'd need to have enough grandmother cells to do vision. The numbers became astronomical extremely quickly. He realized he might have to rethink the problem.

ER: Was the conference the culmination of your work at San Diego?

GH: No. I went back to San Diego for six months a couple of years later. That's when we started on the PDP [parallel distributed processing] books. After San Diego, I went back to England. Jerry Feldman organized meetings more or less every year after that. Those were pretty important in keeping people going. They were very small meetings. It would be Terry and me and Feldman and Fahlman and Dana Ballard and maybe half a dozen other people. After a couple of years, Hopfield came to one of these meetings, so that would probably be '82, summer of '82.

He gave a talk about energy functions. I suddenly realized that they solved the problem that David Willshaw had been thinking about years earlier, which was how you could have an iterative net and have some idea of what it would do and guarantee that it would settle down. They also solved the problem that Marr and Poggio had worked on. Marr and Poggio actually had a net that had symmetric weights in it. They were trying to understand how it would behave. They had failed to notice that there was a Lyapunov function, so they tried analyzing the net by analyzing all the sorts of little configurations of weights you could have. They just hadn't understood about this energy function.

As soon as Hopfield gave that talk, I realized that what you wanted to use these nets for was to solve constraint-satisfaction problems. You wanted to let the energy function correspond to the objective function you were minimizing. I'm not sure Hopfield had really understood that. He was using these nets for memories at that point, 1982.

At that same little meeting in Rochester in 1982, Terry was there. Terry told me about Scott Kirkpatrick's work on simulated annealing. I didn't know about it. Terry decided that simulated annealing might be a good thing to do in a Hopfield net so that you didn't get trapped in local minima. We'd both realized that would be great if you were trying to do constraint satisfaction and if you wanted to escape from local minima and get much better global interpretations.

I remember sitting through one of the talks and trying to figure out what the decision function for a neuron would have to be if you were to implement Kirkpatrick simulated annealing in a Hopfield net. It was a sort of squashing function. I remember that since I'd realized that the decision rule had to be a stochastic squashing function, I got all excited because I thought, "Well, neurons look a bit like that, so that must be what they're doing."

There was a period then for a couple of years when I was absolutely convinced that that's what the brain was up to. I'm no longer convinced of that. It seemed like such a nice theory—that the brain must be solving these constraint satisfaction problems by using this noisy settling to find a minimum in an energy function. I always joked about our local minima.

To begin with, we didn't think about learning; we were just interested in constraint satisfaction. We'd obviously understood that there was a learning issue, but the exciting thing was it could do this kind of constraint satisfaction. That was in the summer of '82.

I had a job in Cambridge [U.K.] at that point, so I went back there. I had programmed the idea up on a VAX and got it to find little paths through mazes. We wrote a paper and sent it to *Nature*, who rejected it.

It wasn't until the Christmas of '82, by which time I'd moved to Carnegie Mellon, that I really started thinking about how to learn the weights. It looked very tricky. I remember I had to give a talk, a sort of research seminar, at Carnegie Mellon in either February or March of '83, and I was really scared about it because I'd just moved there. I wanted to give a really good talk about something. I wanted to talk about this simulated annealing in Hopfield nets, but I figured I had to have a learning algorithm. I was terrified that I didn't have a learning algorithm. I was really seriously lacking a learning algorithm for these things.

Luckily, I had absolutely nothing else to do at Carnegie Mellon. They said in my first year I didn't have to do any teaching, and so I had nothing to do but sit there and worry about the fact that I didn't have a learning algorithm. I sat there and worried for months and months about the fact that I didn't have a learning algorithm. Around Christmas time, I realized you could view these things as doing Bayesian inference, so I understood the relation between what was going on in these stochastic networks and Bayesian inference. But I still didn't understand the learning algorithm.

Then by sheer good luck, as I was worrying about not having a learning algorithm for these things when they had hidden units, I remembered the stuff I'd done much earlier in Edinburgh on learning for these single units and the information-gain objective function, so—I guess basically by good luck—I wrote down the right objective function. I tried lots of objective functions, but among them I tried the right one. I wasn't very good at doing mathematics, and so I remember Terry and I were talking on the phone all the time, and I would go and visit him a lot.

I remember on one occasion calling him up and telling him, "How about trying this objective function, and see what the derivatives looked like?" Maybe the derivatives would come out nice and simple for this one because this was a good objective function to use—because this was kind of the right thing in information theory terms. I remember him calling back and saying, "No, the derivatives didn't come out right."

I thought, "Oh dear." Then I decided I'd differentiate it myself, so I sat down and did the maths, and it's like a whole page of mathematics. I got it so they came out right after a while, and I got these very simple derivatives.

I called Terry back, and he agreed that, yeah, it came out right, so we finally found the learning rule for Boltzmann machines. We'd known there was going to be a simple learning rule because we understood that the energy was linear in the weights and the log probability was linear in the energy so that the log probabilities were linear in the weights. We sort of

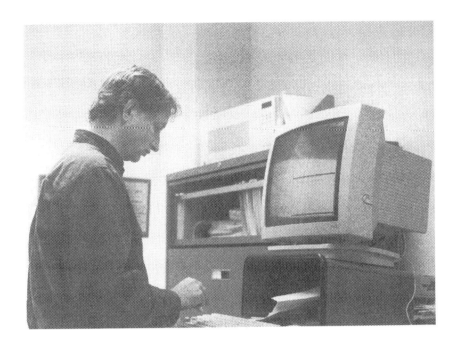

knew this meant that it was going to be easy to manipulate log probabilities by manipulating weights, so there had to be some decent way to do it, but it was quite a while before we wrote down the right objective function.

Then we got very excited because now there was this very simple local-learning rule. On paper it looked just great. I mean, you could take this great big network, and you could train up all the weights to do just the right thing, just with a simple local learning rule. It felt like we'd solved the problem. That must be how the brain works.

I guess if it hadn't been for computer simulations, I'd still believe that, but the problem was the noise. It was just a very very slow learning rule. It got swamped by the noise because in the learning rule you take the difference between two noisy variables—two sampled correlations, both of which have sampling noise. The noise in the difference is terrible.

I still think that's the nicest piece of theory I'll ever do. It worked out like a question in an exam where you put it all together and a beautiful answer pops out.

ER: Terry was at Johns Hopkins at this point?

GH: Terry was at Johns Hopkins.

ER: So you were going back and forth?

GH: We were going backwards and forwards.

ER: How did you end up at Carnegie Mellon?

GH: It was a result of that conference that Jim and I organized. I got to know Scott Fahlman there. I was interested in getting back to the States, and Fahlman was interested in the neural net stuff and basically got me a job at

Geoffrey E. Hinton

CMU. It was partly because of [Allen] Newell also. Although he was somewhat anti a lot of this stuff, he was very eclectic. He was very broadminded. He realized that sooner or later there was going to be a connection between what went on in the mind and what went on in the brain. Carnegie Mellon was a big place. Newell was in favor of having people do all sorts of things there, so he was basically in favor of having someone who worked on neural nets there. He could see it coming back into fashion. Even though it wasn't what he did, and he didn't really believe in it, he had enough insight to realize that it was going to come back into fashion again. So he was in favor of getting somebody like that, and Fahlman sort of pushed my case. That's how I ended up at CMU.

I was very impressed by the fact that Newell was open to getting somebody in an area that he didn't believe in. It's very rare to see that in academics.

JA: Did you ever convince him?

GH: No, no, I never did. At one stage we tried to write a paper together about information processing in the brain. It never got very far. He'd also been very impressed by the work on speech recognition in the '70s at CMU and the fact that the system that worked the best was the Harpy system, not the Hearsay system.

The Hearsay system was an AI system that used a working memory—the facts fitting right into working memory, and demons looking at working memory, and all that stuff. Sorry, they didn't call them "demons"; they called them "production rules." The Harpy system was a Markov model; I think you could call it that. It was a totally dumb system, in AI terms.

It was really a battle between having complicated representations, but no automatic learning rule, and having really dumb representations, like a stochastic finite-state automaton, but a proper learning rule. It turned out in the competition that having a proper learning rule, a way of estimating the parameters, just overwhelmed having better representations. Having good representations and no way to decide what they are isn't as effective as lousy representations and a good way to decide what they are.

Newell understood that when he wrote a paper about this battle and about how people in AI should take note of it. It must mean something. I think it was partly because of this puzzle that he was interested in getting a neural network presence. Indeed, he'd gotten the message then in a way that other people in AI still haven't.

ER: How long did you stay at CMU?

GH: I was there for five years. It was by far the most productive period in my life. I did very little there except work. It wasn't a particularly happy five years, but I got an awful lot of work done.

ER: That was the five years that neural nets were bursting onto the scene, so there was a lot more acceptance in the air.

GH: Much more, yes. There's one other curious piece of history that I left out. I went back to San Diego, in '82 I guess. I was back there in the first half of '82. Paul Smolensky was a postdoc there then. I talked a lot with him. Dave Rumelhart came up with this idea of backpropagation. He wasn't the first to come up with it, but ...

I first of all explained to him why it wouldn't work, based on an argument in Rosenblatt's book, which showed that essentially it was an algorithm that couldn't break symmetry. If you had a deterministic learning rule, and you started off with two identical hidden units, they would stay identical, so the deterministic learning rule was no good.

Now, as you know, the standard way of doing learning is to have random initial weights, or you could just put a little bit of noise in the learning rule —either would be fine. So Dave Rumelhart pointed out that we didn't need to worry about symmetry.

The next argument I gave him was that it would get stuck in local minima. There was no guarantee you'd find a global optimum. Since you're bound to get stuck in local minima, it wasn't really worth investigating.

Nevertheless, Dave programmed it up and did a few things with it. I think he showed it could learn X-OR [exclusive OR]. Paul Smolensky and I programmed it up. Then I tried to use it to get a very obscure effect. I couldn't get this very obscure effect with it, so I lost interest in backpropagation. I managed to get this very obscure effect later with a Boltzmann machine. I'd realized that if you've got a net to learn something, and then you add noise to the weights by making it learn something else, it should be much faster at relearning what it had previously learned. You should get very fast relearning of stuff that it previously knew, as compared to the initial learning.

We programmed a backpropagation net, and we tried to get this fast relearning. It didn't give fast relearning, so I made one of these crazy inferences that people make—which was, that backpropagation is not very interesting. This was a completely crazy reason for losing interest in it. but I was also discontented with it because of the problem about finding only local minima. I hadn't really accepted at that point that this was the best you ever were going to be able to do.

Later on, when I knew about Boltzmann machines, Terry and I initially looked for a learning algorithm to find the global minima. After a while I realized that wasn't really feasible; I thought, "Well, you know, like backpropagation maybe we'll just find a local minimum."

That's what the learning algorithm did. The weights basically just found a local optimum. When Boltzmann machines turned out not to be very good in practice because they were so slow, I kept on at them for quite a while. After we first got them working, I spent over a year trying to get them to work properly, cooking up all sorts of little tricks—like weight decay because by keeping the weights small, you could make sure you didn't get big energy barriers. We tried lots of other tricks, but we never got them to work very well.

I remember at one point discovering that if you get a Boltzmann machine and you train it, it would do quite well at modeling some function. But if you keep on training it, it will get worse and worse. We called this "going sour." The networks would go sour. We just couldn't understand why they went sour. I would print out reams and reams of paper showing the performance of the network and showing what the weights were, and I remember having a stack of paper about three inches thick because I couldn't believe these networks would go sour. I couldn't believe that as you learn more and more, you would get worse and worse.

It took me weeks and weeks to realize that what was going on was the learning algorithm was based on the assumption that you could reach thermal equilibrium. As the weights got bigger, the annealing was failing to reach thermal equilibrium; it was getting trapped in the local minima. So the learning algorithm was then doing the wrong thing. That's why we had to introduce weight decay—to stop that happening.

Anyway, after over a year of fiddling around with such things to try to make them work properly, I finally decided they really weren't going to work. In despair, I thought, "Well, maybe, why don't I just program up that old idea of Rumelhart's, and see how well that works on some of the problems we've been trying?"

So I gave a little presentation to my research group about Rumelhart's idea. They'd all been thoroughly indoctrinated by then into Boltzmann machines. There were about ten students there. I explained this back-propagation idea of Rumelhart's and said, "You know, would anybody just like to program it up? It would only take a day or so to program it, just so we could see how well it worked and compare it with Boltzmann machines."

I remember at the end of the meeting nobody was prepared to program it. They all said, "You know, why would you want to program that?" We had all the arguments: "It's assuming that neurons can send real numbers to each other; of course they can only send bits to each other; you have to have stochastic binary neurons; these real-valued neurons are totally unrealistic. It's ridiculous."

So they just refused to work on it, not even to write a program, so I had to do it myself. I went off and I spent a weekend. I wrote a LISP program to do it. I almost blew it because the first thing I tried it on was a 8-3-8 encoder; that is, you have eight input units and three hidden units and eight output units. You want to turn on one of the input units and get the same output unit to be on.

In a Boltzmann machine, since the units are binary, the states of the three hidden units have to be the eight different binary codes, so you know what the hidden units will look like when they've solved the problem. So I ran backpropagation on this problem and looked at the weights of the hidden units. They didn't have the right structure of weights. I decided it wasn't really working; it wasn't solving the problem. I never bothered to look at the error measure, which had gone to zero. I just looked at the weights because I knew what the solution should look like. It didn't look like that.

I thought, "Oh well, it turns out backpropagation's not that good after all." Then I looked at the error, and the error was zero. I was amazed. Of course, with real-valued hidden units it's much easier to solve the problem. There are many different ways of solving it. Then I tried it on a bunch of other things, and it worked amazingly well on all of the things we tried. It worked much better than Boltzmann machines.

So I sent mail to Dave Rumelhart saying, "You remember that algorithm of yours? It seems to actually work." I don't know if Dave was already experimenting with it again then, but over the next few months we tried it on lots of things. Dave was trying it on things in San Diego, and I was trying it on things in Pittsburgh. That was at the stage when we were just completing the PDP books, so we'd already agreed on what was going to be in the books. The final chapters were being edited. We decided we'd just slip in an extra chapter on backpropagation, so it was a late addition to the book. But I was always a bit disappointed. I mean, intellectually, backpropagation wasn't nearly as satisfying as Boltzmann machines. It's not just because I didn't think of it. I think it's because it didn't have the nice probabilistic interpretation.

ER: I don't know if anybody will ever figure out who really thought of it first. We have Amari, we have Werbos ...

GH: I think there's about a half dozen different people who thought of it—different versions of it—and I wasn't one of them.

ER: What made you leave CMU?

GH: It was a mixture of things. It was Reagan's America back then. I didn't like the politics. I managed to survive for a long time at CMU without taking any military funding, but toward the end of my time there I ran out of money, and I had to take ONR [Office of Naval Research] money and I didn't like that. So it was sort of a political reason—I guess not liking the way American society was organized and not liking having to take military money to do research.

I might have been able to put up with that, but I also got married then, at the end of my time at CMU. My wife didn't like all those things even more. She really didn't want to live in the States, so we looked around for somewhere we would both be happy to live. We decided we'd both be happy to live in Vancouver, so that's why we're in Toronto.

I had a friend in Vancouver. I got in touch with him to see if there were any jobs going in Vancouver, and I learned about the Canadian Institute for Advanced Research, which was providing money to buy people off their teaching. Then I learned that Toronto actually had a better department than Vancouver, and my wife wanted to come to Toronto when we learned more about Toronto. Someone I'd known in San Diego, George Mandler, got in touch with people in psychology at Toronto for me. I ended up getting a job that was mainly in computer science, but partly in psychology. With this funding from the Canadian Institute for Advanced Research I didn't have to do much teaching.

ER: When did you come to Toronto?

GH: '87. I went to Carnegie Mellon in '82, and I left in '87. And, yes, when I was still at CMU, I got interested in trying to show that backpropagation could do some difficult problems, as opposed to just things like X-OR. I realized that phoneme recognition was an important problem that people had tried lots of things on, including hidden Markov models.

One very lucky thing happened to me at CMU. Early on when I was there, I had a graduate student called Peter Brown, who knew a lot about speech recognition and knew all about hidden Markov models. He told me about hidden Markov models while I was doing Boltzmann machines. I wish I'd understood more about them then because I only very, very slowly really understood them.

The reason hidden units in neural nets are called hidden units is that Peter Brown told me about hidden Markov models. I decided "hidden" was a good name for those extra units, so that's where the name "hidden" comes from. By the end of the time I was at CMU, and he'd gone back to IBM, he had some data that he'd used for his thesis on phoneme recognition, where he used very fancy hidden Markov models.

I decided to see if we couldn't beat his performance by using back-propagation, so Kevin Lang and I developed a variety of backpropagation called "time-delay neural networks" for doing phoneme recognition. That worked pretty nicely. It was one of the earlier examples of backpropagation doing well at a tough task that people had tried other good methods on. It wasn't as spectacular as something like Terry Sejnowski's NETtalk. On the other hand, that's not a very tough task.

JA: Was that was your first try at a practical application?

GH: The first practical application I did was that phoneme-recognition study with Kevin Lang. I've done more since then but not that many. I'm not really that interested. I'm much more interested in how the brain does it. I'm only interested in applications just to prove that this is interesting stuff to keep the funding flowing. To do an application really well, you have to put your whole heart into it; you need to spend a year immersing yourself in what the application's all about. I guess I've never really been prepared to do that.

When I got to Toronto, I got more interested in relating what was going on in neural networks to statistics. Also, when I was doing backpropagation, I was still convinced that unsupervised learning was what the brain really did, particularly for perception. Very early on, as soon as I got backpropagation working, I realized—because of what we'd been doing with Boltzmann machines—that you could use autoencoders to do unsupervised learning.

You just get the output layer to reproduce the input layer, and then you don't need a separate teaching signal. Then the hidden units are representing some code for the input.

In late 1985, I actually had a deal with Dave Rumelhart that I would write a short paper about backpropagation, which was his idea, and he would write a short paper about autoencoders, which was my idea. It was always better to have someone who didn't come up with the idea write the paper because he could say more clearly what was important.

So I wrote the short paper about backpropagation, which was the *Nature* paper that came out in 1986, but Dave still hasn't written the short paper about autoencoders. I'm still waiting.

What he did do was tell Dave Zipser about the idea of autoencoders and doing unsupervised learning. Dave Zipser told Gary Cottrell, and they produced a paper on autoencoders. I never did write that paper about autoencoders. Luckily, I thought more about it. A few years ago, I realized that you should think about it in information theory terms. With Rich Zemel I developed a way of doing unsupervised learning based on autoencoders.

In an autoencoder, the hidden layer in the middle is meant to learn codes for the input. There's a way of thinking about it all in communication theory terms. It initially seems very bizarre. You have a sender and a receiver, and they both get to see the input vector. The sender has to tell the receiver what the input vectors are. One way the sender could do it is by just sending the raw input back to the receiver. That would take lots of bits. You would need a very big bandwidth channel to do that. Another way it could be done is the sender could decide on some way of encoding the inputs, which is what the hidden layer's going to do anyway. Then, the sender could tell the receiver what the code is for each input vector and also tell the receiver, "When you try and reconstruct the input vector from that code, here are the errors you'll get."

These are going to be codes, not quite perfect codes, but slightly incorrect codes for things, in the sense that when you reconstruct from these codes, you get an error, so what the autoencoder net is trying to do is make those reconstruction errors small. By trying to make the reconstruction error small, what you're really doing is minimizing the amount of information that has to be sent to explain to the receiver what the reconstruction errors are, because small things are cheaper to send.

As soon as you view it in those terms, you realize there's something missing in a standard autoencoder: to send the input to the receiver, you have to send both the code and the reconstruction error. The standard learning algorithm is just minimizing the cost of sending the reconstruction error, but it also ought to be minimizing the cost of sending the code.

So, in a standard learning algorithm, in the standard autoencoder, you assume that it's free to send the activities of the hidden units to the receiver. You can think about it as, "Take the input vector, turn it into activities in the hidden units, and send those activities to the receiver." The receiver uses those activities to reconstruct the best bet it can for the input vector, and then you additionally have to send the errors to fix up that best bet.

The standard algorithm just minimizes the additional information you have to send to fix up the best bet, but it doesn't minimize the amount of information you have to send to communicate the activities of the hidden units. You can keep that small by having only a few hidden units. You can think of principal components in statistics as a good autoencoder with only a few hidden units. Not much information is required because there's only a few of them.

It's still a bit worrying because you have to send real numbers. Even though there's only a few of them, there might be quite a bit of information on them. What you really ought to be doing is simultaneously minimizing the reconstruction error and the number of bits it would take to communicate the activities of the hidden units. That's much easier to do if you view the hidden units as stochastic binary units, like in the Boltzmann machine, than if you view them as real-valued units, like in normal backpropagation. So Rich Zemel and I developed a system where you have hidden units that are stochastic binary units, and you train up the whole system so as to minimize the amount of information that would have to be communicated to tell a receiver about the input vector by first telling the receiver about the activities of the hidden units and then about the reconstruction error. You're simultaneously minimizing the information in the activity of the hidden units and the information in the reconstruction error.

We showed that that does some nice things. It's a more powerful kind of learning than principal components—or somewhat more powerful, anyway. Subsequently, with Peter Dayan, we generalized that to multilayer systems, with multiple layers of hidden units. That's what we now call a Helmholtz machine. [See P. Dayan, G. E. Hinton, R. M. Neal, and R. S. Zemel. 1995. "The Helmholtz Machine." *Neural Computation* 7:889–904.]

The nice thing is that for the multilayer system, there's a very very simple learning rule that minimizes the information. It's very like Boltzmann machines in that there's a very simple local-learning rule that allows you to learn these multiple layers of representation. The one big difference from Boltzmann machines is that this system seems to work quite well. It works reasonably quickly.

JA: You aren't estimating probabilities?

GH: No, you are estimating probabilities. The underlying theory of it is much more complicated than Boltzmann machines, but the learning rule is very simple. The underlying theory differs from Boltzmann machines in that you're not assuming that you reach thermal equilibrium. If you reach thermal equilibrium, you get one kind of mathematics. If you don't go all the way to thermal equilibrium, but just approximate it, you get a bound rather than an equality. You can work with these bounds instead of equalities, and by working with bounds you get an algorithm that's far more efficient than if you have to settle to an equilibrium so that you get the equality.

One way of summarizing it is that in a Boltzmann machine the mathematics is simple because you assume the network has settled to thermal equilibrium, and now you have an equality. In Helmholtz machines, the mathematics is messy, but the system works much faster because you don't assume that it has to settle to thermal equilibrium.

ER: And you call them Helmholtz machines because …

GH: Because as a physical system settles to thermal equilibrium, it's minimizing a quantity called Helmholtz free energy. At thermal equilibrium, that quantity is minimized. In these new systems, the Helmholtz free energy doesn't settle all the way down to the minimum value. It turns out that the Helmholtz free energy of a physical system is exactly the same as the number of bits that are needed to communicate the input vector by first communicating the code and then communicating the reconstruction error.

There's a precise mathematical equivalence between physical systems that haven't quite reached equilibrium and methods of coding images by sending hidden vectors and then reconstructing things from the hidden vectors. That's one reason they're called Helmholtz machines; for the physical system, the underlying quantity is the Helmholtz free energy.

The other reason they're called Helmholtz machines is that these systems have a generative model of data. That is, from the hidden vector you communicate, you must be able to regenerate the data. Helmholtz believed in generative models. Helmholtz's investigations into perception led him to believe in generative models that allow you to extract the most likely causes of the data. It turns out that one technical way to get an algorithm that does all that is by using the Helmholtz free energy, which he invented in physics.

I want to go and dig him up and explain this to him.

JA: He would have loved it.

GH: Well, he might have seen flaws in it. He was very smart, but I think he would have found it at least intriguing that you could use Helmholtz free energy this way in perception.

ER: I was wondering if you would be interested in making some comments on the state of neural networks today.

GH: I think one very satisfying thing that's happened in the last five years is that people developing neural network algorithms have learned a lot more about statistics. There's been a kind of unification between the computational statisticians who are investigating new algorithms and the neural network people. Those two communities now talk to each other quite a lot. I think that's very important because it's the statisticians who've traditionally investigated this idea of how you estimate things from noisy data.

There's been a lot more use of the underlying algorithm in hidden Markov models; the EM algorithm is used much more in neural nets now. There's been a lot of transfer of ideas from statistics into neural networks. I think there's also transfer the other way. I think it's a very fruitful interaction, so that's something very good that's happened.

Something I am rather disappointed about is that we still haven't got a clue what learning algorithm the brain uses, but let me say one more encouraging thing. Traditional AI always saw itself as very, very separate from neural nets. Neural nets was this weird sort of stuff that used real numbers. People doing expert systems and also thinking about knowledge represention, particularly Judea Pearl, have come up with these things called "belief nets." They're used quite widely now for expert systems because they do correct probabilistic reasoning. Early on in the development of expert systems people came up with silly ways of using things that resembled probabilities because they realized you have uncertain knowledge. They have to deal with uncertainty somehow. They were so resistant to the idea of actually allowing probabilities in that they were much happier to buy into other ways of dealing with uncertainty.

It turns out that those other ways aren't nearly as good as using probabilities. If you want to deal with uncertainties, you want to use probabilities. Now, within standard AI, belief nets are taking over. It turns out that belief nets are very like Helmholtz machines. They have a generative model of the data, a probabilistic generative model.

One of the big problems is that the researchers presently get all the parameters in their belief nets by talking to an expert. You'd really like to estimate the parameters from data, so you've got a learning problem with belief nets. You can view Helmholtz machines as one way of trying to deal with the learning problem in belief nets.

I think what it amounts to is this. A belief net is a generative model of data, so you think about the data as having been generated from some underlying process. In neural net terms, we assume the top-down connections that come from some underlying representation have produced the data. Neural nets have traditionally been recognition devices that go from the data to the underlying representations. What's happening in a Helmholtz machine is you have both top-down connections that are a generative model and bottom-up connections that are a recognition model. The nice thing about a Helmholtz machine is you can use each set of connections for training the other. The top-down connections are used to train the bottom-up connections and vice versa. You get this very simple delta learning rule.

Just as over the last five years we've seen a unification with statistics, where there are transfers of the ideas from statistics into neural nets, I think what we're going to get in the next five years is a big unification with AI, where there are transfers of ideas between the AI people doing belief nets and neural net people who are interested in learning belief nets. I predict that's going to be a big growth area.

JA: Are you looking at that area yourself?

GH: Yes, of course. A journalist sometime ago asked me, "What do you think the hottest new idea in neural nets is?"

I said, "Helmholtz machines."

And he said, "But that's what you're working on."

So I said, "Well, any researcher who says that the hottest new idea is not what he's working on has got to be stupid. If you think it's the hottest new idea, then why aren't you working on it?"

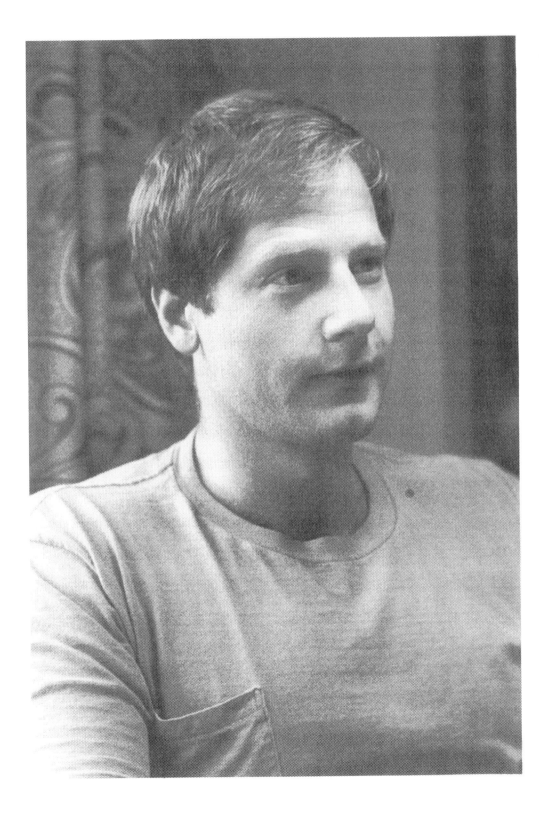

17 Bart Kosko

Bart Kosko is Professor of Electrical Engineering at the University of Southern California, Los Angeles, California. He is the author of the Hyperion nonfiction book Fuzzy Thinking, *the Avon novel* Nanotime, *and the Prentice-Hall textbook* Fuzzy Engineering.

July 1993, Portland, Oregon

ER: Why don't we begin with your date of birth and where you were born?

BK: I was born February 7, 1960, Kansas City, Kansas, in a region called Strawberry Hill, a Slavic community.

My father was Russian. He was a building contractor. My mother was Serbian. She was a housewife. I grew up in a Serbo-Croatian culture. My first musical instrument was a mandolin, an approximation of a *brac*, which is a Slavic instrument. My cousins were in the Tambouritzans, a balalaika-type orchestra but with Yugoslav instruments. I thought everybody spoke a little Serbo-Croatian or Russian. I ate that kind of food, lived that sort of lifestyle to some degree, and knew about the feud between the Croats and the Serbs.

ER: There was no academic interest in the family?

BK: No academic interest. I come from a long line of peasants. My grandparents all came over from the old country in Eastern Europe. They came over poor, and all ended up in a Slavic region. Slavs, Poles, Russians, Dalmatians, Yugoslavs, Czechs—the whole group in Strawberry Hill.

ER: So there was a rather intense family scene?

BK: The Yugoslav side of the family was very much family oriented. It was very positive. The Kosko side, the Russian side, was a little more aggressive—much more in the spirit of The Brothers Karamazov.

ER: Did you have brothers and sisters?

BK: I have one brother. He is three years older. All during high school he was the intellectual. I was always off doing other things, more in the arts and nature. I was an outdoors kid at the time and hunted and trapped and gathered wild ginseng. He got the scholarships first and then went to school. We all went through the hippie era.

ER: I'm curious what your earlier childhood was like.

BK: I grew up very early. I grew up in large part as part of a Kansas City street gang. My brother was the youngest member of it and he was three years older. I grew up very early. I had my first sexual experience with a girl when I was four. A deep dark secret. I didn't find out that my brother and his friends had had their experiences at the same time until I was twenty-five. So we were part of a group of bad boys in the street gangs in Kansas City. Some of those kids grew up to become complete hoodlums. I don't know if they're in jail or not. When I was in second grade, for whatever reasons, my father thought it was a good idea to move out into the country to a farm. That's where we lived for a fair amount of time. That was the best part of my life—out on the farm, wide open, minimal government intervention.

I've always had a problem with the government. When I was three the government took our house through eminent domain to build Freeway 635 for the Kansas City Airport. That was a shocking thing to tell a little kid: "Your house is going to be torn down and destroyed." But when I was seven or eight years old, I found myself on the farm, hunting and fishing and animals. It was bucolic. It was just wonderful. Wide open. My father was a very open-minded man.

That all ended for me when I was ten and the house burned down. A few months after that, my father died. I began living with other people then. My brother and I split up. I still stayed largely in the farm community. We had another farm after that very briefly in the same area. Through high school I stayed in the city of Lansing, Kansas, outside of Levenworth in the northeastern corner. My high school never had more than 400 people in it.

ER: Were you with your mother during this period?

BK: Sometimes with her, but often split up, living with other people.

ER: Relatives?

BK: More often friends. I had different friends during high school. I went through various phases at this point and went through the hippie phase very early, when I was young, and got deep into drugs when I was twelve. That began for me in part when I became a 12-year-old amateur herbalist under the influence of Euell Gibbons, *Stalking the Wild Asparagus.*

It was Kansas, so you would start smoking some local pot (called K-pot or Kansas ditch weed) and then try different kinds of herbs. My brother was deep into chemistry at this point. I remember we read a copy of Aldous Huxley's *Doors of Perception.* I was at the time around twelve years old.

We wanted to try mescaline and did. I had some very mind-opening experiences with LSD. I was deep into the hard rock music. Then I had a bad trip when I was fourteen. A very bad acid trip, a paranoid trip, and I got completely out of it and was turned off to the whole culture, including rock music.

For whatever reason I got deep into classical music at that time. I had some training in the mandolin and I switched that over immediately to a violin. I got book on orchestration and I began to study that. By the time I started high school I was writing my first little violin concerto. I got some supervision at the local college from a music professor there and got deep into music.

So at a farm school in Kansas I saw myself as the next Beethoven and started writing a lot of works—small works, big works. Within a year, members of the Kansas City Philharmonic had performed my first string quartet and piano trio. And so during high school I'd come home at night, and every night before I'd go to bed, I'd make sure that I wrote some music. I learned the discipline of creativity. I would not go to sleep until I had written at least a few bars of some musical project. By the time I was sixteen, I was reasonably good. By the time I was seventeen, I'd won the Young Composer's contest. Then I started getting scholarships. The best one was from USC. And out to USC I went.

ER: So music was always a kind of central organizing principle in your life?

BK: I began with music. The big intellectual event for me happened when in my senior year in high school I learned physics, and I lost my faith in God. This was a big crisis for me. Physics pushed God right out of my head and replaced it with physics. There was an alternative description of the universe. I was deep into Newtonian mechanics. I had a professor, rather an instructor, Bill Geier. Since Lansing, Kansas, is next to Fort Levenworth, many people cycled through the military school there—high-caliber instructors who taught pro bono and stepped in to teach at the local farm schools. This fellow did that for me. He came in to teach our physics class. When I stood in graduation line and I had my robe on, he walked up to me and said, "Here is your graduation gift."

It was May 1978, and it was a copy of that year's Pulitzer Prize winner by Carl Sagan, *The Dragons of Eden,* which speculates about the origins of human intelligence. This was the first book I'd ever read on the brain.

So now I'd lost God, and I was deep into physics as a substitute and got this book and read it cover to cover in a day. He handed it to me then, I think, rather than earlier because this was a Bible belt town. Many would have considered this a radical book. It made me think. It was the first time I ever understood the idea of neural networks and synapses in the brain.

And it had a mechanistic view of mind. I'd long since become a materialist in my philosophical point of view. Here at last were some speculations on how that might actually be brought about. That was my first acquaintance with neural networks. I'm happy to say that many years later, when I wrote my first textbook on neural networks, I wrote thanks to Carl Sagan, and he was nice enough to write a kind response in return and we began a friendship.

When I went away to USC under a music scholarship, I was already working on my first symphony. I had a contract to record. I got it on the basis of an orchestral overture to the *Count of Monte Christo.* When I came to USC I wanted to be the next Richard Wagner. I wanted to make films and score them and write them. I wanted to be the artistic superman of the day. I had no concept of how any of these things worked. I didn't know that USC, for example, is located in the ghetto. I thought of L.A. as filled with movie stars and all those sorts of things a farm boy in Kansas would think about Los Angeles.

So I got out to USC on a full scholarship to the top music school on the West Coast. The first thing I did was take placement exams. These were for undergraduates and I passed them. Understand, at the time I was very advanced in my musical work, had several copyrights, and was orchestrating my first symphony, so they had me take the Ph.D. exams. And I passed those.

The faculty did not know what to do with me because the music that they taught was atonal, and what I like is very tonal. It would tend to be placed more like in the late-nineteenth century in the sense of harmonic romanticism and the expanded orchestra. They were not interested in that. So we fought. The way it played out was that they got me into the graduate course in film composing, which was what I wanted to do anyway, and they let me keep the scholarship for a year, provided I got the hell out of the music program. So I did.

All of a sudden, before classes had started, this guiding principle of my life —this goal, the music—was cut out from beneath me. Now I was drifting, my hobbies had been philosophy and science. They advanced from hobbies to degrees. The four years of undergraduate school led to two degrees— one in philosophy and one in economics. Those in turn have led to the two fields I work in now, fuzzy logic and neural networks. The philosophy led to fuzzy logic and the economics led to neural networks.

ER: You said that you had read widely in philosophy and science before you got to USC. You referred earlier to Aldous Huxley and *Doors of Perception*. Was that what first made you start thinking about philosophy?

BK: I think you think about philosophy when you think about the two big ideas of "goodness" and "Godness." "Does God exist?" and "Is this right?" These were the questions of metaphysics and ethics. Is the universe just? Is that particular action just? It had nothing to do with psychedelics.

My brother came back periodically. He was at Northwestern at the time. He had just taken the latest course in philosphy or math, and we'd debate these sorts of questions. That was the age of *Zen and the Art of Motorcycle Maintenance.* We'd sit around smoking pot or eating magic mushrooms and talking about metaphysical questions. Although we lived on a farm, we had some terrific drug parties out there. Thinking back, it was one of the best parts of my life, but I saw my relationship to the government was very much like my relationship to God. It was one I questioned and one I lost faith in. Most scientists question God while they still cling to government.

Life in Kansas, now that I look back on it, was very good. I think of Kansas now and see it as wide open. A place to do my own thing in my own way, make a lot of mistakes, pursue a lot of paths. The whole drug culture was a part of that.

ER: What made you choose economics?

BK: That's an interesting question because if you're really going to be a fanatic about philosophy, you have to have a political philosophy, so the first thing a young man in philosophy encounters is Marxism. It seems the most radical. The first book I read on it was *Das Kapital*. I read that before I read the *Communist Manifesto*. Having lived on a farm and worked so much with the supply and demand processes, I wasn't impressed with the labor theory of value. I was impressed though with the revolutionary spirit, as I think most young people are. That's what brings them to Marxism—to what makes them man the barricades—not the labor theory of value.

At the same time I found that the collectivist-type arguments really weren't for me. I was looking for a social philosophy, and this is where I stumbled upon libertarianism. This idea has two goals: maximal personal and economic freedom.

Now that I look back upon it, I think that that may be where I got the idea for the fuzzy cube because there's a fuzzy square used to define your political position. It has two axes. One axis is from 0 to 100 percent for political liberties, and the other axis runs from 0 to 100 percent for economic liberties. You slice up the square into four pieces. One quadrant that says "low political freedom" and "low economic freedom" is the populist position—an Archie Bunker position, a government-control position. Another quadrant that says "high economic freedom" but "low personal freedom" is the conservative position, the Rush Limbaugh position. The other quadrant, diagonally opposite from that, says "high personal freedom" and "low economic freedom." That's the modern position, the bourgeois, the petty socialist, the modern liberal—or Bill Clinton, for example.

That leaves the last quadrant, which says "high economic and high personal freedom," and that's the libertarian position. I saw that drawing and realised that's me up there in the far corner. The real question is, "What's the optimal size of government?" I think the answer is zero—somewhere between monarchy and free-market anarchy. I don't think government—or socialized science—is destiny.

I started taking courses in microeconomics. I thought at first that a minimum wage was a good idea. Why not raise it by 50 percent? Why not raise it by a thousand percent? Minimum wage, rent control, tuition subsidies. They all sounded good to me at the time. I was poor. I was working on work-study all my time at USC. But these notions collapsed with a supply-and-demand analysis, so I found myself increasingly in that upper box of the fuzzy political square, arguing for a government for a monopoly on power, that was truly limited.

At the time I thought the limit could in theory go to zero and maybe some day would. That was really the essence of Marxism. The real vision of Marxism was that the state would wither away. In fact it tended not to wither but to grow and grow and grow. The ultimate Marxist state was a very libertarian-looking thing, with complete wealth, complete freedom from the state, and so forth. The issue was the means of achieving that rich stateless society.

I saw that we all wanted to end up in that upper quadrant in that final corner of complete freedom. At the time that I was getting deeper into the libertarian philosophy, I was also being forced to register for the draft. That tends to sharpen one's position on these issues. I was in the first draft pool. The cut-off line began for those born January 1, 1960. I was born February 7, 1960. That made me think a lot about the ideas behind a free-market or volunteer draft.

The case for a volunteer military seemed very clear. In case after case I saw that the alternatives were whether to have the government provide a monopoly service or have competition for a given service. It had nothing to do with the nature of the service itself, whether it was protection by way of the courts, or police protection, or in the end even national defense. The effects of philosophy and economics on me were to further erode my belief in the state. Again like a lot of people, I lost my belief in God with science. With more science and philosophy, I lost my belief in the state. I have little sympathy for atheist scientists who kneel before the state and spend much of their time hunting state subsidies. They have betrayed science and corrupted themselves. They do not live up to their social marginal product.

Now what happened is that part of my work at USC was in political philosophy. My instructor there was John Hospers, who was the first Libertarian presidential candidate. He was at USC and wrote an acclaimed book called *Libertarianism*, the first explicit book on the subject. Right away I became a campus libertarian. My friends and I took charge of the Speaker's Committee. I remember, for example, we made Ted Kennedy speak outside in the rain one day. We brought in speakers and kept out others. I remember we brought in G. Gordon Liddy but he turned us off with his big-government conservatism.

The other thing that I did was write essays. At this time, when I was nineteen, I tried to become a professional writer. I even wrote soft-core porn stories under a pseudonym. It was very hard work. I took courses in the graduate program for writing at USC to train myself for writing. I started making some extra income and I learned the discipline of writing. I started writing essays—essays about the military draft, the abolition of victimless crimes, the nature of liberty. I would run those in the *Daily Trojan* [USC's student newspaper]. Then I sent copies to my friends and comrades at other universities—at KU, Northwestern, at different schools. They would run the essays under their own names, and they would respond to the questions themselves. That was their obligation. I remember at one point I was hitting an audience of more than 100,000 people. That's a very powerful feeling when you're twenty years old.

When I got into philosophy a little more deeply, I started with political philosophy. The modern philosophy is the philosophy of science and the works of [Willard Van Orman] Quine and the logical positivists. Every statement is either true or false. It is meaningful if and only if it is an empirical or testable statement or a logically trivial statement—in other words it is meaningful just in case it is either a statement of math or science. Questions of ethics or other questions may have personal meaning to you but they have no cognitive content.

My heroes were the members of the Vienna circle of logical positivism in the 1930s, from Rudolf Carnap to Quine. Quine even came and visited us at USC in the philosophy department. I began taking courses in symbolic logic. So I had lost my faith in God and I turned to science. I tried fanatically to find some kind of foundation to stand on. I very soon realized that the language of science is math and that the structure of math is logic, and the essence of logic is basically these Aristotelian assumptions of the black and the white. I remember, for example, running across the books of Ayn Rand and her big propagandistic novel called *Atlas Shrugged*. The three acts of the drama are labeled the three so-called laws of Aristotelian thought: "A equals A," "A or not A," and "not the case of A and not A."

I began to question these laws of Aristotle. This was to me the next big changing point of my life. I got deeper and deeper into logic and was taking graduate courses in symbolic logic while still an undergraduate. Suddenly I had a crisis. I couldn't find a single statement of the world, about the world —the descriptive world, the world of factual truth—to which logic applied. I couldn't find a single statement that was either 100 percent true or 100 percent false: "The grass is green." "The sky is blue." "The dirt is brown." These statements were matters of degree, but by logical law they had to be true or not true. They had the same status as the statement "2 equals 2" or "2 equals 3." This was a great crisis for me. I saw a mismatch between a grey world and a black-and-white science.

Then I stumbled on multivalued logic and that to me was a big breakthrough. I thought this was a central issue, trying to get language to match fact. That led very quickly to my fuzzy research. Now, at the same time, in economics I got deeper into the study of free markets. This was the beginning of the Reagan revolution, so the free market was becoming very popular. But there are certain theorems that a lot of people don't know about. One of them is called the Coase theorem. For this, Ronald Coase was given the Nobel prize in economics a few years ago. It says that if transactions' costs in exchange are zero or small, and if property rights are well defined, then the market outcome is Pareto optimum or is efficient. "Pareto optimum" means it's a kind of social equilibrium where it's impossible to make somebody better off without making someone else worse off. It's almost like an ideal Marxian state. So you can view the economy as a big game, an exchange game. If you fall in a state of Pareto optimality the you'll never move out of it. The Coase theorem was bouncing around the halls of both the econ. school at USC and its law school.

The other theory that was very hot at the time and that brought me back to biology was the theory of sociobiology. This was one of these grand, sweeping, worldview theories. The selfish human. We're just gene machines. The chicken is the egg's way of making more eggs. We're DNA's way of making more DNA. I began to look into this. I read E. O. Wilson's big text-book on sociobiology. That was a lot of work. Population biology, ecology —there are many things packed into that book. I started writing my first technical paper on the marijuana market. I viewed that market as a socio-biological type of game that can achieve what's called an ESS or an evolu-tionarily stable strategy—another notion of global equilibrium. That's close to a Nash equilibrium in game theory or the Pareto optimality in the Coase theorem.

I thought more and more about the social systems that emerged through so-called invisible hand mechanisms—for example, language or morals or markets. No one invented languages. They evolved. These mechanisms include most social institutions, general market outcomes, Supply-equals-demand equilibria, and so on. The concept began to fill my head that the more agents enter the game, the quicker and in some sense the better the equilibrium you reach. So between sociobiology and the new mathematical economics and my political enthusiasm for free markets, I was driven deeper into the mathematics.

I was good at logic. When I'd taken calculus earlier, I was at first self-taught and never had much enthusiasm for it. I hadn't run with it as I'd run with music. So when I was twenty, right before Christmas break, one day I went to the book store and bought for $1.50 an old calculus text. I took it with me over Christmas break and began working each problem in each chapter. I thought it was easy and trivial and simple. I kept working these problems like an exercise workout, with the same daily discipline. Pretty soon it was like when I'd worked with physics or with musical theory. I got deep into it and began to think and guess in terms of it. This was when I woke up mathematically.

So when classes resumed, and the new semester came around, I enrolled in an advanced calculus class and got the only A in the course. That began a new line of training for me in mathematics. I pursued it too with religious zeal.

I had to learn topology, so I got the *Schaum's Outlines* books and did some background work and got my first notion of topology, very general notions of connectedness and compactness and smoothness. I studied the trans-formations of one system into another so that I could grasp the works of Gerard Debreu, who won the Nobel prize in economics in 1983. The key book for me was Debreu's *A Theory of Value*. The entire equilibrated econ-omy reduces to a fixed point of the system, the Brouwer fixed point. You can picture it in terms of, again, a unit square if you view the positive diagonal as the locus of fixed points, where x equals $f(x)$. Then it's impossible to draw a curve from the left to the right without hitting that diagonal at least once. The theorem says that a continuous function of a compact convex set into itself always has a fixed point. Debreu had the clever idea of showing the economy in terms of market-clearing functions and setting them up in terms of the compact convex set of price vectors (a simplex). Each price vector is like a probability vector. The components all add up to one. The system maps into itself. Debreu showed there had to be one such price vector that decentralized the economy. That, in effect, was Adam Smith's invisible hand. I thought that this was a clever proof of laissez faire capitalism. It falls right out of the Brouwer fixed-point theorem and the Kakatuni fixed-point theorem that extends it.

I got deep into such things and then ran into the works of neural theorist Morris Hirsch. His book, *Differential Topology*—I couldn't really handle it, and I still have a hard time with it, but increasingly research in economics dealt with what are called generic systems, properties that hold almost everywhere. The more agents you have, the more likely you might see something like you see with neural systems—that is, exponentially fast convergence to equilibrium. It was this idea, systems equilibrating, that got me into neural networks. At the same time I was working with evolutionarily stable strategies of game theory. The idea was to extend that idea to CSSs, or culturally stable strategies. I did that with my marijuana paper, which I wrote in a couple of days but which took me many years to get published.

Another thing that helps concretize my ideas is trying to write them down and get them published. The idea of the invisible hand, the convergence of systems, Debreu's work, Arrow's dictatorship theorem, the Coase theorem —all these things convinced me that we could construe broad social structures in economic terms. Somewhere, someday, I don't remember how or when, I thought of the brain in the same way. Why couldn't the brain act like a big economy?

It was in that context that I ran across an obscure paper by Stephen Grossberg, very hard for me to read, about competition as an organizing principle for biological systems. Competition ruled not just at the broad level of the Darwinian slug out, but even down at the level of the structure of the brain. I have to give Grossberg credit for bringing me into the neural field. In some sense it began with Carl Sagan. But it was with Grossberg that I saw the mathematics for the first time. He had theorems that tied agent behavior to brains.

Around this time then I wrote my own paper called "Equilibrium in Local Marijuana Games," which was a game played among growers, ripoffs, and narcs. I wrote that paper after watching a Ted Koppel program on ABC's *Nightline* on the growing of marijuana. There were narcs trying to raid the pot patches. The narcs found that as these narc raids went up, the rip-offs went up as well. That was the game played between growers and rip-offs. So in modeling that phenomena, I had my first mathematical result. I derived a global equilibrium for the entire grass game. Given any combination of agents—any mix of growers, rip-offs, and narcs—the game would always converge, exponentially quickly and independent of initial conditions, to a stable outcome.

I had just graduated from USC and had no money. I was accepted into graduate school in math at UCSD. During that summer I remember I checked out more than one hundred books at the USC library because I now spoke the mathematical language. I read books on traffic theory and books on engineering and as much as I possibly could on population biology. I laid out my first novel on sociobiology. I was writing a little fiction along those lines and did publish some stories.

I tried hard to get my marijuana paper published. The only place I thought I could do that was in *High Times*. They accepted it, but rather than paying me for the article they offered me advertising space. That was really not the sort of thing that I do, so it didn't get published at that time. It took many years. It didn't appear until 1991, and I changed it along the way, but the essence remains, the result that I derived when I was an undergraduate. It is still one my favorite results—my mapping from TV to math.

In my last semester at USC, when I was taking various math courses, I wanted to understand general relativity. It was just an intellectual goal. To do that, you need to understand differential geometry, the calculus of curvature, calculus on manifolds. They offered a course on it that semester with a fellow named Mark Kac. He was one of the editors of *The Annals of Probability*.

I remember when Mark walked into the class. He was a big man, big powerful presence, white hair, bright red tie. He said, "I'm here to tell you the truth and only the truth, but not the whole truth because that would scare you." I was very taken with the man. I began pursuing differential geometry much more than I otherwise would have, and I became something of his protégé. He was new at USC, and I was just about to leave USC. He wanted to see as many people as possible go into pure math. Within a month or two he was writing letters of recommendation for me. That's how I got into UCSD's math department.

I was offered a scholarship in the economics program at USC, but I wanted to pursue math. I was into the idea that math was the language of science, that this was the new religion or at least the bedrock of the Information Age. I couldn't learn enough of it. So through the help of Mark and others. I made it to UCSD. I remember we'd have many discussions about the nature of probability. He was a rabid probabilist and called himself an operationalist. That led me to believe that what exists was what you could measure. Mark had worked with Richard Feynman and others on the foundations of quantum mechanics. If you asked him, "Is the moon there if you're not looking?" he would say, "No."

I thought, "Now here's a guy I have great respect for, saying something that is clearly false, clearly outrageous, and yet there's a reason why he says that." I'm very suspicious of probability, not just because of its general problems, but also because probability looked a lot like God. It was used to explain a lot of things, and you could never catch it in the act. You could never find the real thing. You find at most its footprints.

I remember asking Mark about multivalued logic, and he pooh-poohed it. We talked instead about what was called "the measure theory of probability." So when I was twenty-two and at graduate school at UCSD in mathematics, and a TA in calculus, I began to pursue measure theory, or the formal theory of probability. My economic development went on hold.

At the time, I was very poor. I had no money and a minimal scholarship in the math department. This was at the height of the recession, in 1982–83. I raced through and got a master's very quickly, in one year, and got a job. I sent out seventy resumes.

The only job I could get was at General Dynamics. I had mixed feelings about this. I mean, here was a libertarian about to go to work for the largest defense contractor in the world. Yet it was very seductive. They were paying me $30,000, and I had never had anything like that. I had earned maybe $5,000 a year, if even that. So I got $30,000 to be, in effect, an artificial intelligence consultant, a mathematical internal consultant. I could continue Ph.D. work gradually on the side. I had to take it. I'd always been poor, and I wanted to have my first home and all those sorts of things.

So before I knew it I was at General Dynamics. I started work on July 11, 1983. I began the security interviews and all the things that you have to do to work there. Again, I felt the omnipresence of the state that had plagued me since I was age three. But the one thing that was very good at General Dynamics was they had a library at the Convair Division, where I was in San Diego. They had unlimited technical resources. They changed the copying machine policy because I copied so many articles.

The first thing I got into there was fuzzy logic. I had stumbled across that term "fuzzy" in an article by Ronald Yager. Before, I'd always heard the field described as "multivalued" or "vague." I read the works of Lofti Zadeh and checked out all the books I could find on it and ordered other books on the subject. I went to seminars and just devoured works on that field and related ones. I looked more at artificial intelligence. I found interesting the problems of AI. But there was little mathematical basis there.

It was at this time at General Dynamics that I began looking at neural networks in detail. I wanted to apply the economic notions I'd worked out to military planning. Somewhere along the line I ran across the words "dendritic tree," and so it was time to start looking at neural networks. I got some primers on neurobiology. Before long, I ran across Stephen Grossberg's book, *Studies of Mind and Brain*, which had just come out. I had a hell of a time reading that. I still have a hell of a time reading that book. Yet it remains my favorite book in the field.

For me, these two fields that were to play such a heavy role in my life began to come together. The first research type thing I did in '83 was to come up with something called a fuzzy cognitive map. Now, the term "cognitive map" has been used by many people in psychology and also in political science as a way to relate causal events. The idea is pretty obvious, just to allow fuzzy causal events as well. So if this node goes up, then that connected node goes down to some degree. The nodes themselves can stand for fuzzy sets—like the strength of a government, or political activism, or these kinds of abstract notions to which all events belong to some degree.

My application stemmed from the problem of how you put values on a target. I was working on some smart weapons at the time, largely the Tomahawk cruise missile. There was the problem of launching several Tomahawks at different targets. It is a relative evaluation problem. It's the problem of the target value of a bridge. The bridge is worth a lot before the tanks go over it. It's worth very little once they've gone over.

We looked at expert system decision trees, and they didn't really handle the problem. Then I tried cognitive maps. I wrote my first fuzzy paper using them. The analysis suggested that the maps really should have feedback, but the minute you put in feedback, then there were closed loops and no more tree structure. Then the doors of AI shut, and you couldn't do inference. The question was, What can you do with feedback cognitive maps?" There was just one idea: "The hell with graph search. Why not just let the thing spin around, and see if, like an economy, it would cool down and equilibrate?"

This was a type of feedback neural network I was playing with. It was the year after the Hopfield paper came out. I read that and other papers. I started to see the neural connection, though I was still thinking of the cognitive map in terms of causal prediction, which lies at the heart of much of philosophy. Hume said that causality is an illusion. When you say, "A causes B," really it just means "if A, then B." Causality is a constant conjunction of events, I wanted to see if we could have an adaptive causal structure. Data change the causal links in a cognitive map.

The problem I had with the Hume idea—which was a correlation idea, really a Hebbian idea—was that it grew spurious causal links. The idea that came to me was that of John Stuart Mill who said that causality is a *concomitant variation* of events. A simple way to deal with variation is as a change, as a derivative, and as a product or concomitance you just multiply. This is where I came up with my first neural contribution, what I later called the differential Hebbian law, or the differential synapse. I designed it at first for causal prediction on a cognitive map with no intention of a neural connection. Much later, I saw the work of Harry Klopf, who did apply a similar idea to neural networks.

I began to study how a cognitive map might behave and saw how to exploit its matrix and nonlinear structure. I read a book edited by Jim Anderson and Geoffrey Hinton and saw that you could reduce a lot of neural networks to linear algebra, followed by some nonlinear operations. I worked that out for cognitive maps.

At about the same time, I was proving my first theorems on the foundations of fuzzy set theory. By now I was caught up in the debate between fuzziness and probability. Most people just said fuzziness was probability in disguise. I wanted to see whether that was true. I expected that it might be, or that it might be the other way around, since I sat in the fuzzy world. At this point, I had met Lofti Zadeh and many of the founders of the field. Lofti took me on, in effect, as a long-distance graduate student and steered me into electrical engineering, which is why I moved from UCSD to UCI and UC Berkeley. I could find no interest at UCSD in this at all.

My goal was to recast fuzzy theory from the foundations. So I thought that it might proceed like this: In the most general case, you have a set of objects and all possible subsets of those objects, what's called the power set. If you have n you have 2^n subsets. I wanted to work with the set of all possible fuzzy subsets, which is infinite, even if n is finite. That's the big sigma-algebra. It's all in the algebraic structure of the sets. The big advance was when I saw that that sigma algebra had the structure of a unit hypercube—it was like Jim Anderson's Brain State in a Box. Maybe that was a triggering event in my life, or maybe it was the libertarian cube. I don't know what it was. I remember thinking that a Rubik's Cube has eight corners, just as a set of three objects has a power set with eight objects in it. Any point inside a Rubik's cube corresponds to a fuzzy set of three elements, where each element belongs to some degree.

About this time, 1984, I ran into Robert Hecht-Nielsen. He and I were part of the neural underground in San Diego, the neural fuzzy underground. He had designed a processor called a fuzzy associative memory. It really wasn't fuzzy, but it did have some outcomes where output values could take on a spectrum of values. Robert and I became friends at once. We never fitted in at UCSD. We were never members of the PDP [parallel distributed processing] group. And when we tried to get in later, we were always persona non grata perhaps because we were in industry. The UCSD folks did not allow me to present my neural theorems there. They instead allowed my friend Professor Clark Guest to present them for me. So Robert and I were on our own.

Robert was at TRW then. He ran the AI lab. Very soon I moved to a smaller company called VERAC; the V stands for nothing, but the rest is Engineering Research Analysis Corporation. I soon became manager of adaptive systems. Also, I ran a local neural network interest group. We'd invite various people to speak—for example, David Rumelhart and David Zipser. It was very much of an underground movement.

Now, to step aside here from the technical issues, there was also a political development. Something happened in 1985. I thought at the time that the most important conference series was the IJCAI and AAAI series of artificial intelligence conferences. That's where I met, physically met, Lofti Zadeh. I saw AI experts pummel him on the panel on uncertainty. I watched Lofti

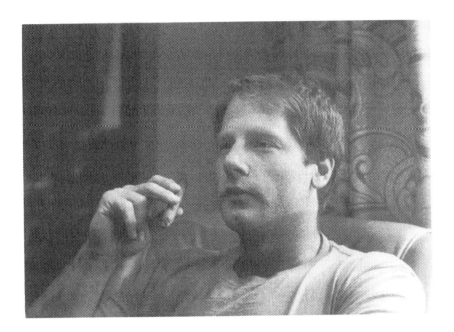

Zadeh try to sell fuzzy logic to the AI experts in the section called "Management of Uncertainty in Expert Systems." They didn't buy it, they only joked about it. At the same time, I would scan the "Proceedings" and seldom see a neural paper. Robert and I were both trying to get our papers published—in my case neural and fuzzy, in his case just neural. It never worked.

I remember the 1985 AI conference at UCLA. This was at the height of the AI movement. I'd done some work with the Symbolics Company, one of the developers of the LISP machine. I'd developed a program for the government called ADBM, an Adaptive Distributed Ballistic Management System, which tried to organize the SDIO System [Strategic Defense Iniative Office, often called Star Wars] like a big free-market system in the sky. The folks at Symbolics Graphics had worked out a videotape that was very popular and that soon brought me, the libertarian, to the headquarters of the Strategic Defense Initiative to explain the system. From that point, I began to see that the way we pursued mission planning in the military was purely centralized or socialistic. The DOD remains the world's largest command economy.

The turning point was in 1985 at the AI conference. This was the peak AI conference in terms of attendance and certainly in terms of enthusiasm. It was held in our backyard at UCLA, and my fuzzy friends and neural friends were there. Robert Hecht-Nielsen and I went up to L.A. Of course they rejected our papers, but what we saw there made a deep impression—just the panache of the AI community. The two competing vendors of LISP machines —LMI and Symbolics—both had separate limousine services that would take you to the Beverly Wilshire, another very large downtown hotel. There was all the food and drink that you wanted. There was a big Malibu party from Symbolics. It was very posh—the structure of the tutorials, the plenary talks, the way the venture capitalists were running around trying to fund the field. And somewhere in there the idea began to emerge, sort of at a subliminal level still: why not do something like this for the neural or fuzzy fields?

That same year, after the AI conference, in the summer of 1985, the president of my company VERAC happened to be the IEEE [Institute of Electrical and Electronics Engineers] San Diego chairman of the computer society. He said, "How would you like to be chairman next year, in 1986? The only requirements are that you say, 'I do,' and that you be an IEEE member."

I wasn't a member. So he wrote me the letters and I became a member and I said, "I do."

So when 1986 rolled around, I had a vote on the executive committee of the San Diego IEEE section. At the same time, I was teaching a course at UCSD at night on fuzzy theory, in which I was developing a lot of my fuzzy ideas to the point where I was giving out homework problems on them. Often I would create a new theoretical idea, like the idea of fuzzy entropy, and within a week I'd already assigned homework problems on it to the students and for myself to explore. This was in early 1986.

Then I did something. The local section of the IEEE had about $30,000 in the treasury. They felt that each year they were eating that up by about $5,000. So they were slowly going broke. They needed something to raise revenues. I had the idea, "Why don't we get a bunch of these AI vendors together and throw a miniconference? We'll call it the AI Slugout. We'll have LMI compete with Symbolics and bring in all the smaller vendors that are selling AI machines." These included Sun Microsystems, Silicon Graphics, and other companies that had AI packages, the AI software tools people, and so forth. So at UCSD I rented Mandeville Auditorium for $1,000, courtesy of the IEEE, and brought together several of these vendors.

In April 1986 we had the AI Slugout. It was on a Sunday afternoon. I'll never forget it. The curtain hadn't been drawn; it was to start at 2:00. I went behind the scenes, and there were at least twenty people, most of whom were major vendors. The two biggest ones refused to show up, Symbolics and LMI, but the smaller vendors showed up, and we had a show. I peeked outside the curtain, and there were exactly six people in the audience. There were far more vendors than attendees, so I told the vendors that the program had been delayed about half an hour. I ran outside with my friends, and we began to grab anybody walking by and tell them they had to come see this artificial intelligence conference. We got maybe fifteen, twenty people. That got a critical mass going. Other people began trickling in. We put up a small sign, and at one point the crowd reached almost as many as a hundred people.

The local IEEE section judged it a success. I had the vendors contribute $200 apiece. The net result was we not only paid for Mandeville Auditorium, but we made a profit. In the eyes of the local IEEE section, this was a big stamp of credibility for me.

We'd been talking, always talking, about perhaps having a conference someday as a major revenue enhancer. They weren't sure about what. They were talking about having maybe something in manufacturing, where there already was a conference, and trying to cosponsor it. In the first week of June 1986, I believe, *Business Week* ran our famous article on neural networks. In it were pictures of Robert Hecht-Nielsen bending over his neural machine at TRW and John Hopfield standing with his arms folded in front of a picture of a neural network. Everybody was talking about it. Robert had thrown the first neural short course in the fall, which largely neural researchers attended, and had scheduled another one for later in that summer. I was about to begin a course at UCSD on neural networks.

I sat at the monthly IEEE meeting. I had brought a copy of *Business Week* with me and said, "Have you all seen this?" I showed the pictures of Robert and John Hopfield. I said, "We have a very large neural effort here in San Diego, such as the PDP group."

At this point the Rumelhart PDP books were not out, but we'd all seen advance copies of it and talked to members of the group. Every week, *EE Times* had run articles on neural networks. I had some of those with me, so I said, "Why don't we throw a neural network conference?"

I put forth the motion, got a second, and won approval to explore the issue. I called Robert Hecht-Nielsen and bounced the idea off him. He seemed enthused. I think we had lunch some time after that to talk about it. The next big step was when I brought Robert and his golden mouth to the next board meeting of the San Diego IEEE section. Robert and his magnetic personality convinced them that not only could we do it, but we could do it with panache just like the AI guys did at IJCAI-85 at UCLA.

That was the plan. We would structure this just like the big, glossy 1985 AI conference. We would have the tutorials, the plenaries, the luminaries. We'd do it right in a big hotel. We'd have a party, a banquet, the whole thing, and most of all, we'd use the mailing list of the AI community. We would schedule the conference two to three weeks before the big AI conference. We'd beat them at their own game. Sure enough, the AI community sold us their mailing list, and we had kept copies of the brochures and proceedings from previous conferences and completely copycatted what we viewed as our competition.

Now the problem, of course, is that a local section, a city section of the IEEE has no authority to throw an international conference, not even a region-wide conference, and yet we'd gone ahead and done it. The IEEE is a volunteer organization. If somebody has the initiative to do something, it's very hard to stop him.

By the fall of 1986 we had already printed a preliminary brochure. We went around to the many feuding factions in neural networks. The feuds were really beginning to heat up now. The PDP books were out. There were different camps, and we felt the only thing to do was have a level playing field. Libertarian capitalist that I am, I suggested that we offer a very lucrative tutorial fee, but conditional. The deal was, if the conference didn't make money—and nobody thought it would make money at this point—the tutorial presenters got nothing. If it did make money, they could make as much as $15,000 if they brought in enough audience. So there was a risk in the package, something that critics later ignored.

Many of the leaders of the neural field who we asked to participate and to give tutorials literally hated each other's guts but now had a joint, common self-interest in this conference. We wanted something on a very broad scale in San Diego, something again that looked a lot like the AI conferences. The idea I learned from Marxist politics is that you don't just criticize a field. You don't just shoot holes in somebody's boat. What you do is you build a second boat, and then you shoot holes in the first boat. That was the idea. The problem was that we didn't have nearly the money that you need to fund this big conference. In terms of marketing, it was all bootstrapping. We had to commit to a hotel, the entire Sheraton. The only way we could get it was to commit to the entire thing, to fill it up. That meant we had a legal liability of more than half a million dollars, maybe as much as a million dollars. The San Diego section, with just $30,000 in the bank, had just put itself on the line for more than half a million dollars.

We began to line up more and more of the scientific talent. I was technically the general chair, but we called it the organizing chair. We had Stephen Grossberg be honorary chair, but de facto general chair. We brought in all the major players in the neural field. We had various schedules and cut-off dates and appointments. By late January, when my daughter was born—January 30, 1987—about that time, we were at the first cut-off date, and we had done some linear prediction of attendees. We thought we'd have several hundred people enrolled by February 1. I think there were less than twenty.

Then came the calls to close down the conference, including calls from some members in the local IEEE in San Diego. People were getting scared. Worse, people had begun to hear about the conference in the IEEE: "Who the hell were these people in San Diego who have put the IEEE on the hook for a half-million dollars? And the reputation of the IEEE? Who the hell is a twenty-six-year-old puke named Bart Kosko? How many conferences has he managed? Who's Robert Hecht-Nielsen?" And so on.

Critics circulated petitions to close the conference. This occurred as late as a month before we threw the conference in June of 1987. It was very much a classic success story. The great bulk of attendees registered in the last two or three months. Then we knew we had a smashing success. The rest is neural history. We had the conference, about two thousand paid attendees, and the San Diego section, which had broken a lot of IEEE rules, had become the richest section in the history of the IEEE. All of a sudden, the game changed. And, of course, there was the risk package for the tutors. I made a lot of money; everybody made a lot of money. Engineers and academics criticized us in some bitter mix of real concern and raw envy.

I also want to give credit where due. Right before the conference was held, in the spring of 1987, there was an emergency meeting about what to do about this conference. The executive director of IEEE, Eric Hertz, who happened to be a former head of the San Diego section, flew in and met with me and my other Ph.D. advisor, Professor Alan Stubberud from UC Irvine, who had been the chief scientist for the Air Force and was about to become director of region six of the IEEE. We met, and Merrill Buckley was there, who was about to become president of the IEEE. Merrill wanted to close us down, but Eric Hertz stood up for us. He put his job on the line to Buckley, who was, I think, on the governing board of the entire IEEE, and said, "Do you want to fire me or not?" Buckley backed down, and the conference survived.

But something I'll never forget, when it was all over, when Robert and I were talking with Eric Hertz, he told us the golden law of bureaucracy: "It's easier to get forgiveness than permission." He was going to let us go this time, "but don't ever pull something like this again."

So it was a success. After the conference in June and the formation of the INNS [International Neural Network Society], the field congealed to a sort of stable state as we now know it. At that point, there came the question, "What would be the next conference?" The reason the IEEE had done it and had in the end endorsed it, was that they knew there was going to be a lot of money when they saw the final attendance. It became a big dog fight. Different societies in the IEEE wanted a piece of the action. The IEEE is a massive bureaucracy, and it in effect took over the conference.

At the same time, Steve Grossberg's INNS set up the first INNS annual meeting in Boston. It looked like something of a competition would emerge. So the real interesting drama was how there ever came to be an ICNN [International Conference on Neural Networks] '88 because the IEEE had formally cancelled it. During the summer of 1987, the IEEE wanted to proceed with the next annual conference. It was a question of who would run it. There were many fights about this. The one thing they agreed upon is that Bart Kosko and Robert Hecht-Neilsen would have nothing to do with it. We could live with that. The problem was we felt they were about to kill the goose that laid the golden egg. They were going to let the conference series die. That we could not live with.

So in September or October 1987, Robert and I asked IEEE what the status was, and they said, "We've killed it. No one can reach a consensus."

This was totally unacceptable, so Robert and I decided to do it again. Supposedly, there's an Al Capone saying: "Do it first, do it yourself, and keep doing it." I appeared as program chair for 1988 and Robert as general chair. We had our say. It wasn't just ego, although there was certainly a lot of that. It was more than that. The IEEE had shut down the conference. Robert and I said, "To hell with this. We're going to the 1987 NIPS [Neural Information Processing] conference and sign up as many people as we can for the next ICNN conference in '88."

We asked Teuvo Kohonen to be the honorary chair. He agreed. We set out with the same structures we had before, went down the list, filled out the slots, found the people we'd like to invite and those we had to invite. By fall the IEEE had circulated letters, and different members had circulated letters to every major society, asking them not to support Hecht-Nielsen and Kosko in this endeavor. There would be no ICNN '88.

Robert and I really took a big risk here because if we failed we would be the Milli Vanilli of neural networks. Robert at this point was head of his own company HNC [now HNC Software Inc.]. We signed up most of the major neural researchers, just as we'd done before. I think Steve Grossberg didn't want to do it because he thought it would interfere with the INNS annual meeting, but nevertheless we signed up most of the major people. We would have had serious egg on our faces if it didn't come to pass.

Once we had a slate, with all the intellectual fire power to do it the next year, and the hotel reserved because we had the reputation from the previous conference, and the management structure, what happened is that my former Ph.D. advisor, my good friend and mentor Alan Stubberud, was about to become region six director of the IEEE. He was also now a boss at the National Science Foundation, which carries a lot of weight in the socialized academic community. There was a great screaming match held in his office at NSF [the National Science Foundation] between Robert Hecht-Nielson, who argued for the conference, and the current president of the IEEE, Troy Nagle, who opposed it. They hammered out a basic deal in which the local San Diego section got some cut of the a future conference series, and the IEEE got theirs. This was the basis of what continued as the ICNN series. In the following July, I guess it was, we had the conference. I was program chair and Robert was general chair. We gambled and won.

ER: I think you've given us a very complete history.

BK: So that's how the conference series began. To get back to technical developments, for me one of the big achievements of my career is the thing called the BAM, or the bidirectional associative memory. That was in 1985, back in those times when I was very much taken with the idea of global stability, Hopfield-style networks, the ball rolling into the energy well. At the same time, I thought the neatest idea in neural networks was Grossberg's Adaptive Resonance Theory [ART] that you learn only if you resonate. But to me the weakness of the adaptive resonance paradigm was that global stability was not part of it. You might be searching through an awful lot of grandmother cells before you resonated finally and learned the pattern.

At the same time I was fooling around with fuzzy associative memories. These were fuzzy matrices that mapped fuzzy vectors or points in the unit hypercube into other points in the hypercube. I remember pushing a vector through a matrix and getting out a different-size vector on the other side and then pushing that back through the other way. When I pushed the output vector back through, I had to use the transpose or flip the matrix over and then a fixed point developed there. That was an interesting property.

I wondered what whould happen if you did this with a regular matrix, with linear algebra operations, and did the usual thresholding. You push vector A through the matrix, and out pops B, and then you transpose the matrix, push vector B back through, and out pops A. I did it, and lo and behold, it always stabilized. It seemed for any matrix that was always the case. So this was one of those moments, those epiphanies of scientific discovery, where now you have a theorem to prove. I quickly proved a simple version for a discrete, additive BAM, showed the global stability—that is, that *any* matrix always stabilizes in a BAM.

I got excited by this. I also applied it to an autoassociative matrix, a Hopfield net, but in the Hopfield case you had to update one neuron at a time. In the BAM, you update the entire vector at a time.

I did many extensions of it. If this result was that robust, you should be able to change the weights slowly, and then you would have what I thought was something more like adaptive resonance theory, in the sense that you have both the neurons changing and synapses changing. You could extend the idea to what I called an ABAM, or adaptive BAM, and have a Hebbian learning law. The system always converges to fixed points. If you use the competitive learning law, it would still work. Now you have something that's similar in contour to the ART model. I kept extending results and finally got into a random domain. As long as you have a system perturbed by a noise of *finite* variance, the system will always cool down. In effect, the learning is structurally stable. It is robust.

That was one line of research. Along the way, I found a learning law that I think is a more important idea, the idea of combining competitive learning with differential Hebbian learning—in other words, using not just a competition signal, but the signal velocity. The question had always been, "How could a neuron or synapse compute a derivative?" It's a very complicated calculation and very unstable numerically. But if you have pulses, as you have with real neurons, then it falls out very simply. The derivative is just the pulse minus the expected signal value. So you can estimate the derivative at any moment by whether there's a pulse. If there is, it's a positive derivative. If there's not, it's a negative derivative. That's a biologically plausible mechanism.

By this point I'd also worked out a lot of theorems on the foundation of fuzzy sets, all housed in the geometry of a hypercube. It was my approach to try to see things in math because if it's a real structure, you can always picture it. One inspiration was the Brain State in a Box neural model, where the allowable state space of a neural system is bounded and is in effect equivalent to a unit hypercube. There ought to be a neural connection. The next level was to go from a cube to two cubes and mappings between the cubes. This was the idea of a fuzzy associative memory. If that mapping changed with time, then you had an adaptive fuzzy associative memory—or, if you like, a neural fuzzy associative memory. So each fuzzy rule defined one of these little mappings from one cube to another. If the air was cool, then it turned down the air conditioner a little. If the air was cold, then it turned it down a lot. Each one of those rules is a mapping. The fuzzy system has all those rules firing in parallel as it converts inputs to outputs.

I began to pursue this, building it from cubes to multiple cubes. By this point, late '80s, Hal White had proven that feed forward neural networks could approximate any function if you used enough neurons. I was convinced you could do the same thing with fuzzy systems. I found a very simple proof. If you view a rule as a patch in the state-space geometry, mapping from the input, trying to estimate the function that maps from input to output, that's just a curve that would go through some high-dimensional space. You could cover the graph of that curve with patches and average the overlapping patches, and that gives you back a fuzzy system. The catch is exponential rule explosion—the curse of dimensionality. In my dissertation I'd worked with this averaging process. I'd developed my fuzzy integral. The dissertation was called "The Foundations of Fuzzy Estimation Theory," and I did it with Stubberud and Zadeh.

I went back to that work and extended it to this problem of function approximation. I was teaching the subject at USC. I had a class where I introduced, libertarian that I am, a market incentive. I offered $1,000 prize money that came from a hightech company. Whoever developed the best neural fuzzy project would win the prize and get some local press. Students produced a neural computer-dating service, and the usual applications to robotics, and lunar landers, and a wide variety of fuzzy applications. Some were bawdy, some very clever, some were done on video tapes. Each time I'd teach a class, I would do a video countdown from the previous class. It was a place to try out new ideas. The Discovery Channel's "Beyond 2000" tapped the project presentations in 1993.

I was convinced that I saw a quick proof that you could approximate any function with a fuzzy system. Unlike the neural proof, this was a little more constructive because the patches were rules. We had geometrized a piece of knowledge as a rule, and we could estimate those patches with neural networks. The rules could not only find the first patch, but tune it. In time, we found that a one, two punch of unsupervised learning to estimate and supervised to tune was the best combination. We tried it out for a class and applied it to Bernie Widrow's truck "backer upper." Widrow showed that you could back up a truck and trailer in a parking lot into a loading dock with a neural system. We showed you could also do that with a small set of fuzzy rules and then showed you can convert any neural system into an epsilon-equivalent fuzzy system, which has similar input-output characteristics, but with the fuzzy system you can open the black box, and you have a set of structured rules.

For me, all this brought together the lines of research that began with Carl Sagan's *Dragons of Eden,* the works of Debreu, the economics, the libertarianism, the philosophy; all came together in what I call the FAT theorem, the fuzzy approximation theorem. It says you can always approximate any continuous or measurable function on a compact set to any degree of accuracy with a finite set of fuzzy rules. These rules can be very general but they tend to be exponential in number. I now prefer to pick these as ellipsoids, or regions of attractability in mathematical analysis. I also proved that optimal fuzzy rules cover the extremes or turning points in the graph of a function. They patch the bumps.

ER: Maybe we should talk a little bit about how you got into doing your recent book, *Fuzzy Thinking.* It's for the general reader. It tries to describe these ideas, make them more accessible, and has almost a Buddhist point of view.

BK: I was a writer all along. I always did freelance writing, a lot of political writing—very little of which paid. So in pursuing the libertarian writing and my writing of fiction, most of which has been done under a pseudonym, I got into the discipline of writing every day. I write every day and I exercise every day. I get up in the morning and pay my quota to myself. I write a certain quota of words and exercise, and then I go to the university to do whatever it is that I do.

In that way I turned out my first textbook, a very large book, *Neural Networks and Fuzzy Systems,* with a lot of my work and the work of other people. I edited a volume called *Neural Networks and Signal Processing,* and now there is a third book coming out called *Fuzzy Engineering,* part of a three-book package from Prentice-Hall.

Along the way I also began writing essays on the philosophy of neural networks and fuzzy systems in the tradition, I thought, of the old philosophers, who would learn as much science as they could—stand at the periphery of science—and then speculate. That had always been the nature of metaphysics and ethics and the like in the past.

An editor asked me to write a a series of essays for *AI Expert,* an AI magazine, in 1989. The managing editor called me up and asked me if I was interested in having a regular monthly or bimonthly column. We decided we'd call it "Meditations," and it could be about anything I wanted. I sent him several topics, and we agreed that the first essay would be an article entitled "In Defense of God" because after having lost my faith in the God of shepherds, I gradually regained belief in a math God of sorts. I wrote that essay and sent it in, and, of course, there was a change of editor; a very anti neural-fuzzy editor took over. The editor had to send the article for review to other people for an outside opinion. They did publish the essay "In Defense of God," but that was it. I would get no series.

But in time that essay secured me a contract for the popular book *Fuzzy Thinking.* A sci-fi reader read it, and some other people, and it led to a profile in the *L.A. Times Magazine.* Different editors and agents read that article, and around and around it went. They wanted a book talking about God and neural-fuzzy speculation.

Here was the argument about God. The strongest arguments against God had always been the fact that God could never be defined. That is, you can't say *what* he is. So you can't say *that* he is. The one thing that neural networks taught me is what we call "recognition without definition." You could recognize the pattern of a face without having the ability to define it. Surely dogs and animals have this property. They can't articulate anything but they sniff out and see patterns just fine.

This idea is a negative one—that the inability to define God is in itself not a sufficient reason not to believe in him. There are other reasons you may not believe in God: the fact that your prayers don't work is the most popular, or AIDs spreads, or the worst get on top and stay there, or science is enough, or whatever the reason happens to be. But just because you can't define God, that itself is not sufficient. That was point number one.

The second thing that both disturbed me and delighted me was that science seems to track math, but doesn't have to. The classic example is that Maxwell puts forth some equations for electricity and magnetism. You manipulate the equations and then, poof, out pops light or rather the wave equation for light. You get a wave equation as a mathematical prediction, and sure enough, we find that experience verifies this. The same thing occurs with the general relativity equations or the so-called Einstein Curvature equation: what immediately falls out is a wave equation, hence the prediction of gravitational waves that travel at the speed of light.

For some reason, science tracks math, but logically it doesn't have to. That impresses me. It seems to me that God, the power, whatever you want to call it, is the he, she, or it that wrote the math. The idea of the Math Maker. This is the one we take orders from. I think if this continues—if we take orders from a Pythagorean theorem and a million others—for a thousand, a million, a trillion years then the idea of the math blueprint in the sky will be clearer. We tend to recognize that pattern even though we can't define it.

That was the content of the essay, the last line of which is, "There may be no God but the Math Maker and science is His Prophet." That idea of speculating at the periphery of science intrigued some editors.

I had other essays. I'd written essays on the Buddha. I saw a sort of historical duality here between Aristotle and the Buddha, between "A or not A" and "A and not A." To Artistotle, the pink rose is either red or not. The Buddha says it's both red and not red to some degree. So around that historical boxing match, I cast a book, *Fuzzy Thinking*, whose thesis is that everything is a matter of degree. If we look at the world through a set of gray glasses we might see the mismatch between precise black-and-white math and science and a grey world.

ER: If you were advising someone just getting started in the neural network field, as you probably do as a professor, what is it that you tell him or her?

BK: Learn as much math as you can. But what sells a field or a career is a vision. What sold Marxism was a vision of the state withering away and the complete freedom that would follow. Some people want to become the next Steven Jobs or Bill Gates. A major in information science, neural networks, or fuzzy systems may be the means to do that. Other people want to understand our meat brains or build the Commander Data of the future.

I like to ask researchers where they get their ideas. The only answer I've heard that makes any sense is, "You vary your input if you want to vary your output." Do lots of things. If you've gotta take drugs, take drugs. Take long walks, meditate, watch a lot of movies, learn a new language, read different books, argue the other side of the debate—anything you can to vary your stimuli. And then you have to, as they say, "keep the ass in the seat." You actually have to sit down and write. Do it in a disciplined way. I think if people have a certain minimal training in mathematics, the problem will take care of itself because neural networks are inherently interesting, and I believe they will stay interesting well into the next century.

ER: Where are neural nets now? What do you think the future looks like?

BK: I'm very skeptical of subsidized science. If I look at the fields of AI, neural networks, and fuzzy logic, I see an inverse relationship between government funding and commercial products. I've heard estimates that in the past 40 or so years, something like $100 billion dollars went into AI, and we all know there's hardly a product to show for it.

There's been at least $100 million or more put into neural networks, and finally some products have come out. We gambled on the first conferences. We thought there would be products in three, four, or five years. Enthusiasm might lead to products. Finally some products did appear: pap smear recognizers, bomb detectors, process controllers, and so forth. It's taken a long time.

As for the fuzzy systems, there was, in effect, zero research investment and now billions of dollars in product.

Let me just tell you a little story. In 1987, after the success of the first neural conference, Robert and I were at the first NIPS Conference in Denver. We were soliciting, signing up people, to talk and to chair the sessions of ICNN '88. One of those people was Carver Mead. There was a meeting about what should be done to get more money from the government. That was the question. Only one person had a dissenting view, and it was Carver Mead. He put forth a Gresham's Law. Gresham's law in economics says that bad money chases out good. His view was that bad researchers chased out the good ones. We ought not get any money at all from DARPA [the government's Defense Advanced Research Projects Agency]. I was very impressed by that idea; there's a lot of wisdom to it. When you pick winners, you tend to end up supporting dinosaurs. Imagine if the state picked winners in Hollywood as it tries to pick them in science.

I'm suspicious of government funding and worry about appealing to government agencies. Yet this is something we did. The first conferences had government panels, and each government agency had someone get up and talk about the money they could give out. I think the best thing that could happen to neural networks, happened. That was the collapse or contraction of the aerospace industry, the end of the cold war. That helped take off the training wheels that the field had begun to support itself with.

ER: Do you see the future as in some way bound up with fuzzy systems?

BK: To some degree. First off, there is the interplay between the two systems, the intertranslatability between neural and fuzzy systems. I realize, and it breaks my neural heart, that I want to use the neural systems now largely just to tune a fuzzy system, but you can use either one as approximators. There is this problem with the neural system: when you learn something new, you may forget what you've already learned. In a fuzzy system, you can open that black box, study the rules, and see how they're changing. The problem is rule explosion. A neural system sees abstract patterns in the data, and those patterns are fuzzy sets—a concept like "cool air," for example, or the setting of the motor speed to "a little" or "a lot." In the next step, it begins to reason or associate those patterns into fuzzy rules. But the system itself, which turns inputs to outputs, is a fuzzy system. So I think, at least from an applications point of view, for many years the way to go is a neural fuzzy system.

I think an area of future application is neural fuzzy systems in the small, at the nano level—the so-called "nanobot." Viral swarms of little computers that can recognize the abstract pattern of a cancer cell or an AIDS virus and eat it and convert it into healthy nutrients for the other cells and, in time, repair the cells one cell at a time. If you can fix up a smashed up car a part at a time, why can't you resurrect the body a cell at a time? In the bigger picture, we can reduce death to a problem of molecular engineering.

Maybe the neural-fuzzy nanobots will help bring us back from death. I intend to find out. As of now I'm about the 350th person signed up to be cryonically suspended upon death. I've gone for whole body suspension. Most of my colleagues have gone for head only—the idea being that if nano-science could resurrect the brain, its synaptic structure, it could also regrow the body from the head stump, from the information in the DNA. It was really my final conversion to materialism through neural networks that drew me to the belief that *I am my synapses.* If I can resurrect those, repair those, and fill in missing links with some clever averaging algorithm, I may come back. Cryonics also acts a crude default strategy in case we do not live long enough to transfer our synaptic patterns of "self" to a computer chip. It's a hell of a thing to live in a meat machine that has no back up. I would not bet my life on cryonics. But I am more than happy to bet my death on it.

Glossary

No one, and that includes the editors of this book, could read all these interviews without encountering unfamiliar words, terminology, jargon, and technical vocabulary. Brain theory is a field with a long, sometimes glorious, history, and it has accumulated many ideas, concepts, and techniques, all described with a specialized vocabulary. Moreover, many of our interviewees sometimes used their own terminology, especially when describing the history of their own research.

We felt it was necessary to provide definitions of some of the more common and more important specialized terms that appear throughout the book. At the same time, there are simply too many words that are sure to be unfamiliar to one or another reader to list them all in a glossary. Therefore, we decided that we would provide a short glossary of the terms we felt were general enough, or important enough, or appeared often enough, or were odd enough to require a little explanation. We are not including terms that were used infrequently or that are idiosyncratic to one speaker. When encountering such an undefined term, two things can be done. First, in fact, an exact definition is rarely necessary to get the gist of what the speaker is talking about. Second, to get fuller explanations of all of the terms, we suggest going back to the original technical literature. We asked our interviewees to provide a single reference that best represented their work. Other information can be obtained from the *Neurocomputing* and *Neurocomputing 2* collections of papers mentioned in the Introduction, or from any reasonably comprehensive textbook in neural networks. We mentioned the text from one of the editors (James Anderson, *An Introduction to Neural Networks*, 1995, Cambridge, MA: MIT Press) as one source of explanations of most of the ideas presented here. Another excellent, large, comprehensive and much more mathematical introduction to neural networks can be found in the text by Simon Haykin, *Neural Networks*, Macmillan, 1992 (2nd edition, 1998).

ACM   The Association for Computing Machinery, a large professional organization.

action potential   The most striking characteristic of a neuron, discovered early in the history of physiology. When a neuron is excited above a threshold value, the cell changes properties ("fires a spike") so the voltage inside the cell goes from negative to positive and then quickly (1/2 millisecond) returns again to negative. The action potential is traditionally described as "all-or-none," that is, either there or not there rather than graded. The action potential travels along the axon, often for considerable distances, without change or attenuation.

Adaline   An "ADaptive LInear NEuron" designed by Bernard Widrow to implement the LMS algorithm around 1960. During the dark days when neural networks were unpopular in the 1970s, Widrow re-acronymized it as the "ADaptive LINear Element," but it did the same thing as before.

adaptive maps   A learning algorithm that builds a topographic map of input patterns, so that similar patterns tend to be near each other on the map. Properly done, this technique can perform useful clustering and preprocessing for many purposes. Topographic maps are common in cerebral cortex and seem to be a useful computational technique widely used in the real brain.

AI   See *Artificial intelligence.*

algorithm   A series of explicit rules and procedures for accomplishing a task.

ARPA   Advanced Research Projects Agency. Government agency known for supporting high risk-high reward projects. ARPA has an impressive record, for example, developing what has become the Internet. For reasons impenetrable to outsiders, ARPA changes its name to DARPA periodically. (See *DARPA.*)

ART   Adaptive resonance theory. ART and its many variations perform categorization and clustering. Originated and investigated by Stephen Grossberg and Gail Carpenter.

Artificial intelligence   Universally known by its initials, AI. As an independent discipline, AI developed in the 1950s and '60s. During the 1960s AI and neural networks were competitors for influence and funding but now their areas of interest overlap to a degree, though there is still some tension between them. The most general goal of AI is given by its name: to make smart machines. The techniques used may have nothing to do with those used by a biological nervous system, but sometimes they may.

association   Since Aristotle it has been observed that much of human cognition depends on forming somewhat arbitrary links between different events. For example, the familiar animal species dog is arbitrarily associated with different sound patterns in different languages: "dog," "chien," "Hund," etc.

attractor state   Nonlinear dynamical systems often have attractor states. In a "fixed-point" attractor, as time progresses and the network state evolves, the system may reach a point where the state no longer changes. A physical analogy would be a rock rolling down hill into a valley. The bottom of the valley would be an attractor state since the rock will not move further. These stable states correspond to local energy minima, or minima of a Lyapunov function. Another possibility for an attractor state is repeating "limit cycles" where the system state evolves toward a closed oscillation which attracts nearby states.

autoassociation   In autoassociation, a pattern is associated with itself, that is, both the input of the network and the output are the same pattern. This permits reconstruction of the whole pattern from a fragment of it. A number of nonlinear neural networks use this architecture. An autoassociative architecture seems very restrictive but in fact is quite general. (See *heteroassociation.*)

autodidact   Self taught. The most notable example mentioned in this book is Walter Pitts.

autoencoder   An autoencoder is a multilayer neural network where the goal of learning is to reproduce the input state as accurately as possible at the output. The hidden layer has fewer units than the input and output layers, therefore the output is an approximation of the input. A well-known autoencoder problem is the "8-3-8" problem with eight input and output units and three hidden units. All input units are zero except there is a single "1" at one of eight input positions and the correct output pattern should have a "1" in the same position in the eight output units. One way to solve this problem is to observe that a binary representation of the numbers from 1 to 8 only requires three values, therefore three hidden units should be able to learn the correct transformation, and indeed, learning algorithms like backpropagation can find solutions to this problem.

backpropagation   By far the best known supervised neural network algorithm. "Backprop" is very good at learning accurate input-output associations using gradient descent error correction and has a number of valuable practical applications. A typical backprop network has multiple layers: an input layer, and output layer, and one or more hidden layers. The output error for an input pattern is computed and then propagated backwards and used for gradient descent error correction from the output layer to the hidden layers to the input layer. Any neural network text can provide details.

basin of attraction   In a nonlinear dynamical system, the set of points that move to a particular attractor when the system settles into its final state.

Bayesian inference   An approach to analyzing complex systems where prior probabilities are incorporated into the computation. The Bayesian approach is particularly useful for analyzing low-level vision, where a multitude of possible arrangements of objects in the world can give rise to the same image on the viewer's retina. Given the observed image, and statistics about the world estimated from prior experience, the Bayesian computation tries to give the most probable actual situation corresponding to the observed retinal image.

bifurcation   At a bifurcation in a dynamical system, a small change in the value of a parameter can lead to a qualitatively different evolution of the behavior of the system. An example might be the development of chaotic oscillation.

binary units   Model neural elements that have only two states. These two states can be variously described as one or zero, plus one or minus one, or, with much greater philosophical weight, "true" or "false." A famous 1943 McCulloch and Pitts paper was based on (a) the binary, all-or-none nature of neural activation, i.e., either quiescent or firing an action potential, and (b) the analogy between "all-or-none" and "true or false." This led to a very influential early model of the nervous system based on the idea that neurons were computing the truth or falseness of logical predicates.

binding problem   How does the brain bind together the different features of a complex object so that it can behave like a single unitary object in our mental life? For example, the activity of cells coding "red" cooperate in the perception of a stop sign in one context whereas activity of the same cells coding red in a different context are part of the perception of a firetruck. The units alone are ambiguous, yet our perceptions and object identifications are selective, stable, and precise.

bionics   Word formed by the combination of "biology" and "electronics." This name was used in the 1960s for research in what would now include neural networks.

Boltzmann machine   A technique capable of finding the global energy minimum in a complex neural network by combining stochastic binary units with simulated annealing. The network state has much added random noise (high system "temperature"), which is slowly decreased. The system state is more and more likely to be found in the lower energy states as the noise decreases (lower system "temperature"). Eventually, the system state spends almost all its time in the lowest energy state. When combined with a statistical learning rule, the Boltzmann machine gave rise to one of the first practical learning algorithms for multilayer networks.

Boolean algebra   Formal techniques for calculating with discrete logic.

bug detector   A famous 1959 paper by Lettvin, Maturana, McCulloch and Pitts called "What the Frog's Eye Tells the Frog's Brain" (reprinted in *Neurocomputing 2*) described a class of retinal cells that responded strongly to small, convex, moving objects. These units were called "bug detectors" by the neuroscience community. Besides their importance for neurobiology, their discovery led to an active search for other kinds of "detectors" since it suggested that a model for brain function might be based on more and more selective cells. The most extreme version of such a model assumes that the brain contains what are called "grandmother cells" (see entry).

cerebral cortex   The outer layer of the mammalian brain. Essentially a two-dimensional folded sheet of cells, about the size of a dish towel in humans. The cells (gray matter) are extensively interconnected by fibers comprising the white matter. Cognitive science is the continuation of cortical neurophysiology by other means.

coarse coding   A distributed coding technique. Units that are unselective and respond to a wide range of parameter values can give rise to a highly selective overall system response.

credit assignment problem   In a complex interacting system—a neural network, a chess game, a bureaucracy—when a good outcome occurs it is often hard to tell exactly what was responsible for it. Conversely, is it not clear what gets the blame if there is a bad outcome. If you don't know where to put praise or blame, it is hard to make the system learn to do better.

cybernetics   A field of applied mathematics and engineering particularly associated with Norbert Wiener. The name is derived from the Greek word for "steersman" and it has become associated with the mathematics of control and information.

DARPA   Defense Advanced Research Projects Agency. Same as ARPA (see entry).

data representation   See *representation*.

DEC   Digital Equipment Corporation. A large computer corporation. They now prefer to be called "Digital" for short, but are much more widely known by the monosyllable "DEC."

distributed representation   A form of data representation in the brain that assumes that neurons are somewhat unselective. A complex input stimulus therefore gives rise to the discharge of many neurons. Advantages of distributed representations include ability to generalize, robustness, and ease of formation of broadly selective units. Disadvantages include the binding problem. (See *grandmother cells*.)

dynamical system   A mathematical system that evolves in time. The changing system state is characterized by a trajectory in state space. Dynamical systems are often described by a set of differential equations.

EEG   Electroencephalogram ("brain waves"). Small electrical potentials recorded from the scalp. EEG has some medical uses, but has never fully lived up to its scientific potential.

energy function   The behavior of some neural networks can be characterized by an "energy function." This function mathematically takes the same form as energy in a physical system, though this quantity is not actual physical energy. As the system evolves in time, system "energy" decreases. See *Lyapunov function*.

equipotentiality   A theory about organization of the cerebral cortex associated with Karl Lashley. It proposed that cortex was unspecialized and function was widely distributed. If part of the brain was lost, the deficit was proportional to the amount lost, and not to the exact location of the loss.

evoked potentials   Event-related potentials from the nervous system. For example, a flash of light produces a characteristic potential at an electrode near visual cortex. These potentials are small and variable, and when analyzing them potentials from multiple events often must be averaged to reduce noise.

excitation   Making a neuron or a group of neurons more likely to be active, or be active at a higher level than before.

exclusive-OR   Often abbreviated "X-OR." A logic function that played an important role in the history of neural networks, since the simplest neural networks have trouble learning it. The Exclusive-OR of two predicates A and B is True (a) if A is True or (b) if B is True. Exclusive-OR is False if (a) neither A nor B is True or if (b) Both A and B are True. ("Either A or B but not both A and B.")

Faraday cage   A space completely surrounded by conductors, say, a cube of copper screening. Outside electrical interference is highly attenuated inside a properly designed Faraday cage, so one is often used in laboratories for recording of small neuroelectric potentials.

firing frequency   The number of action potentials a neuron fires per second.

fortification illusion   A visual hallucination often accompanying or preceding a migraine headache. In the most common form, a jagged, somewhat semicircular broad line of shimmering colors moves slowly outward from the center of gaze, taking several minutes to cross the visual field. The jagged line, apparently composed of short bright colored line segments at right angles to each other, bears a fancied resemblance to the jagged walls of a fort.

Fourier analysis   A method for analyzing a signal as the sum of components of particular frequencies. (See *linear system*.)

fuzzy logic   An engineering and computational technique of considerable utility based on the observation that in the real world events or properties are rarely absolutely either one thing or another but usually fall somewhere in between. It is hard to apply traditional formal logic with only "true" or "false" values allowed to such situations.

Gaussian distribution   The normal distribution of statistics, or the "bell-shaped" curve.

global minimum   Suppose we have a complex system with an objective function such as a measure of system error. Every set of system parameters, say, the weights in a neural network, gives rise to a different value for error. The set of error values plotted against the system parameters defines a surface. Such a surface may have many low points, local minima, where movement in any direction causes the error to increase. The minimum with the lowest value of the function is the global, or overall, minimum. A local minimum in the United States might be a mountain valley; the global minimum: Badwater in Death Valley.

gradient descent   A technique for finding the minima of a complex high-dimensional surface. If we always head downhill, eventually we will come to a point where every direction we move is uphill. However, the slope of the hill may be steeper in one direction than in others. If we always move downhill in the direction of the steepest slope, we should get to a minimum quickly. Many neural network learning rules (LMS, backpropagation) perform gradient descent on the error surface. This technique is sometimes called "steepest descent." Gradient descent usually finds a local minimum. To find the global minimum it is sometimes necessary to move in the wrong direction, upward, to get over a ridge to reach the next valley. Simulated annealing is one way of accomplishing this.

grandmother cells   An extreme form of selectivity in data representation. The name is a mildly pejorative caricature. The notion is that the concept, idea, and memory of "grandmother" corresponds to the activity of a single neuron—the "grandmother cell"—somewhere in the brain. Advantages of grandmother cells are their conceptual clarity and lack of a binding problem. Among other disadvantages are lack of ability to generalize and the observation that there are probably more things to learn in this world than there are grandmother cells to learn them with. (See *distributed representation* and *bug detector*.)

Hebb synapse   Some variant of a Hebb synapse is the most commonly used learning rule in neural networks. It is named for Donald Hebb, who proposed it in the 1949 classic *The Organization of Behavior*, though similar rules were proposed earlier, most notably by William James. The rule says that a synapse coupling two neurons increases in strength if both neurons are excited at the same time, that is, coincidence of activation of the two neurons is required for learning, not just activation of one or the other by itself. There is now strong biological evidence for the existence of some version of Hebb synapses in the mammalian brain.

heuristics   Techniques that make a system work better or more reliably even though it is often not fully understood why.

heteroassociation   A neural network associator where the input and the output are different patterns. (See *autoassociator*.)

hidden units   In a multilayer network, a middle layer of units that is neither an input layer nor an output layer.

Hodgkin and Huxley   Scientists who first accurately described and modeled the dynamics of the nerve cell axon (the squid giant axon) and received a Nobel prize for their work. The Hodgkin-Huxley equations are a set of coupled, nonlinear differential equations that predict the behavior of the axon.

Hopfield nets   A simple recurrent nonlinear neural network composed of binary units. Hopfield nets are autoassociative networks that can be shown to be minimizing an energy function as they evolve in time. Their behavior is similar to some well-studied physical systems, for example, spin glasses and the Ising model. Their simplicity and rich behavior attracted the interest of a number of theoretical physicists in the mid-1980s.

hypercolumn   A concept proposed by David Hubel and Torsten Wiesel for visual cortex. The set of all units in cortex that look at a particular point in visual space. The idea is that every point in space should be fully analyzed with units sensitive to all orientations, both eyes, etc., and this set of cells form the hypercolumn.

IEEE Institute of Electrical and Electronic Engineers. A large and influential engineering professional society.

inhibition Making a neuron or a group of neurons less likely to be active, or be active at a lower level.

lateral inhibition An active unit is wired so as to inhibit neighboring units and so reduce their activity. First described quantitatively in the Limulus eye, but something similar had been conjectured to exist by Ernst Mach as an explanation of Mach bands. A major function of lateral inhibition appears to be to increase contrast at edges.

limit cycle A dynamical system attractor state where the system state becomes attracted into a closed orbit. (See *attractor state*.)

linear system A system that obeys the principle of superposition. Briefly, if we have a linear system L, suppose input f gives rise to an output g. Suppose input f' gives rise to an output g'. A system is linear if we use the sum of the inputs, $(f + f')$ as input to L and the output is given by the sum of the outputs due to each component of the input, that is, $(g + g')$. Many important physical systems (electromagnetic waves, for example) are linear and it is possible to understand the way they behave by using a number of straightforward techniques. For example, a technique like Fourier analysis can take a complex input signal and break it down into simpler components, sine and cosine waves, which can then each be processed independently. Once the processing of the separate components is finished, the overall system output is generated by summing the component outputs.

linear associator A simple neural network associator, using the Hebb rule and linear computing units.

linear separability Suppose we have two sets of patterns that can be described mathematically as sets of points in a space. The two sets of points are said to be linearly separable if a line or hyperplane exists that separates the points. Perceptrons can only learn to separate linearly separable pattern classes, a major limitation.

line detectors In primary visual cortex, most units do not respond to simple light or dark, but to oriented line segments, that is, to complex features of the image.

Limulus eye *Limulus polyphemus*, popularly known as the horseshoe crab, is a common invertebrate on the east coast of the United States. The eye of *Limulus* is a model small visual system that performs neural computations in a way similar in important respects to the vertebrate visual system. Lateral inhibition was first observed in the *Limulus* eye.

LMS algorithm Least mean squares algorithm. Also known as the Widrow-Hoff algorithm. When a neural network is trying to learn a set of input-output relations, every set of weights has an associated error. The goal of the LMS algorithm is to adaptively reduce the error to the smallest value possible. It does this by using a gradient descent technique. The power of the LMS algorithm is that the learning rule used to implement gradient descent is simple and the technique is very robust.

local learning An often assumed constraint on the form learning can take in a neural network learning algorithm. For example, the Hebb synapse only depends on information available in close physical proximity to the synaptic junction.

Los Alamos A U.S. government national laboratory in New Mexico. The laboratory was founded during the Manhattan Project to design and construct the atomic bomb.

Lyapunov function A complex system can have associated with it a Lyapunov function. The "energy" defined for a neural network is an example. The Lyapunov function can be used to predict that some system states will be stable.

Mach bands A famous optical illusion described by Ernst Mach and largely due to lateral inhibition in the human eye. A smoothly graded edge of light intensity seems to be flanked by an illusory dark band and light band. The mechanism normally helps sharpen edges and make them more prominent.

Markov models A set of psychological models where the present state is a function only of the immediate past state.

matrix A two-dimensional array of numbers that can transform one point in a space into another. The mathematics of vectors and matrices is called linear algebra and plays a prominent role in neural networks and brain theory.

McCulloch-Pitts neurons Proposed in a famous 1943 paper by McCulloch and Pitts. Model neurons that can be either in an on state or an off state. These two states can also be considered as "true" or "false" states. This assumption lead to a model of brain computation based on units that computed logic functions. (See *binary units*.)

MOSIS A VLSI custom chip fabrication service. This service is popular with educational institutions since classes can get chips made through support from DARPA and NSF.

multivalued logic An alternative approach to logic that assumes a statement can be other than true or false. For example, a proposition might be "true," "false," or "uncertain." Fuzzy logic is one version of multivalued logic.

nearest neighbor model A pattern recognition technique where new inputs are given the classification of the nearest classified pattern. A simple, powerful, and highly effective algorithm, based on the observation about the way the world is constructed, things that look and act similarly are likely to be given the same classification. (If it looks like a duck, and quacks like a duck . . .)

negative feedback A powerful control technique used in everything from stereo amplifiers to the nervous system. A sample of the output of a system is subtracted from the input so as to compensate for error and distortion and make the output pattern as true a copy of the input pattern as possible.

neuromodulators Chemical signals that control, often in complex ways, the behavior of large groups of neurons. Neuromodulator effects range from the control of excitability and enhancement of learning in a structure to a major change in the pattern of neural responses in an entire nucleus.

neurotransmitters Chemicals used for synaptic transmission. There are many neurotransmitters which can be small molecules (acetylcholine, dopamine, glutamate) or large protein molecules (endorphins).

NIH National Institutes of Health. The major U.S. funding source for biomedical research. Notoriously conservative and somewhat hostile to brain theory.

NIMH National Institute of Mental Health. One of the National Institutes of Health whose primary concern is with mental illness, behavioral science, neuroscience, and related fields.

noise Noise, like weeds, is what you don't want where it happens to be. Often a matter of definition, particularly for neural networks, where sometimes noise is based on what you happen not to be thinking about at the time.

nonlinear Systems that do not obey the principle of superposition, i.e., not-linear. (See *linear*.) This definition is similar to and as arrogant as the distinction between vertebrates (1% of species) and invertebrates (99%) of species. Formal logic is a good example of a highly nonlinear system. Consider the logic function inclusive-OR of two predicates A and B. Inclusive-OR is true if either A or B is true. It is not twice as true if both A and B are true. As an additional example, the logic function exclusive-OR of A and B (See entry) is false if both A and B are true. We have techniques to analyze linear systems in great detail but often have great difficulty analyzing nonlinear systems.

nonlinear dynamical system   A nonlinear system evolving in time.

NSF   National Science Foundation. The major U.S. civilian funding agency for science except for health-related research. (See *NIH*.)

Oak Ridge   A U.S. national laboratory located in Tennessee. Formed during the Manhattan Project to help design and construct the atomic bomb.

objective function   A mathematical expression used to describe the state of a complex system, for example, a neural network. A measure of error between the actual output and what the network would get if it worked perfectly might be an objective function, or a cost associated with a process. The function of learning is often described as minimizing an objective function, for example, reducing the error measure to as small a value as possible.

ONR   Office of Naval Research. A U.S. military funding agency with an impressive record of supporting innovative basic research.

PDP books   The very influential two-volume set of books that introduced and described neural networks to a wide audience in 1986. (D. E. Rumelhart, J. L. McClelland and the PDP Research Group, *Parallel Distributed Processing*, Volume 1. *Foundations*. Cambridge, MA: MIT Press. J. L. McClelland, D. E. Rumelhart and the PDP Research Group, *Parallel Distributed Processing*, Volume 2. *Psychological and Biological Models*. Cambridge, MA: MIT Press.)

perceptron   An influential learning neural network, proposed by Frank Rosenblatt in the late 1950s. This model gave rise to the first major burst of enthusiasm for neural networks. According to neural network lore, Marvin Minsky and Seymour Papert terminated interest in neural networks by pointing out eloquently that simple perceptrons could not compute some things it would be nice to compute, for example, exclusive-OR.

perceptron convergence theorem   One of the first formal proofs that a learning machine, the perceptron, could learn something interesting. The proof showed that a perceptron could learn to separate patterns if the examples of the patterns were linearly separable.

pixel   A single "picture element" in a digitized image.

positive feedback   The output of a system is returned to the input with a positive sign, so the amplitude of the output grows. A squealing public address system is the paradigmatic undesirable example of positive feedback, but positive feedback has a number of very valuable uses in both electronics and neural networks.

protein folding   A protein starts as a linear string of amino acid residues which proceeds to fold up in what can be a very complex structure. Predicting the final configuration of the protein is very difficult and of great practical importance.

receptive field   Many neurons are selective and respond to only some kinds of sensory inputs. For example, a visual neuron may respond only to patterns of light and dark falling on a small area of the retina, the receptive field. A neuron responding to touch may have a receptive field of only part of a finger, or a small patch of the skin.

recurrent nets   Nets that have inputs based to some degree on their own activity, either based on their activity at past times or based on feedback from their current state.

reinforcement learning   Reinforcement learning concerns itself with cases where only information about success or failure of the entire computation is available. In a situation of any complexity it is very hard to know where or when the system did the right thing that led to a successful outcome. (See *credit assignment problem*.) A number of interesting and important learning algorithms based on reinforcement have been developed.

representation   In neural networks, probably the most important single decision made by a neural network designer: how the input and output data are represented in the pattern of activities shown by the neurons in the network. In AI, a representation describes features of the entities in the computation, how they interact, and how they are structured.

saccade The eyes move around a scene from location to location in extremely quick movements called saccades.

Schrodinger equation An amazingly general, powerful, and simple equation describing the behavior of many quantum mechanical systems. Called the "God equation" by MIT undergraduates.

sigmoid An S-shaped curve. In neural networks, this curve is typically monotonically increasing, roughly linear in the center and bends toward the horizontal at top and bottom bounded by upper and lower limits on unit activity.

simulated annealing A mathematical technique that can be used to find the true global minimum of a complicated function. Controlled but decreasing amounts of noise, related to temperature in physical systems, are added to the mathematical system. As "temperature" drops, the system is more and more likely to be found in the global minimum. Named by analogy with annealing a hot metal, where rate of temperature decrease has important effects on the ultimate properties of the metal.

spike An action potential. Called a "spike" because of its shape on an oscilloscope screen.

spin glass A physical system that was used as an inspiration for the Hopfield net.

stereopsis The ability to combine information from the two eyes to see objects in three dimensions. Depth perception.

STM Short-term memory. "Short-term" is variously defined to range from seconds to hours. Short-term memory is usually held to have very different properties from long-term memory, for example, limited storage capacity.

stochastic binary neurons Probabilistic neurons with only two states, say, on and off. Instead of having their state absolutely determined by their inputs, sometimes the state of the unit will be in agreement with what its inputs say it should be and sometimes it will not be in agreement. Although it seems counterintuitive to add "noise" to a deterministic system, in fact such neurons can be used to find better solutions to problems than noise-free units. (See *Boltzmann machine*.)

supervised learning Assumes the existence of a "supervisor" who knows in detail what the right answer to a network computation is supposed to be. The more detailed knowledge that is available about the error between what the network was supposed to do, and what it actually did, the better job a learning algorithm can do to adjust the network so as to reduce error.

synapse The connection between biological neurons. Synapses are very complex structures. Some are capable of modification with experience.

system state A complete description of a complex system at an instant in time. For example, in a neural network, it would be the activity of all the units at a particular time. Often represented as a vector.

threshold A neuron does not fire a spike or action potential unless it is excited enough so its membrane potential rises above a critical, threshold value.

topographic maps In the cerebral cortex, many sensory systems represent information with a strong spatial arrangement. For example, in primary visual cortex (V1) there is a map of visual space on the surface of cortex. In somatosensory cortex, there is a map of the body surface.

TRW A large company known for its aerospace and defense work.

unit A single computing element in a neural network. Modeled originally on biological neurons, but very much simplified.

unsupervised learning Learning without feedback as to correctness or incorrectness of response. An unsupervised learning system might learn a set of patterns and, based on the pattern statistics, decide that there are "really" only a certain number of significantly different events giving rise to the input patterns. In cognitive science, a "concept forming" system has sometimes been cast as an unsupervised learning problem. Intrinsically more difficult and less well defined than supervised learning, but also often more useful and realistic.

V1   The first visual cortical area, receiving input from the retina by way of the lateral geniculate body in the thalamus. V1 is large, and located at the back of the head.

VAX   A famous computer model particularly popular in the 1980s. Made by Digital Equipment Corporation (DEC).

vector   A one-dimensional array of numbers. Geometrically, a vector represents a point in what may be a very high-dimensional space. The most common interpretation of a vector in neural networks is the pattern of activity shown by a group of neurons.

visual cortex   Region of the cerebral cortex involved in processing vision. In the human brain, V1, the primary visual cortex, lies at the back of the head.

VLSI   Very-large-scale integration. The "chip" technology that lies behind modern computers.

VOR   Vestibulo-ocular reflex. Reflex compensatory eye movements that tend to stabilize the retinal image as the head moves. The neural pathways involved can be shown to be adaptive and have been used as a model system to study neural plasticity.

wavelets   A class of functions used to analyze signals. Wavelets (and the related Gabor functions) have frequency selectivity, in that they respond to some frequencies more strongly than others, but also respond best to signals at a particular location.

weight   The strength of connection between two units in a neural network. Weights in a network are an abstraction of the synaptic coupling between two biological neurons. Weights are usually assumed to have a single value. Synaptic coupling between neurons is far more complex.

white noise   Random noise characterized by equal energy in all frequencies. The hiss between stations on the radio is a familiar example of approximately white noise.

Wickelfeature representation   A method of coding information about letters based on ideas of Wayne Wickelgren. Used in an important and controversial model of past tense learning by Rumelhart and McClelland in the PDP books.

Widrow-Hoff algorithm   See *LMS algorithm.*

WTA network   A winner-take-all neural network. At the end of a WTA computation in a group of units, only one unit remains active (the winner) and the rest of the units are inactive.

X-OR   See *exclusive-OR.*

Index

Topographic mapping in the brain, 32, 261
Truck-backing problem, 67–69, 407
TRW, 299–300, 399, 402
Turing, A.
  and biological dynamical processes, 32, 111, 118
  and McCulloch, W., 102
  Turing machines, 12, 103, 111, 214–215, 217
  the Turing test, 91

UCLA (University of California at Los Angeles), 27, 29, 217, 230, 247–248, 250–253, 271, 299, 330, 400
UCSD (University of California at San Diego), 113, 229–230, 254, 271–272, 274, 276–283, 301, 309, 323–324, 329–330, 370, 372, 376, 378, 396–397, 399, 401–402
UCSD meeting (1979)
  influence of, 255, 279, 321–322, 330, 370–372, 374
  organizing the meeting (by Anderson, J. A. and Hinton, G.), 255, 276, 370
  Parallel Models of Associative Memory (Hinton and Anderson, Eds.), 255, 321, 370, 398
University of California, Berkeley, 27, 31, 69, 282, 370
University of Chicago, 2, 25, 104–105, 110–111, 117
University of Illinois, 1, 3, 78–80
University of Maryland, 349–351, 369
University of Massachusetts, 225–229, 231
University of Rochester, 8, 279, 322, 372
University of South Dakota, 269–270
University of Toronto, 378–379
University of Washington, 150, 154
Unsupervised learning. *See also* ART; *glossary definition*
  with autoencoders, 379–380
  in category learning 366–367
  in fuzzy system, 407
  in radar network, 260
  in "universal recoding" map, 186
USC (University of Southern California), 230–231, 232, 250, 389–392, 394, 396, 407

VAX computers, 88, 324, 373
Vietnam War, 63, 339–340, 349
Vision. *See also* Character recognition; Cortex, visual; Visual hallucinations; Hubel, D.; Wiesel, T. N.; Migraines; Stereopsis, models of

color vision, 136–137, 193–194
computer vision, 36, 135, 190, 322, 329–330, 369
dyslexia, as a visual problem, 18–19
eye movements, 234–235
fortification illusion, 119–120
rog visual system
  bug detectors, topology of response, 17–18
  Pitts W., reaction to research by Lettvin, J. Y., 10
  Rana computatrix, 232
  retina, and AI, 12
  structure, 108
  "What the Frog's Eye Tells the Frog's Brain," 10, 17–18, 108, 215, 223–224, 249, 344
illusions, and, 109, 119–120
imagery, as reflection of cortical anatomy, 118–121
perception, 19, 231, 233, 275
  action oriented, 224
  of connectedness, 254–255
  multistable, 259
  of objects, 208, 233, 256–257
  prototype formation, 257–258
Vision (Marr), 115, 231–232
Visual hallucinations, 117–120, 150. *See also* Epileptic seizures; Migraines
VLSI (very large scale integration). *See also* Mead, C.
  analog, 15, 134
  digital, 131–132
von der Malsberg, C., and visual cortex models, 84, 120, 180, 367
von Neumann, J., 98, 109, 169, 219, 335
  and early interaction between computers and neural nets, 12, 26, 102
  and funding of Lettvin, J. Y., 8
  on probabilistic logic and reliability, 99, 101–102, 216

Wall, P., 8, 101, 220–221
Werbos, P. J., 61, 68, 179, 180, 183, 200, 286, **335–358**, 334, 348, 378
  background, 335–336
  backpropagation
    application in energy model, 355
    early work, 338, 341, 342, 347
    first application, at MIT, 348
    through time, 356
  on DARPA project, 349–351
  at Department of Energy (DOE), 351–355
  and Deutsch, K., 342, 346–347

Printed in the United States
by Baker & Taylor Publisher Services